# Reading, Understanding, and Applying Nursing Research

A Text and Workbook

# Reading, Understanding, and Applying Nursing Research

## A Text and Workbook

second edition

**James A. Fain,** PhD, RN, BC-ADM, FAAN
Associate Dean for Academic Programs/Associate
Professor, University of Massachusetts Worcester
Graduate School of Nursing
Worcester, Massachusetts

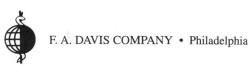

F. A. DAVIS COMPANY • Philadelphia

F. A. Davis Company
1915 Arch Street
Philadelphia, PA 19103
www.fadavis.com

Printed in the United States of America

Last digit indicates print number: 10 9 8 7 6 5 4 3 2 1

*Publisher:* Joanne Patzek DaCunha, RN, MSN
*Developmental Editor:* Peg Waltner
*Production Editor:* Scott Filderman
*Cover Designer:* Louis J. Forgione

As new scientific information becomes available through basic and clinical research, recommended treatments and drug therapies undergo changes. The author(s) and publisher have done everything possible to make this book accurate, up to date, and in accord with accepted standards at the time of publication. The author(s), editors, and publisher are not responsible for errors or omissions or for consequences from application of the book, and make no warranty, expressed or implied, in regard to the contents of the book. Any practice described in this book should be applied by the reader in accordance with professional standards of care used in regard to the unique circumstances that may apply in each situation. The reader is advised always to check product information (package inserts) for changes and new information regarding dose and contraindications before administering any drug. Caution is especially urged when using new or infrequently ordered drugs.

**Library of Congress Cataloging-in-Publication Data**

Fain, James A., 1953-
   Reading, understanding, and applying nursing research : a text and workbook / James A. Fain.—2nd ed.
     p. ; cm.
   Includes bibliographical references and index.
   ISBN 0-8036-1112-9 (alk. paper)
   1. Nursing—Research. I. Title.
   [DNLM: 1. Nursing Research—methods. WY 20.5 F162r 2003]
   RT81.5.F35 2003
   610.73'07'2—dc21

2003046170

To Linda and our children, Lauren, Jillian, and Timothy

# preface

Research plays an integral part in determining the roles and responsibilities of nurses. Involvement in research can range from conducting an independent research study to critically appraising the research literature. Enhancing knowledge of research and practicing research skills can help nurses increase their appreciation of how research influences the quality of patient care.

This second edition of *Reading, Understanding, and Applying Nursing Research — A Text and Workbook* provides several new features that will assist undergraduate students, RNs returning to school, and practicing nurses in critically appraising research reports. This edition continues to emphasize how to read research reports, evaluate them critically, and apply the findings to practice by providing more examples of nursing research throughout the book. Steps of the research process are illustrated with excerpts from studies that have been published in nursing literature.

This edition continues to organize content into three parts. In Part I, *Nature of Research and the Research Process,* the importance of nursing research is presented. In addition, suggested research activities of nurses are presented in several documents. In Part II, *Planning a Research Study,* specific aspects of the research process are discussed; providing students with information they need to understand inductive and deductive reasoning along with the formation of research questions and hypotheses from a conceptual model or theoretical framework. Two new chapters were added to Part II, *Applying Appropriate Theories and Conceptual Models* and *Evidence-Based Practice.* The first new chapter explains how theories and models provide the primary mechanisms by which students learn to organize research findings into a broader conceptual context. The second new chapter helps students understand how to track down the best evidence to guide specific approaches to patient care by introducing them to several major databases. In Part III, *Utilization of Nursing Research,* suggested strategies for evaluating and critiquing research reports are introduced along with guidelines for utilization of research findings.

Specific objectives of this edition are to provide students with (1) an understanding of the steps of the research process, (2) a sound ethical knowledge base, (3) the skill to critically evaluate a problem and purpose statement, (4) the knowledge of what specific statistical procedures can be used to answer various research questions and/or hypotheses, (5) the knowledge of randomized clinical trials as a methodological "gold standard" and why use of other types of design is so often necessary in nursing research, and (6) a sense of confidence in their ability to read research reports.

Student learning objectives are presented at the beginning of every chapter, along with a glossary of terms, summary of key ideas, and learning activities. Another new feature in the second edition includes a more detailed guide on "how to" critique research studies. Each chapter in Part II includes a subheading titled "Questions to Consider When Critiquing." More examples of published research from actual journal articles are included in each chapter to help students gain proficiency in reading research reports. This approach is aimed at helping students improve their skills in reading and understanding research reports. Finally, more information is presented on why reliability and validity and other psychometric properties are important if research results are to be valid.

The quality of patient care depends largely on the quality of nursing research. The ability to understand components of the research process and to integrate scientific knowledge with practice to make informed judgments and valid clinical decisions is critical. *Reading, Understanding, and Applying Nursing Research* provides the skills necessary to help students understand what researchers are trying to communicate in published research reports. As consumers of nursing research, the emphasis is on assisting the student to understand and evaluate research reports being discussed. *Reading, Understanding, and Applying Nursing Research* provides a clear and practical presentation of these skills.

JAMES A. FAIN

# acknowledgments

Sincere thanks are extended to the many individuals who contributed to the development of this textbook. Specifically, I wish to acknowledge those individuals who have been most closely involved in the production of this textbook. Thanks to the publisher at F. A. Davis Company, Joanne P. DaCunha, MSN, RN, whose support and patience from the beginning were essential. A special thanks to Peg Waltner, freelance editor assigned to the textbook, for her careful reading of the entire manuscript and helpful comments and suggestions for improving the exposition.

Undertaking such a project would have been impossible without the support, help, and contributions of special individuals. For their assistance in contributing several key chapters, I would like to thank Cheryl Tatano Beck, DNSc, RN, CNM, FAAN; Suzanne C. Beyea, PhD, RN, CS; Paula T. Lusardi, PhD, RN, CCRN, CCNS; Courtney Lyder, ND, APRN, CS, GPN; Leslie H. Nicoll, PhD, MBA, RN; Gail E. Russell, EdD, RN, CNAA; and Donna Schwartz-Barcott, PhD, RN.

Finally, I would like to thank my wife, Linda, and children Lauren, Jillian, and Timothy, along with the many students over the years who have contributed directly and indirectly through their interest and support.

JAMES A. FAIN

# contributors

*Chapter 11:* SELECTING A RESEARCH DESIGN: QUANTITATIVE VERSUS QUALITATIVE
Paula T. Lusardi, PhD, RN, CCRN, CCNS
Clinical Nurse Specialist, Intensive Care & Intermediate Care
Baystate Medical Center
Springfield, Massachusetts

*Chapter 12:* PHENOMENOLOGICAL RESEARCH
Gail E. Russell, EdD, RN, CNAA
Associate Professor of Nursing
University of Massachusetts, Darthmouth
College of Nursing
Darthmouth, Massachusetts

*Chapter 13:* ETHNOGRAPHIC RESEARCH: FOCUSING ON CULTURE
Donna Schwartz-Barcott, PhD, RN
Professor/Director, Graduate Studies in Nursing
University of Rhode Island College of Nursing
Kingston, Rhode Island

*Chapter 14:* GROUNDED THEORY RESEARCH
Cheryl Tatano Beck, DNSc, RN, CNM, FAAN
Professor of Nursing
University of Connecticut School of Nursing
Storrs, Connecticut

*Chapter 15:* INTERPRETING AND REPORTING RESEARCH FINDINGS
Courtney Lyder, ND, APRN, CS, GPN
Professor of Nursing
University of Virginia School of Nursing
Charlottesville, Virginia

*Chapter 17:* RESEARCH UTILIZATION
Leslie H. Nicoll, PhD, MBA, RN
Editor, *Computers, Informatics, Nursing & Journal of Hospice & Palliative Nursing*
University of Southern Maine
College of Nursing and Health Professions
Portland, Maine

Suzanne C. Beyea, PhD, RN, CS
Darthmouth Hitchcock Medical Center
Hanover, New Hampshire

# consultants

Nagia Ali, PhD, RN
Professor
Ball State University
Muncie, Indiana

Sean Clarke, RN, PhD
Assistant Professor
University of Pennsylvania
Philadelphia, Pennsylvania

Rosalee Seymour, RN, EdD
Associate Professor
East Tennessee State University
Johnson City, Tennessee

Jacqueline M. Stolley, PhD, RN, CS
Professor
Trinity College of Nursing
Moline, Illinois

# contents

Part 1  **Nature of Research and the Research Process**   1

    1. INTRODUCTION TO NURSING RESEARCH   3
    *James A. Fain, PhD, RN, BC-ADM, FAAN*

    2. UNDERSTANDING THE RESEARCH PROCESS AND ETHICAL ISSUES IN   15
    NURSING RESEARCH
    *James A. Fain, PhD, RN, BC-ADM, FAAN*


Part 2  **Planning a Research Study**   41

    3. SELECTING AND DEFINING THE PROBLEM   43
    *James A. Fain, PhD, RN, BC-ADM, FAAN*

    4. APPLYING APPROPRIATE THEORIES AND CONCEPTUAL MODELS   63
    *James A. Fain, PhD, RN, BC-ADM, FAAN*

    5. UNDERSTANDING EVIDENCE-BASED PRACTICE   75
    *James A. Fain, PhD, RN, BC-ADM, FAAN*

    6. FORMULATING HYPOTHESES AND RESEARCH QUESTIONS   87
    *James A. Fain, PhD, RN, BC-ADM, FAAN*

    7. SELECTING THE SAMPLE AND SETTING   103
    *James A. Fain, PhD, RN, BC-ADM, FAAN*

    8. PRINCIPLES OF MEASUREMENT   123
    *James A. Fain, PhD, RN, BC-ADM, FAAN*

    9. DATA COLLECTION METHODS   143
    *James A. Fain, PhD, RN, BC-ADM, FAAN*

    10. ANALYZING THE DATA   165
    *James A. Fain, PhD, RN, BC-ADN, FAAN*

    11. SELECTING A RESEARCH DESIGN: QUANTITATIVE   191
    VERSUS QUALITATIVE
    *Paula T. Lusardi, PhD, RN, CCRN, CCNS*

    12. PHENOMENOLOGICAL RESEARCH   219
    *Gail E. Russell, EdD, RN, CNAA*

    13. ETHNOGRAPHIC RESEARCH: FOCUSING ON CULTURE   243
    *Donna Schwartz-Barcott, PhD, RN*

    14. GROUNDED THEORY RESEARCH   265
    *Cheryl Tatano Beck, DNSc, RN, CNM, FAAN*

Part 3  **Utilization of Nursing Research    287**

15. INTERPRETING AND REPORTING RESEARCH FINDINGS    289
   *Courtney Lyder, ND, APRN, CS, GPN*

16. CRITIQUING RESEARCH REPORTS    307
   *James A. Fain, PhD, RN, BC-ADM, FAAN*

17. RESEARCH UTILIZATION    327
   *Leslie H. Nicoll, PhD, MBA, RN*
   *Suzanne C. Beyea, PhD, RN, CS*

part

1

# Nature of Research and the Research Process

# Introduction to Nursing Research

James A. Fain, PhD, RN, BC-ADM, FAAN

## LEARNING OBJECTIVES

*At the end of this chapter, you will be able to:*
1. Describe the importance of nursing research for nurses.
2. Explain how the scientific method is applied in nursing research.
3. Describe the nurse's role as a consumer of research.
4. Identify strategies for executing research responsibilities.

## GLOSSARY OF KEY TERMS

**Empirical data.** Documented evidence (data) gathered through direct observation rather than a researcher's subjective belief.

**Nursing research.** A systematic process of investigating problems to gain knowledge about improving care that nurses provide.

**Nursing science.** The body of knowledge that is unique to the discipline of nursing.

**Qualitative research.** An approach for generating knowledge using methods of inquiry that emphasize subjectivity and the meaning of an experience for the individual.

**Quantitative research.** An approach for generating knowledge based on determining how much of a given behavior, characteristic, or phenomenon is present.

**Replication.** The ability of researchers to repeat a study using the same variables and methods or slight variations of them.

**Research consumer.** Readers of nursing research whose objective is applying findings to nursing practice or using the findings to conduct further research.

**Research team.** A group that collaborates to conduct a research project, from determining the initial research question through communicating the results.

**Rigor.** Striving for excellence in research, which involves discipline, scrupulous adherence to detail, and strict accuracy.

**Scientific inquiry.** The process of analyzing data critically that have been gathered systematically about a particular phenomenon.

**Scientific method.** A systematic research process that involves the following steps: selecting and defining the problem, formulating research questions or hypotheses or both, collecting data, analyzing data, and reporting results.

**Triangulation.** Use of quantitative and qualitative methods to collect data about a particular phenomenon.

**Ways of knowing.** An assortment of methods used to acquire new knowledge.

Understanding nursing research is more than learning a method of inquiry. **Nursing research** is a process that allows nurses to ask questions that are aimed at gaining new knowledge to improve patient care. Whether nurses practice in an acute-care facility, long-term rehabilitation setting, or community agency, quality care is expected to reflect assimilation of knowledge into practice. In addition, nurses are responsible for assuming an active role in developing a body of nursing knowledge. Nurses must examine how research can best be incorporated into their everyday practice. In this chapter the value of nursing research is discussed, and the application of the scientific method in nursing is described. The role of the research consumer and guidelines for participating in research are also addressed.

## THE IMPORTANCE OF RESEARCH IN NURSING

The challenges confronting the health-care system compel practitioners in all specialties to justify their clinical decisions. The discipline of nursing is no exception. Nurses participate in research activities to develop, refine, and extend nursing science, which is a unique body of nursing knowledge. Nursing research is systematic inquiry designed to develop knowledge about issues of importance to nursing.[1] As an academic and professional discipline, clinical practice is an integral part of nursing's activities, along with educating clinicians and administration of nursing services. Therefore, research in nursing encompasses systematic inquiry into each of these areas. Nurses who base their clinical decisions on scientifically documented information act in a professionally accountable manner and help define the identity of nursing and promote excellence in practice through knowledge development.

"Clinical decisions" and "actions based on research findings" mean that nurses engage in research-based (evidence-based) practice. Such practice is informed by the best available evidence as it relates to patient care. Research-based nursing practice refers to clinicians making an effort to integrate research findings into clinical thinking and decision making.[2,3]

Nursing is a discipline with its own body of knowledge that focuses on knowing and understanding individuals and their health experience. No other discipline is as concerned with the individual and how health is experienced. By designing relevant research, nurse scientists contribute to the development of specific nursing knowledge that aids problem-solving in patient care.

The importance of nursing research is an established reality; it is no longer necessary to justify its value. Instead, nurses must focus on improving their understanding of the research process and fostering the development of research designs that provide the information needed to explain, change, and expand nursing practice.

## WHAT IS RESEARCH?

Research is a systematic inquiry into a subject that uses various approaches (quantitative and qualitative methods) to answer questions and solve problems. The goal of research is to discover new knowledge and relationships and find solutions to problems or ·questions.[2] Research is sometimes referred to as synonymous with problem-solving. This is incorrect because research deals with discovering or generating new knowledge, whereas problem-solving refers to using current knowledge. Previous research generates knowledge used in problem-solving. If use of existing knowledge is found to be inadequate, problems can be posed as research questions in need of scientific investigation. New knowledge is then applied to deal with future problems.

What is knowledge? Knowledge is information acquired in a variety of ways. **Ways of knowing** are various methods used to acquire new knowledge. For example, you may say that you *know* your friend John, *know* that the Earth rotates around the sun, *know* how to give an injection, and *know* pharmacology. These are all examples of knowing: being familiar with a person, comprehending the facts, acquiring a psychomotor skill, and mastering a subject matter.[4] Knowledge can be gained from a variety of sources such as tradition, authority, trial and error, personal experience, intuition, logical reasoning, and use of the scientific method.[1] Use of the scientific method is of primary concern to nursing as a science. As consumers of research, nurses need to know how information is gathered and organized in a research or scientific context.

## THE SCIENTIFIC METHOD

Achieving the research goal of discovering new knowledge and relationships requires understanding the scientific method. Students hearing the word *science* often think of laboratories, experiments, intellectual skills, and mathematics. They believe scientists are individuals with a tremendous amount of knowledge, drawing on years of experience. While this might be somewhat true, science is a method of knowing and acquiring new knowledge.

**Scientific inquiry** is a process in which observable, verifiable data are systematically collected from our surroundings through our senses to describe, explain, or predict events.[1] The **scientific method** involves selecting and defining a problem, formulating research question(s) or hypotheses or both, collecting data, analyzing data, and reporting results. Two characteristics that are unique to the scientific method and not associated with other ways of knowing are objectivity and the use of empirical data.[1,2] Objectivity is defined as an ability to distance the research process as much as possible from the scientist's personal beliefs, values, and attitudes. The scientific approach is applied in such a way that other scientists will have confidence in the conclusions. The term **empirical data** refers to documenting objective data through direct observation. Findings are grounded in reality rather than personal bias or the subjective belief of the researcher.

The scientific method involves testing of ideas, hunches, or guesses. For example, a nurse may have an idea that patients who receive preoperative teaching will have a healthier postoperative recuperative period. A physician might guess that people who are more internally controlled will lose more weight than those who are externally controlled. Both examples are only guesses or hunches. A systematic, planned approach to data collection, analysis, and evaluation is necessary to see if such guesses or hunches hold up. The value of using the scientific method is that the method can be replicated by other researchers.

**Replication** is the ability of researchers to repeat a study using the same variables and methods or slight variations of them. Replication is an important concept in research. An essential characteristic of a research study is that it should be replicable so that research findings can be verified. Repeating a study increases the extent to which the research findings can be generalized, providing additional evidence of validity.

Nursing research is the systematic application of the scientific method to the study of phenomena of interest to the nursing profession. For example, systematic investigation of patients and their health needs is of primary concern to nursing. The results of such an investigation add to the body of knowledge that is unique to nursing. A major difference between scientific research and nursing research is the nature of the material studied. Nursing research primarily involves studying people, and people do not behave consistently, as do chemicals in a laboratory. In a laboratory setting it is much easier to explain, predict, and control the situation. Rigid controls that are imposed and maintained in a laboratory setting are impossible to achieve in the practice setting. Likewise, ethical considerations do not allow the range of experimentation with people that is possible with animals.

Scientific inquiry is sometimes referred to as **quantitative research.** The notion of objective observations made by the researcher, along with the ability to generalize the findings to other populations, constitutes a scientific approach. Quantitative methods are well developed and have been used extensively and effectively in nursing research. Quantitative research methods emphasize measurement, testing of hypotheses, and statistical analysis of data.[1,2] Quantitative nursing research uses traditional quantitative approaches such as experiments, questionnaires, and surveys to advance nursing science. When the research question addresses an individual's subjective experience, different methods must be used to study that type of phenomenon.

**Qualitative research** is an approach to structuring knowledge that uses methods of inquiry that emphasize verbal descriptions and the meaning of the experience for the individual.[5] Qualititative research methods emphasize understanding of phenomena from the individual's perspective. Participant observation, in-depth interviews, case studies, ethnographies, and narrative analyses are the tools to gain new knowledge in qualitative research. Regardless of the methods used, researchers have the responsibility of conducting a study with rigor and skill. **Rigor** is the striving for excellence in research that involves discipline, scrupulous adherence to detail, and strict accuracy.[4]

**Triangulation** refers to the use of both quantitative and qualitative methods to collect data about a particular phenomenon.[5] The term can also refer to various combinations of research designs or instruments used in the same study. A combination of psychosocial instruments, interviews, and observations can be used to describe a particularly complex phenomenon. The two approaches are complementary and provide an accurate representation of reality.

## RESEARCH AND THE ENTRY-LEVEL NURSE

The scope of research activities for which nurses are responsible is
lated in several documents. In *Guidelines for the Investigative Functi*
a publication of the American Nurses Association, an outline is provided of research
competencies that are expected of nurses graduating from associate, baccalaureate,
and graduate degree programs in nursing. Suggested research activities of nurses at
various educational levels are presented in Table 1.1. These guidelines provide
direction for nurses to initiate research activities that can be carried out individually
or in collaboration with other nursing professionals.

The role of researcher is classified on a continuum by the degree of participation
in the conduct of research. At one end of the continuum are nurses who are
consumers of research. The role of the **research consumer** includes the ability to
read and evaluate research reports. Nurses are increasingly expected to maintain, at
least, this level of involvement with research. Developing skills to read and understand research critically takes time and repeated practice and requires knowledge of
the research process. At the other end of the continuum are nurses who conduct
research and actively participate in the design and implementation of a study. As
members of a **research team,** nurses can collaborate on the development of an idea
and actually participate in the design and production of a study. Today, nursing
research is undertaken by many nurses with advanced degrees who are working in
the clinical setting. Several research-related activities[2] in which nurses may participate are listed in Table 1.2.

Participation in research activities is shared by nurses at all levels and requires
knowledge of the research process and the ability to determine what constitutes
good research. Developing the skill of reading and evaluating research reports
allows nurses to feel confident that the findings of a study are accurate and will
provide an improvement in nursing practice.

### Guidelines for Scientific Integrity

Every nurse scientist has the responsibility of promoting the integrity of **nursing
science.** In this pursuit, nurse scientists are guided by principles that include respect
for the integrity of knowledge, collegiality, honesty, trust, objectivity, and openness.
These principles are universal and relevant for each phase of the research process.
The nature of nursing and the problems of interest to nurse scientists allow for a
variety of methods that are appropriate for investigating nursing problems. Although
different methods may highlight specific issues and questions, the underlying principles of scientific integrity remain the same.

The Midwest Nursing Research Society developed guidelines[7] that build on and
complement the American Nurses Association's *Human Rights Guidelines for
Nurses in Clinical and Other Research.*[8] Major areas addressed in the Midwest
Nursing Research Society guidelines include data access/management and publication practices. Principles that guide the actions of researchers with respect to data
access/management are presented in Table 1.3.

## TABLE 1.1 INVESTIGATIVE FUNCTIONS OF NURSES AT VARIOUS EDUCATIONAL LEVELS

### Associate Degree in Nursing

1. Demonstrates awareness of the value or relevance of research in nursing
2. Assists in identifying problem areas in nursing practice
3. Assists in collection of data within an established structured format

### Baccalaureate Degree in Nursing

1. Reads, interprets, and evaluates research for applicability to nursing practice
2. Identifies nursing problems that need to be investigated and participates in the implementation of scientific studies
3. Uses nursing practice as a means of gathering data for refining and extending practice
4. Applies established findings of nursing and other health-related research to nursing practice
5. Shares research findings with colleagues

### Master's Degree in Nursing

1. Analyzes and reformulates nursing practice problems so that scientific knowledge and scientific methods can be used to find solutions
2. Enhances quality and clinical relevance of nursing research by providing expertise in clinical problems and by providing knowledge about the way in which these clinical services are delivered
3. Facilitates investigation of problems in clinical settings by, for example, contributing to a climate supportive of investigative activities, collaborating with others in investigations, and enhancing nurses' access to clients and data
4. Investigates for the purpose of monitoring the quality of the practice of nursing in a clinical setting
5. Assists others in applying scientific knowledge in nursing practice

### Doctorate Degree in Nursing or a Related Discipline

1. Provides leadership for the integration of scientific knowledge with other types of knowledge for the advancement of practice
2. Conducts investigations to evaluate the contributions of nursing activities to the well-being of clients
3. Develops methods to monitor the quality of the practice of nursing in a clinical setting and to evaluate contributions of nursing activities to the well-being of clients

### Graduate of a Research-Oriented Doctoral Program

1. Develops theoretical explanation of phenomena relevant to nursing by empirical research and analytic processes
2. Uses analytic and empirical methods to discover ways to modify or extend existing scientific knowledge so that it is relevant to nursing
3. Develops methods for scientific inquiry of phenomena relevant to nursing

*Source: American Nurses' Association Commission on Nursing Research: Guidelines for the Investigative Function of Nurses. American Nurses' Association, Kansas City, MO, 1981.*[6]

## Scholarly Publications and Practices

Disseminating research findings is an integral part of the research process. Scholarly publications are documents that communicate to other professionals the methods and achievements used in academic study and research investigation. The growth of

## TABLE 1.2  RESEARCH-RELATED ACTIVITIES

- Participating in a journal club in a practice setting that involves regular meetings among nurses to discuss research articles
- Attending research presentations at professional conferences
- Evaluating completed research for possible use in the practice setting
- Assisting in data collection research; e.g., distributing questionnaires to patients or observing/recording patients' behaviors
- Collaborating on the development of an idea for a research project
- Participating on an institutional review board that examines ethical aspects of a proposed study

## TABLE 1.3  SCIENTIFIC INTEGRITY GUIDELINES

### Data Access

1. All co-investigators on a team have access to data, as agreed on at the outset of the research, and all assume responsibility for safeguarding data confidentiality.
2. When doing so does not violate confidentiality of subject information, scientists should provide data to the journal editor, if requested, to enable a more complete evaluation of manuscripts.
3. Following publication of results, scientists may be expected to provide sufficient information to enable other qualified scientists to replicate the study.
4. Different considerations apply before publication. Research materials and data are considered privileged until they are formally disseminated. Disclosure or sharing of data prior to peer review and publication is not required.
5. Sharing of results with the news media should be done following completion of peer review.
6. Any discoveries/inventions from research leading to patents are governed by policies of the institution.
7. Investigators are encouraged to provide other researchers, including graduate students, with access to their data for purposes of secondary analysis.

### Data Management

1. Data are collected according to stated protocol.
2. Potential sources of bias in design and conduct are identified and minimized.
3. It is recommended that original data be preserved for a period of 5 to 7 years or longer, as there is reasonable expectation that the original data will continue to be the basis of ongoing research, publication, or both. Exceptions involving considerations for human subjects may be negotiated with the institutional review board.
4. Specific teams should develop and agree on procedures appropriate for the project.
5. Scientists have the responsibility to ascertain that data are reported accurately, including the decision rules used for collecting and analyzing data.
6. If an error is discovered, it is corrected and made public.
7. The principal investigator is responsible for ensuring that data are of high quality and that steps are taken to prevent intentional withholding or selective reporting of data that may be contrary to investigator expectations.

*Source: Reprinted with permission of the Midwest Nursing Research Society from Guidelines for Scientific Integrity, Glenview, IL: Copyright © 1996. Midwest Nursing Research Society, 4700 W. Lake Avenue, Glenview, IL 60025-1485.*[7]

and support for nursing research are reflected by the impressive number of journals devoted to the publication of nursing research studies. These research journals (with their abbreviated titles from Index Medicus) include *Advances in Nursing Science (Adv Nurs Sci), Applied Nursing Research (Appl Nurs Res), Image: Journal of Nursing Scholarship (Image: J Nurs Scholarship), Nursing Science Quarterly (Nurs Science Q), Nursing Research (Nurs Res), Research in Nursing and Health (Res Nurs Health), Scholarly Inquiry for Nursing Practice (Scholarly Inquiry Nurs Pract)*, and *Western Journal of Nursing Research (West J Nurs Res)*.

In addition to research journals, the consumer of research can find a wealth of relevant scientific knowledge in many of the specialty journals. Some of the more common specialty journals include *American Journal of Maternal Child Nursing (Am J Maternal Child Nurs), Association of Operating Room Nurses Journal (AORN J), The Diabetes Educator (Diabetes Educ), Heart & Lung (Heart Lung)*, and *Oncology Nursing Forum (Oncol Nurs Forum)*. Authorship in any type of journal implies responsibility for the published work and significant contribution to the conception and execution of the paper. A list of guidelines[7] that refer to intellectual honesty and responsibility in publication practices is presented in Table 1.4.

## Promoting Nursing Research

Nursing organizations have responded to the need for support of research activities. In 1986, the National Center for Nursing Research (NCNR) was established under

---

TABLE 1.4  GUIDELINES FOR AUTHORSHIP OF PUBLISHED PAPERS

1. Authors contribute substantially to the published work. This involves assuming responsibility for two or more of the following areas: conception and design, execution of the study, analysis and interpretation of data, and preparation and revision of the manuscript. Others, who provide financial, technical, information, or other kinds of support, may be acknowledged but may not be considered authors.
2. Decisions about conferring and ordering of authorship need to be made in advance, based on the foregoing considerations. Order may be reassessed if contributions change.
3. Status of individuals, such as trainees/students or their rank per se, should not be a determining factor in authorship decisions.
4. The principal investigator, when directing a team on sponsored projects, assumes overall responsibility for all publications resulting from the project, regardless of his or her authorship status, unless negotiated otherwise.
5. All authors should review the final manuscript and take responsibility for the work.
6. Duplicate and fragmented publications should be avoided. When the same or substantially similar content is reported in two or more publications, authors should notify editors, who should inform reviewers.
7. Authors should provide additional information requested by editors.
8. When parties disagree on authorship matters, they are encouraged to seek consultation from colleagues.

---

*Source: Reprinted with permission of the Midwest Nursing Research Society from Guidelines for Scientific Integrity, Glenview, IL: Copyright © 1996. Midwest Nursing Research Society, 4700 W. Lake Avenue, Glenview, IL 60025-1485.*[7]

the Health Research Extension Act and the auspices of the American Nurses Association. The purpose of the NCNR was to conduct a program of grants and awards supporting nursing research and training, to promote health, and to further the prevention and mitigation of the effects of disease. In 1993 the NCNR was awarded the status of an institute in the structure of the National Institutes of Health (NIH) and was redesignated the National Institute of Nursing Research (NINR).

The mission of the NINR is to support basic and clinical research to establish a scientific basis for the care of individuals across the life span.[9] According to its mandate, the NINR seeks to reduce the burden of illness and disability by understanding and easing the effects of acute and chronic illness, to improve health-related quality of life by preventing or delaying the onset of disease or slowing its progression, to establish better approaches for promoting health and preventing disease, to improve clinical environments by testing interventions that influence health outcomes, and to reduce costs and demand for care.

The National Nursing Research Agenda was launched in 1987 to provide structure for selecting initiatives and developing the knowledge base for nursing practice. Senior nurse researchers around the country were invited to the Conference on Nursing Research Priorities (CORP #1) in Washington, D.C., in 1988 to help identify research priorities. During CORP #2, held in Washington, D.C., 1992, key nurse scientists from all areas of nursing practice identified research priorities through the year 1999. The research agenda emphasized linking research to practice, along with providing nurse researchers with an opportunity to interact among themselves and with researchers from other disciplines. NINR research priorities selected from both conferences and research opportunities for the 21st century are presented in Table 1.5.

NINR accomplishes its mission by supporting grants to universities and other research organizations as well as by conducting research intramurally in Bethesda, Maryland. In addition, NINR supports research training and career development to conduct nursing research. Examples of NINR-supported research include[9]:

- **Cancer.** It is possible to predict which cancer patients are likely to experience nausea during chemotherapy and to prevent or ease this unpleasant side effect and improve adherence to the life-saving treatments.
- **End of Life.** Family members involved in making a decision to withdraw support experience extremely high stress levels, which are reduced in the presence of an advance directive.
- **Feeding Tubes.** An inexpensive bedside test equals costly x-rays in accurately determining incorrect insertion or dislocation of feeding tubes used to provide nutrition fluids.
- **Care of AIDS Patients in Hospital Units.** Care of AIDS patients in dedicated units, with higher nurse-patient ratios and closer involvement of nurses and physicians with specialized AIDS experience, significantly lowered mortality rates and increased satisfaction with care.
- **Diabetes.** Teens who typically have trouble controlling their diabetes are able to improve control after training in coping skills, particularly in difficult social situations.

---

TABLE 1.5  NURSING RESEARCH PRIORITIES AS DEFINED BY THE NATIONAL INSTITUTE OF
NURSING RESEARCH (NINR)

---

**First Conference on Nursing Research Priorities (1988)**

• Low Birthweight: Mothers and Infants
• HIV Infection: Prevention and Care
• Long-Term Care for Older Adults
• Symptom Management: Pain
• Nursing Informatics: Enhancing Patient Care
• Health Promotion for Older Children and Adolescents
• Technology Dependency Across the Lifespan

**Second Conference on Nursing Research Priorities (1992)**

• Community-Based Nursing Models
• Effectiveness of Nursing Interventions in HIV/AIDS
• Cognitive Impairment
• Living with Chronic Illness
• Biobehavioral Factors Related to Immunocompetence

**NINR Research Priorities (2000-2002)**

• Chronic Illnesses
• Quality and Cost-Effectiveness Care
• Health Promotion and Disease Prevention
• Management of Symptoms Adaptation to New Technologies
• Health Disparities
• Palliative Care at the End of Life

---

• **Cardiovascular Disease.** A highly effective cardiovascular risk reduction
program about nutrition and exercise has been tested for grade-school
children that is fun and easy to follow and that helps them establish positive
health habits.
• **Pain.** Certain pain relievers for acute pain are more effective in women than
in men, underscoring the importance of gender in considering analgesics.
• **Transitional Care.** Researchers developed a model for the transition from
hospital to home care that has been tested in a variety of patient populations.
A modification of this model, applied to prenatal and infant care, reduced
infant hospitalizations and deaths, resulting in lower overall health costs.

## LINKAGES

The following web sites offer students some helpful information on research, funding possibilities, and network opportunities.

**Agency for Healthcare Research and Quality**
http://www.abcpr.gov/
**Centers for Disease Control and Prevention**
http://www.cdc.gov/

**Eastern Nursing Research Society**
http://www.enrs-go.org/
**Midwest Nursing Research Society**
http://www.mnrs.org/
**National Institutes of Health**
http://www.nih.gov/
**National Institutes of Nursing Research**
http://www.nih.gov/ninr/
**Sigma Theta Tau International**
http://nursingsociety.org/
**Southern Nursing Research Society**
http://www.snrs.org/

## SUMMARY OF KEY IDEAS

1. Nurses are responsible for assuming an active role in developing a body of nursing knowledge.
2. Nursing has its own unique body of knowledge that represents the knowing, experiencing, and understanding of phenomena related to providing patient care.
3. The scientific method is an approach to gaining new knowledge that is a systematic collection of empirical data.
4. Replicating a study increases the extent to which research findings are verified by providing additional evidence of the validity of the findings.
5. The role of the research consumer includes the ability to read and critique research reports.
6. Key nursing research journals include *Advances in Nursing Science, Applied Nursing Research, Image: Journal of Nursing Scholarship, Nursing Research, Nursing Science Quarterly, Research in Nursing and Health, Scholarship Inquiry for Nursing Practice,* and *Western Journal of Nursing Research.*
7. Nurses are responsible for promoting the integrity of nursing science.

## LEARNING ACTIVITIES

1. Select back issues of a research journal and identify several quantitative and qualitative studies. Did the studies satisfy the definition of research as stated in this chapter? Why or why not?

2. Did any of the studies combine both quantitative and qualitative approaches? If yes, were both approaches necessary? Why or why not?

## References

1. Gillis, A, and Jackson, W: Research for Nurses: Methods and Interpretation. FA Davis, Philadelphia, 2002, pp 7–10, 23–28.
2. Polit, DF, Beck, CT, and Hungler, DB: Essentials of Nursing Research: Methods, Appraisal, and Utilization, ed 5. Lippincott Williams & Wilkins, Philadelphia, 2001, pp 4–6.
3. Brown, SJ: Knowledge for Health Care Practice: A Guide to Using Research Evidence. WB Saunders, Philadelphia, 1999, pp 3–4.
4. Burns, N, and Groves, SK: The Practice of Nursing Research: Conduct, Critique, and Utilization, ed 4. WB Saunders, Philadelphia, 2001, pp 11–14, 38–39.
5. Morse, JM, and Field, PA: Qualitative Research Methods for Health Professionals, ed 2. Sage Publications, Thousand Oaks, CA, 1995, pp 16–19.
6. American Nurses' Association Commission on Nursing Research: Guidelines for the Investigative Function of Nurses. American Nurses' Association, Kansas City, MO, 1981.
7. Scientific Integrity Committee of the Midwest Nursing Research Society: Guidelines for Scientific Integrity. Midwest Nursing Research Society, Glenview, IL, 1996.
8. American Nurses' Association: Human Rights Guidelines for Nurses in Clinical and Other Research. American Nurses' Association, Kansas City, MO, 1985.
9. National Institute of Nursing Research (May, 2000). About NINR: Mission statement. http://www.nih.gov/NINR/research/mission.html

# 2

# Understanding the Research Process and Ethical Issues in Nursing Research

James A. Fain, PhD, RN, BC-ADM, FAAN

## LEARNING OBJECTIVES

*At the end of this chapter, you will be able to:*

1. Identify the basic components of the research process.
2. Distinguish between basic and applied research and between experimental and nonexperimental research.
3. Describe the process of ensuring that subjects participating in a study have been protected from violation of human rights.
4. Define informed consent and its key elements.
5. Explain the role of institutional review boards in safeguarding the rights of subjects participating in a study.
6. Explain how to evaluate the ethical implications of a research report.

## GLOSSARY OF KEY TERMS

**Anonymity.** A condition in which the identity of subjects remains unknown, even to the researcher, to protect subjects participating in a study.

**Applied research.** A type of study designed to gather knowledge that has direct clinical application.

**Basic research.** A type of study designed to develop the knowledge base and extend theory without direct focus on clinical application.

**Confidentiality.** Protecting data that is gathered or learned from patients by not disclosing information without their permission.

**Correlational research.** A type of nonexperimental study designed to examine the relationship between and among variables.

**Cross-sectional research.** A study that collects data at a particular point in time and does not require follow-up.

**Descriptive research.** A type of nonexperimental study designed to provide a knowledge base when little is known about a phenomenon; used to describe variables rather than to test a predicted relationship.

**Experimental research.** A study in which the researcher manipulates and controls one or more variables and observes the effect on (an)other variable(s).

**Human rights.** The protection of subjects participating in a research study; includes the right to freedom from injury, the right to privacy and dignity, and the right to anonymity and confidentiality.

**Longitudinal research.** A study that follows a cohort of subjects and collects data over time.

**Nonexperimental research.** A descriptive study that does not exhibit a great amount of control over variables.

**Prospective research.** A study that examines data collected in the present.

**Retrospective research.** A study that examines data collected in the past.

**Risk-benefit ratio.** The relationship between potential harm to subjects and potential positive outcomes of participating in a research study; an evaluation used by subjects to make voluntary informed consent.

**Secondary analysis.** A reanalysis of data collected previously for other purposes that is now being used to create a new research project.

The ability to read and evaluate research findings is important for nurses when practice is based on such research. Learning about components of the research process helps nurses become consumers of research and helps them develop the ability to determine the quality and merit of research reports. The purpose of this chapter is to provide an overview of the research process and of the various types and methods of research. Specific components of the research process are examined in succeeding chapters. This chapter includes a discussion of the accountability of researchers in maintaining ethical standards at all phases of the research process to protect the rights of individuals participating in a study.

## THE RESEARCH PROCESS

The research process involves decision making in order to consider various alternatives and to decide what methods will answer particular research question(s) or test hypotheses. The term *research* is derived from an earlier word that means to go around, to explore, and to circle. Many major decisions that researchers make are conceptual. Ideally, the chosen methodology follows these conceptual decisions logically and coherently. The research process is also flexible. There is no one correct answer but rather multiple possibilities from which researchers must choose, all with their own strengths and weaknesses.

Polit, Beck, and Hungler[1] describe 16 steps associated with the research process; Wilson[2] identifies 10 steps. The use of the word *steps* is misleading; the word implies finishing one activity or task before moving on to the next. Steps in the research process, however, tend to vary in their sequence and number depending on the purpose of the study and the researcher's style. Therefore, it is more useful to think of steps as guidelines.

The research process is circular. When conducting a study, researchers may need to go back and forth to rethink and reconceptualize the problem several times. For example, researchers continually review the literature to keep up with the most current information and refer to other research reports to get ideas for sampling, operational definitions, and research designs. Available instrumentation for measurement also influences the way that researchers think about the problem, even though conceptualization precedes the selection of measures. Another example of the circular nature of research is the use of the results of one study to create questions for the next study. Researchers may find at the end of a study that they have asked the wrong question(s). This observation does not necessarily mean that the time and energy put into the study were wasted. Refining questions is an important part of the process. Sometimes researchers cannot determine the correct question without first researching an incorrect question.

The intent of the research process is not to present a set of rules but to describe the general thinking of the researchers who plan the study. Although many different research models exist, the research process actually consists of standard elements (Fig. 2.1); the order may vary, and the steps may overlap in different research situations. The five general phases of the research process are:

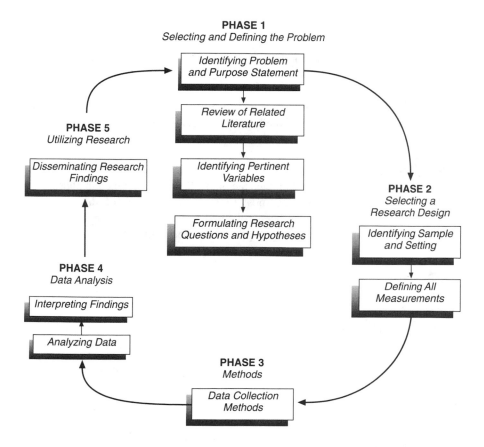

FIGURE 2.1 Model of the research process.

1. Selecting and defining the problem.
2. Selecting a research design.
3. Collecting data.
4. Analyzing data.
5. Using the research findings.

Each of these phases is discussed in detail in later chapters; a brief overview of the process follows.

## Phase 1

This phase involves selecting and defining an area of research that provides an opportunity to advance nursing knowledge. Through a review of related literature, the researcher determines a rationale for conducting the study, a justification of the need to investigate the problem, and a theoretical framework for interpreting the results (see Chapter 3). Research questions, hypotheses, or both, are proposed in phase 1 (see Chapter 6).

## Phase 2

In this phase the researcher designs the study and plans the methods of subject selection, testing, and measurement (see Chapter 8) to ensure that all procedures are defined clearly (see Chapter 11). The choice of the research design is based on how the research problem is conceptualized. These planning tasks act as guides to help with the selection of appropriate methods for analyzing the data.

## Phase 3

In this phase the researcher implements the plans that were designed in phases 1 and 2. Data collection is usually the most time-consuming part of this phase (see Chapter 9). After the data have been collected and recorded, the researcher must organize the information into an appropriate form for analysis.

## Phase 4

This phase involves analyzing, interpreting, and making valid conclusions about the data. Statistical procedures are applied to summarize the quantitative data in a meaningful way (see Chapter 10). During this phase the research hypotheses will be either supported or not supported. Analysis of results leads to new questions that stimulate further study.

## Phase 5

In this final phase of the research process researchers have the responsibility of sharing their findings with other colleagues. Research findings that are not disseminated to other colleagues are of little value to anyone. Reporting of research can take many forms, including journal articles, abstracts, oral presentations, and poster presentations. The research process culminates with interpreting the findings and communicating any new knowledge gained from the research (see Chapters 15 to 17).

## TYPES OF RESEARCH

The research process provides a general strategy for gathering, analyzing, and interpreting data to answer questions or test hypotheses. Classification of research is based on the purpose of a study (see Chapter 3) and amount of control (see Chapter 11). One such classification is basic versus applied research.

### Basic Versus Applied Research

**Basic research** is often referred to as pure or fundamental research. The major purpose of basic research is to obtain empirical data that can be used to develop, refine, or test a theory without immediate concern for direct application to clinical practice. Basic research closely resembles the work done in laboratories and is associated with scientists. Researchers who study how blood cells function or who examine the structure and function of parts of the brain are conducting basic research to better understand those structures. Although the information gained from basic research may be useful later in the development of a particular treatment or drug, the sole purpose of the study is to advance knowledge in a given subject area.

**Applied research,** as the name suggests, is conducted to gain knowledge that can be used in a practical setting. This type of research is usually performed in actual practice conditions on subjects who represent the group to which the results will be applied. Regardless of the type of problem studied (i.e., patient care, education, administration), the research findings contribute to some modification of present practices. Excerpt 2.1 displays findings from a study that examined needs of women after breast biopsy procedures. Through the use of a focus group, nine breast clinic patients provided the researcher with information needs women have after a breast biopsy. Such knowledge is pertinent for nurses to understand and use in planning care for women undergoing breast biopsy procedures.

Most clinical nursing research falls into the category of applied research; nursing has not, for the most part, been involved in basic research. Although the difference between basic and applied research appears to be rather distinct, a continuum actually exists between the two extremes. In many cases, one must have basic knowledge to be able to interpret the findings of applied studies. Many studies provide clinical application as well as new knowledge that contributes to a theoretical understanding of basic behavior.

### Experimental Versus Nonexperimental

Another classification of research is experimental versus nonexperimental. **Experimental research** refers to a study in which the researcher manipulates and

**EXCERPT 2.1**

## EXAMPLE OF FINDINGS FROM AN APPLIED RESEARCH STUDY

The participants identified nine information needs in three categories as the most important. The three categories included the types of benign breast disease, meaning of risk associated with benign breast disease, and diagnostic tests required to evaluate a breast lump. The participants determined that information related to an ambulatory breast biopsy procedure and breast cancer treatment was less important for a breast lump evaluation. The following nine most important needs chosen by the focus group participants does not represent a rank ordering: types of benign breast disease, meaning of risk associated with benign breast disease, what makes a lump suspicious for breast cancer, what are the chances of getting breast cancer, how long can women wait before having a breast biopsy and being in real danger of getting breast cancer, when will the results of the biopsy be returned, how many tests are needed to give a definite diagnosis, what is involved in the mammographic needle localization procedure, and do women need follow-up tests or exams if the biopsy is negative?

*Source: Deane, KA, and Degner, LF: Determining the information needs of women after breast biopsy procedures. AORN J 65:767, 1997. Reprinted with permission. Copyright © AORN, Inc, 2170 S Parker Road, Suite 300, Denver, CO 80231.*

controls one or more variables and observes the effect of manipulation on other variables.[1,2] The notion of manipulation and control refers to the researcher having the ability to administer a treatment (sometimes referred to as an intervention) to some participants in a study and not administering (or administering an alternative treatment) to others. For example, a nurse might be interested in examing the impact of preoperative teaching program with respect to use of pain medication. One group of participants (experimental group) is instructed how to cough and breathe deeply as well as set expectations for the immediate postoperative period, whereas a second group is given a standard brochure on preoperative instructions. Both groups are measured on the amount of pain medication administered during the first 8 hours postoperatively. In this case, the experimental research design tests whether a preoperative teaching program has an impact on pain medication usage. Experimental research is carried out using several types of designs (e.g., experimental and quasi-experimental). See Chapter 11 for a more detailed discussion of research designs.

Dellerfield and McDougall's[3] study is an example of an experimental design. Their study tested the effects of a 2-week, four-session group intervention with older adults, designed to increase memory self-efficacy and memory performance. One hundred forty-five older adults were recruited to participate in the study. Of those, 74 received the intervention (experimental group), and 71 did not (control group). Memory self-efficacy was measured using four subscales associated with the Metamemory in Adulthood Questionnaire; memory performance was measured by the Memory Performance Test. The researcher manipulated the independent variable by assigning some subjects to receive the intervention ($n = 74$) and others not ($n = 71$). The impact of the intervention was assessed by measuring the effects on two dependent variables: memory self-efficacy and memory performance.

Nonexperimental research refers to studies that are more descriptive or exploratory in nature. The researcher is interested in describing what already exists. Descriptive studies answer the question "What is this?" Nonexperimental research is sometimes classified as descriptive and/or correlational. In descriptive research a particular situation or event that already exists is described systematically. No attempt is made to explain or predict what the situation might be in the future or how it might be changed. Descriptive research uses questionnaires, surveys, interviews, or obseerevations to collect data. Sample subjects are chosen who represent the population at large. For example, Hilton[4] in a nonexperimental, descriptive study investigated the intake of folic acid among women between the ages of 18 and 24. A convenience sample of 42 female college students enrolled in a small liberal arts college in western North Carolina was invited to participate and fill out a survey. With the literature suggesting a link between folic acid intake and the incidence of neural tube defects in newborns, the focus of the study was to determine whether young women consume the recommended daily allowance of folic acid. There was no attempt to examine relationships or make predictions.

Correlational research examines the relationship between and among variables. The research collects data on at least two variables for the same group of individuals and calculates a correlation coefficient between the measures. A high number of research studies in nursing are classified as descriptive correlational designs.

Houldin, Jacobsen, and Lowery[5] examined the relationship between self-blame and illness adjustment in women with breast cancer. The study was descriptive in that sociodemographic data, along with scores on the Psychosocial Adjustment to Illness Scale and Global Adjustment to Illness Scale, were reported on women diagnosed with stage I and II breast cancer. The study was correlational in that the study examined the relationship of self-blame as a singular concept (i.e., characterological or behavioral) with adjustment to breast cancer, taking into account perceived control and avoidance.

## CLASSIFICATION OF RESEARCH BY TIME DIMENSION

### Retrospective Versus Prospective Research

*Retrospective* and *prospective* characterize a particular time perspective. Retrospective research examines data collected in the past, typified by review of medical records. In these records, events have already occurred, and variables have already been measured. In Excerpt 2.2, data were collected from a chart review. Charts were selected randomly from a list obtained from medical records, based on inclusion criteria provided by the researchers. Data retrieved from charts included laboratory values of potassium, calcium, and magnesium. In addition, several preoperative demographic data were recorded.

Prospective research examines data collected in the present. Prospective studies are more reliable than retrospective studies because of the potential for greater control of data collection. For example, Gennaro[6] designed a prospective study by examining how employment, income, and out-of-pocket expenses changed in

Excerpt 2.2

## USE OF MEDICAL RECORDS AS A RETROSPECTIVE APPROACH TO RESEARCH

**Design**

This retrospective study consisted of a chart review conducted in the medical records department of a 600-bed urban referral hospital in the southeast with a large cardiovascular surgical program.

**Sample**

The target sample included patients aged 20 to 80 years experiencing CABG for the first time. Patients with current valve replacements or valve repairs were not included. A sample of 40 patients experiencing SVT and 40 patients not experiencing SVT was randomly selected from a list obtained from the medical records department with use of the international Classification of Diseases Code to identify patients undergoing CABG for the first time during the year 1991. The obtained list was not in any systematic chronologic or alphabetic order.

**Instrument**

The data collection sheet was developed based on the review of the literature, available data from the intensive care unit (ICU) flowsheet, and discussion with nurses providing care for patients with CABG. Preoperative demographic information recorded included sex, age, obesity, history of congestive heart failure, cardiac arrest, previous surgery, diabetes, hypertension, valve disease, tobacco use, and SVT. Postoperative data retrieved included laboratory values of potassium, calcium, and magnesium. Fluid measurements recorded included intravenous (IV) intake, including maintenance IV and bolus IV fluids given the first 24 hours after surgery, along with IV bolus doses of potassium, calcium, and magnesium.

*Source: Nally, BR, et al: Supraventricular tachycardia after coronary artery bypass grafting surgery and fluid and electrolyte variables. Heart Lung 25:31, 1996, with permission.*

224 families of low-birthweight infants during the first 6 months after the infant was discharged home. Mothers kept logs of expenses and were interviewed about changes in employment and income at infant discharge from the hospital and at 1, 3, and 6 months later. The sample was monitored for 6 months to see what changes occurred over time. Researchers invest a considerable amount of time when conducting prospective studies.

## Cross-Sectional Versus Longitudinal Research

**Cross-sectional research** collects data at one point in time with no follow-up. The result is a measurement of what exists today, with no attempt to document changes over time in either the past or the future. In Excerpt 2.3, pain perception in elderly subjects who were cognitively impaired was assessed using a cross-sectional approach. In this study, the authors chose to asess pain once, with all subjects being tested at the same time. There was no attempt to monitor these subjects over time.

**EXCERPT 2.3**

## EXAMPLE OF CROSS-SECTIONAL RESEARCH

**Design and Setting**

This cross-sectional study used face-to-face scripted interviews and chart review. Residents were selected regardless of their length of time in the institution, physical condition, or pain history.

**Participant Selection**

Participants were randomly selected by using a list of bed numbers without regard to length of stay or admission date. Inclusion criteria for the study were English-speaking residents, older than 65 years, who were not comatose. Both university and agency human subjects internal review boards approved the study.

**Procedure**

A scripted, interview format was used to obtain cognitive functioning and pain data. The Short Portable Mental Status Questionnaire (SPMSQ) was administered to evaluate and classify level of cognitive impairments. After administration of the SPMSQ, each resident was asked if they had any pain. If after 30 seconds there was no response, the question was asked, "Do you hurt anywhere?"

*Source: Manz, BD, et al: Pain assessment in the cognitively impaired and unimpaired elderly. Pain Manag Nurs 1:106, 2000, with permission.*

**Longitudinal research** follows a cohort of subjects and collects data at different intervals over time. In Excerpt 2.4, the authors state that data were collected over a 9 months. The various data collection points were not identified. An advantage of longitudinal research is the ability to collect data on the same individuals over time. However, there are several practical difficulties associated with longitudinal research. Loss of subjects at different points is a major problem. In addition, longitudinal research studies can be threatened by testing effects, with subjects being tested repeatedly.

Researchers make decisions as to whether they conduct retrospective or prospective studies, based on either causes in the past (retrospective) or present causes for future effects (prospective). In addition, researchers may look for descriptions of events and things that occurred in the past (retrospective), may follow individuals into the future to describe events as they occur (prospective), or may describe what exists today (cross-sectional).

## ETHICAL ISSUES IN NURSING RESEARCH

For many nursing students, the first personal contact with research will be to invite patients to participate in a study or help with data collection. With nursing studies dealing primarily with human subjects, there is a concern for protecting individuals from any harmful effects that might result from participation in a study. As nurses engage in various research activites, it is important that the profession operate from a sound ethical knowledge base. Adequate protection of research subjects may cause

EXCERPT 2.4

## EXAMPLE OF LONGITUDINAL RESEARCH

**Research Methods**

This study was designed to evaluate the feasibility of implementing the DSM intervention in a rual area with African American participants. For this purpose, a longitudinal, quasi-experimental study using a one-group pretest-posttest design was conducted from February 1999 to November 1999. Specific aims were to (1) evaluate the effects of dietary self-management education on physiological outcomes, diabetes self-management, and costs of care; (2) assess adherence to intervention sessions; (3) assess the ability to recruit an African-American sample; and (4) assess the ability to retain rural African-Americans in the study.

*Source: Anderson-Loftin, W, et al: Culturally competent dietary education for southern rural African Americans with diabetes. Diabetes Educ 28:245, 2002, with permission.*

a delay in the proposed schedule or a change in the research design. In either case, such changes are absolutely necessary if the safety of participants is involved.

### Developing Professional Guidelines

Nursing has developed guidelines to ensure the protection of human subjects while research is conducted. The basic documents that have been used to develop guidelines are based on the Articles of the Nuremberg Code (1947)[7] and the Declaration of Helsinki (1964).[8] The Articles of the Nuremberg Code serve as a standard against which to measure the individual rights of subjects participating in experimental and clinical research.

### Historical Events That Helped Shape Guidelines for Human Subject Protection

Before World War II, few guidelines were available to ensure the protection of human subjects participating in research. Although Germany was the most scientifically and technologically advanced country during World War II, the Nazi party exploited people's trust in the medical community and public health by performing unethical experiments on populations they discriminated against. For example, in one series of experiments, Air Force pilots were placed in vacuum chambers that could duplicate the low air pressure and anoxia (lack of oxygen) at altitudes over 65,000 feet. The German Air Force was interested in understanding if pilots could survive at extremely high altitudes, only to find that over 40 percent of the pilots died as a result of anoxia and ruptured lungs. The German Air Force was also involved in investigating survival times after pilots parachuted into cold water. Pilots were immersed for hours in tubs of ice water; others were fed nothing for days but salt water. Still others were kept outside at subfreezing temperatures for hours. Finally, at several concentration camps, Polish women were shot and slashed on the legs. Wounds were stuffed with glass, dirt, and various bacteria cultures and sewn shut. The infected wounds were then treated with experimental anti-infective agents. In all instances, no attempts were made to relieve the tremendous suffering caused by these experiments. It was not uncommon for one out of every four individuals to die as a result of their involvement in the experiments.[9]

## Nuremberg Code

As a result of the horrifying acts and unethical medical research experiments conducted by Nazi doctors in the name of science, the Nuremberg Trials took place. Several American judges who presided over the final judgment in the Nuremberg Trial were instrumental in developing the Nuremberg Code. The code was developed in 1947 to address protection of human subjects and basic principles of ethical behavior. Sections of the Nuremberg Code are presented in Table 2.1. Articles within the code emphasize adequate protection of subjects from risk or harm, the right to withdraw from experimentation, and adequate qualifications of those conducting research.[7]

## Declaration of Helsinki

In 1964, the World Medical Association met in Finland and developed guidelines for physicians conducting research. In addition to reiterating aspects of the Nuremberg Code, the Declaration of Helsinki outlined two categories of research: research that has a therapeutic value for subjects and research that does not have direct therapeutic value for subjects.

The essence of the Declaration was the need for subjects to be informed of the benefits of the study before consenting to participate in the research. Subjects also

---

TABLE 2.1 SECTIONS OF THE NUREMBERG CODE

1. The voluntary consent of the human subject is absolutely essential.
2. The experiment should be such as to yield fruitful results . . . and not random or unnecessary.
3. The experiment should be based on . . . [prior knowledge] and the anticipated results should justify the experiment.
4. The experiment should . . . avoid all unnecessary physical and mental suffering and injury.
5. No experiment should be conducted where there is an *a priori* reason to believe that death or disabling injury will occur; except where the experimental physicians also serve as subjects.
6. The degree of risk should never exceed . . . the importance of the problem to be solved.
7. Proper preparations should be made and adequate facilities provided to protect subjects against possibilities of injury, disability, or death.
8. The experiment should be conducted only by scientifically qualified persons.
9. During the course of treatment, the human subject should be able to bring the experiment to an end.
10. During the course of treatment the scientist must be prepared to terminate the experiment if he or she has probable cause . . . that a continuation of the experiment is likely to result in injury, disability, or death to the experimental subject.

were to be informed when their participation could be harmful or of little value to them.[8] The Declaration also allowed legal guardians to grant permission to enroll subjects in research and recommended written consent.

After the Nuremberg Code was established and informed consent laws were rewritten, protection of human subject rights was far from guaranteed. The Centers for Disease Control and Prevention conducted studies in the rural South to determine the prevalence of syphilis among blacks while exploring the possibilities of treatment. Tuskegee, a town in Macon County, Alabama, was found to have the highest incidence of syphilis among six counties.

### The Tuskegee Syphilis Study

In 1932, the U.S. Public Health Service (USPHS) began an experiment in Tuskegee, Alabama. The study included 400 black sharecroppers diagnosed with syphilis and 200 black men who did not have syphilis. The study, known as the Tuskegee Syphilis Study, began in 1932 and ended in 1972. The study design called for the selection of black men with syphilis who were between 25 and 60 years of age. Subjects were randomly assigned into two groups, 400 men with untreated syphilis and 200 men without syphilis. As the study began, difficulties arose in recruiting subjects. Consequently, the men were told they were ill and would be offered free treatment. The USPHS did not inform subjects that they were part of a research study on syphilis. Instead, they were told they were being treated for "bad blood."

In 1933, the USPHS decided to continue with the study and treat subjects with mercurial ointment, a noneffective drug. This was in the face of findings in every textbook that clearly advocated treating patients who had syphilis, even in the disease's latent stages. By 1936, first reports were out that men with syphilis developed more complications than did the control group. By 1946, the death rate for men with untreated syphilis was twice as high as for the control group. In 1955, it was likewise reported that more than 30 percent of those autopsied had died directly from advanced syphilitic lesions of the cardiovascular or central nervous system.[10,11] After the study ended, those men who had syphilis, along with their wives and children who had contracted the disease, were given free antibiotics and lifetime medical care. However, the damage to their health, as well as their trust in the medical research community, was beyond repair. In a formal White House ceremony in 1997, President Clinton apologized to subjects and their families who participated in the Tuskegee Study and called for a renewed emphasis on research ethics.

### The Willowbrook Study

The Willowbrook State School on Staten Island, New York, was the focus of unethical research during the 1950s to 1970. The purpose of the Willowbrook Study was to determine the period of infectivity of infectious hepatitis. Subjects were mentally handicapped children who were given either intramuscular or oral doses of hepatitis B virus. If parents wished to admit their child to the school, they were required to sign their child on as a study participant. Parents gave consent for the administration of the hepatitis B virus, but they were not told of the serious consequences, such as flu-like symptoms, skin rashes, and liver damage. During the 20-year investigation, Willowbrook closed its door to new admissions because of overcrowding, yet the research ward continued to admit new residents. Administrators at Willowbrook believed they were conducting ethical research in a category called "natural experiments." The question whether the Willowbrook experiment was an ethical "study in nature" has been debated for years. The belief was that if there was no cure or treatment for a particular disease, then observing its course with the informed consent of participants is a study of nature.[11]

## The Crisis at John Hopkins University

In April 2001, a 24-year-old healthy volunteer and technician at John Hopkins Asthma and Allergy Center consented to participate in a study. The purpose of the study was to gain a better understanding of the pathophysiology of asthma, specifically the mechanism of airway hyperresponsiveness. The study was based on the hypothesis that in normal individuals, lung inflation protects the airways from obstruction through a neural mechanism that might be lacking or impaired in people with asthma.[12]

The protocol involved healthy subjects inhaling a ganglionic blocker, hexamethonium. If ganglionic blockage suppressed the protective effects of deep inspiration on the airways, it would suggest that neural mechanisms helped the airways stay open. Hexamethonium was chosen because it blocks neurotransmission. The drug had been used to treat hypertension, but it removed from the U.S. market in 1972 after the Food and Drug Administration (FDA) found it was ineffective.[12]

In the consent form, hexamethonium was described as "a medication that has been used during surgery, as part of anesthesia; that is capable of stopping some nerves in your airways from functioning for a short period." The section on risks stated that hexamethonium "may reduce your blood pressure and make you feel dizzy especially when you stand up." The consent document was later criticized as having "failed to indicate that inhaled hexamethonium was experimental and not approved by the FDA" and because it was referred to as "medication."[12]

The 24-year-old volunteer was the third subject to receive hexamethonium. Mild shortness of breath and cough developed in the first subject, resolving over a period of about 8 days. The second subject received hexamethonium while the first subject still had symptoms. The 24-year-old volunteer inhaled 1 gm of hexamethonium on May 4, 2001, and developed a cough. On May 9, the volunteer was hospitalized with fever, hypoxemia, and abnormalities on a chest x-ray. By May 12, progressive dyspnea had developed, and the volunteer was transferred to the intensive care unit. On June 2, the volunteer died as a result of progressive hypotension and multiorgan failure.[12]

The crisis at John Hopkins University led to several reviews of clinical research. These reviews were conducted by internal and external review committees convened by the university, the FDA, and the U.S. Office for Human Research Protections. After the death of the volunteer, John Hopkins temporarily suspended all studies involving healthy volunteers.

*Other Scandals Regarding Unethical Research Studies*

Beecher,[13] a well-known Harvard anesthesiologist, describes a series of unethical research studies conducted at major medical institutions across the country. The article made it clear how widespread the problems really were. All of these studies reinforce the important need for institutional review boards (IRBs) to review studies conscientiously and for researchers to act ethically. Rothman[14] cautioned researchers not to take advantage of subjects in particular social predicaments because they will become accomplices to the problem, not observers of it.

## Developing Guidelines for Clinical Nursing Research

The Articles of the Nuremberg Code and Declaration of Helsinki are prototypes for the development of guidelines for conducting research in nursing. The American Nurses Association (ANA) has developed two documents that provide such direction. In *Guidelines for the Investigative Function of Nurses,*[15] general research competencies expected of graduates from associate, baccalaureate, and graduate degree programs in nursing are outlined (see Chapter 1). In *Human Rights Guidelines for Nurses in Clinical and Other Research,*[16] the principles in the Nuremberg Code are emphasized and directed toward voluntary participation of subjects, protection of human subjects, and informed consent. This document focuses on the rights of subjects who are involved in research, along with ethical issues within clinical nursing research settings. A summary of this document is presented in Table 2.2. Adhering to these guidelines reduces the chance of violating the rights of subjects. Key points addressed in the document are summarized in Figure 2.2.

## Protecting Human Rights

The guidelines presented in Table 2.2 provide nurses with principles intended to safeguard human rights. The researcher must consider these guidelines at every stage of the research process, from selecting and defining the problem, selecting a research design, and collecting data to interpreting and publishing the results. **Human rights** involves the protection of human subjects participating in research; the term refers to the following three rights outlined in the ANA guidelines[11]:

1. Right to freedom from injury
2. Right to privacy and dignity
3. Right to anonymity and confidentiality

*Right to Freedom From Injury*

A basic responsibility of all researchers is to protect subjects from harm while they are participating in a study. Subjects have the right not to incur physical or emotional injury as a result of participating. If there is a possibility of any potential injury that could occur, subjects need to know an estimate of the extent of such injury before giving their consent. Providing subjects with an estimate of the poten-

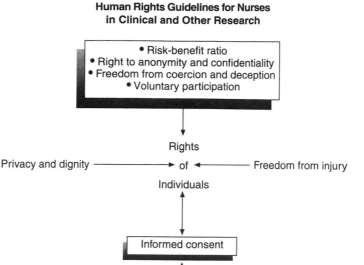

**Human Rights Guidelines for Nurses
in Clinical and Other Research**

- Risk-benefit ratio
- Right to anonymity and confidentiality
- Freedom from coercion and deception
- Voluntary participation

Rights

Privacy and dignity ⟶ of ⟵ Freedom from injury

Individuals

Informed consent

Institutional review
boards (IRBs)

FIGURE 2.2 American Nurses
Association guidelines for protecting human rights.

tial risks in relation to the potential benefits is called the **risk-benefit ratio.** Two
factors emerge when attempting to ensure the right to freedom from injury:

1. Ability of the benefit to justify subjects' exposure to involved risks.
2. The subjects' vulnerability.

The risks to subjects must be justified by the potential benefit to the individual (in
the case of clinical research) or to society (in the case of knowledge produced). In
short, the benefits should exceed the risks. Even then, however, a cancer patient's
risks of increased side effects from multiple chemotherapeutic agents may not
always be justified by advancing society's knowledge of cancer treatment.

The risk-benefit ratio remains a primary objective standard by which we can
judge the ethics of certain research procedures. Calculating this ratio involves
naming and weighing the benefits, as well as considering:

1. How important is the research?
2. How serious are the risks to human subjects involved in the research? Often,
   the benefits of basic research are difficult to identify.

In any case, if potential for harm exists, whether physiological or psychological,
the researcher must explain how the risks will be minimized. Subjects must be fully
aware of the risks, and the nature of the benefits expected from the study must be
convincing.[9]

---

TABLE 2.2 SUMMARY OF GUIDELINES FOR PROTECTING THE RIGHTS OF HUMAN SUBJECTS

1. If research participation (medical, nursing, or other) is a condition of employment, nurses must be informed in writing of the nature of activity involved in advance of employment and if this is not done, nurses must be given the opportunity of not participating in research. Potential risks to others must be clarified in advance of research as well as ways to identify risks and counteract potential harm.
2. *Freedom from risk of injury or harm.* Researchers must estimate risk and benefit involved, and subjects must be informed of any potential mental or physical risk as well as personal benefit and procedures or activities that extend beyond personal need. Nurses must carefully monitor sources of potential risk of injury and protect subjects who are particularly vulnerable as a result of illness or members of captive groups (e.g., prisoners, students, institutionalized patients, and the poor).
   *Right to privacy and dignity.* All proposals, instruments, and procedures involved in the research activity must be discussed with prospective subjects and others participating in the project so that individuals may make an informed decision about whether to participate.
   *Right to anonymity.* The researcher must describe to prospective subjects the methods that protect the identity of subjects and the information obtained under privileged conditions.
3. Guidelines for protecting human rights apply to all individuals involved in a research activity. The use of subjects with limited civil freedom can usually only be justified when there is predicted benefit to them or others in similar circumstances.
4. Nurses have an obligation to protect human rights and a professional responsibility to support research that broadens the scientific knowledge base of nursing for the practice and delivery of service.
5. Voluntary informed consent to participate in research must be obtained from all prospective subjects or their legal representatives.
6. Nurses have an obligation to participate on institutional review boards to review the ethical implications of proposed and ongoing research. All studies that involve gathering data from humans, animals, or charts should be reviewed by healthcare professionals and community representatives.
7. The following practical guidelines are concerned with conducting research: content and function of institutional review boards, institutional sponsorship of outside investigators (e.g., graduate students), and subject recruitment process.

---

*Source: American Nurses' Association: Human Rights Guidelines for Nurses in Clinical and Other Research. American Nurses' Association, Kansas City, MO, 1985, with permission.*[10]

The vulnerability of potential subjects must also be considered when determining the risk-benefit ratio. Certain groups of individuals may be considered vulnerable and at risk for coercion because they are limited in their capacity to enter freely into a study with full understanding of the benefits and risks associated with participation. Vulnerable subject groups may include children, prisoners, and mentally disabled, elderly, sedated or unconscious, and dying individuals. Researchers need to incorporate additional safeguards to ensure adequate protection for these special population groups.

### Right to Privacy and Dignity

The type of data collected may be highly sensitive to the subjects' privacy and dignity. Many questionnaires or surveys require subjects to provide data such as income, marital status, personal activities, opinions and beliefs, and attitudes. In addition, the use of cameras, one-way mirrors, tape recorders, diaries, and patient records may easily be construed as an invasion of privacy. Participant observation is frequently used as a method to collect data in qualitative research studies. Such an approach may not be clearly understood by subjects. In all instances, the researcher is obligated to make sure that subjects clearly understand all procedures, the type of data being collected, and the data collection methods, so that they can make an informed decision about participating in a study.

### Right to Anonymity and Confidentiality

Closely related to protecting privacy and dignity is the right of subjects to remain anonymous and to be assured of confidentiality. The researcher must plan carefully to consider handling, storage, and reporting of data. **Anonymity** refers to keeping individuals nameless[9] and limiting access to information that is gathered about a subject. Anonymity can be facilitated by using code numbers for subjects' identity to prevent others from linking reported information with them. A master code list should be kept locked up, with access to the data limited to those who are intimately involved in the research. In anonymity, even the researcher cannot link the data to the subject.

**Confidentiality** refers to protecting data by not divulging information that is gathered or learned in caring for a patient without that individual's permission to do so.[9,15] This right is extremely important when the information may carry a stigma, such as a diagnosis of HIV or AIDS, evidence of domestic violence, or a prison record.

## Ensuring the Protection of Human Rights

Several procedures can be used to ensure protection of human rights, such as procedures for obtaining informed consent and review of study protocols by an ethics committee, often referred to as an institutional review board (IRB).

### Key Elements of Informed Consent

A basic responsibility of researchers is to ensure that potential subjects understand the implications of participating in a research study and recognize that they have the freedom to decide whether they want to participate. The idea that individuals have the right to decide for themselves is referred to as the principle of self-determination, which is central to the process of informed consent.

Key elements of informed consent are (1) providing potential subjects with sufficient information about participating in a research study and (2) assuring them that participation is voluntary and can be withdrawn at any time without negative consequences. The language is kept simple to make sure that all subjects understand the meaning of informed consent.

Subjects give informed consent before participating in a study by signing a written consent form, which is also signed and dated by the researcher and a witness. The researcher discusses the proposed research study with subjects to provide feedback in response to subjects' questions, concerns, or both. Consent forms should be divided into sections with headings. Medical jargon should be avoided for purposes of clarity and readability; sentences should be short, margins should be reasonably wide, and the pages should not be overcrowded with too much text. An example of a consent form is shown in Figure 2.3. The following information should be conveyed to potential subjects:

1. Title of the study.
2. Personnel engaged in the study (e.g., principal investigator, coinvestigator(s), research assistants).
3. Invitation to participate in the study (e.g., "You are invited to participate in a research study"; not "requested," "chosen," or "eligible").
4. Reason the particular subject is being invited to participate.
5. Clear description of the purpose of the study.
6. Detailed description of procedures of the study (e.g., descriptions of what will actually occur; how much time is required of the subject; whether hospitalization will be required and whether it will *always, sometimes,* or *never* be required as part of the subject's standard care; how much and how often blood will be drawn, if applicable).
7. Potential risks to subjects, including psychological, social, and physical risks (e.g., explanation of steps that will be taken to protect against risks; estimation of likelihood of occurrence, severity, and duration of potential risks, if applicable).
8. Potential benefits of the study (e.g., identification of desired benefit to society, the risk-benefit ratio, statement of whether there are direct subject benefits).
9. Economic considerations (e.g., whether subjects will incur any additional expenses as a result of participation).
10. Confidentiality considerations (e.g., explanation of steps that will be taken to ensure the confidentiality of information that is obtained during the course of the study, such as who will have access to the data and when the data and specimens will be destroyed).
11. Freedom of subjects to ask questions and withdraw from the study at any time without penalty.

Some research subjects may be unwilling or unable to sign a consent form. For example, the elderly may be wary of signing forms, and other individuals may have certain physical handicaps preventing them from being able to sign. The researcher needs to decide the best way possible to document permission. In some cases, an audiotaped or videotaped recording may be used to present information and obtain verbal consent. In the case of children, a parent or legal guardian must sign the consent form. Children (individuals under 18 years of age) are not considered legally competent to provide informed consent. When children are involved in a study, the researcher should obtain informed consent of the parent or legal guardian as well as assent of the child. Assent of a child refers to a child's affirmative agreement to participate in a research study. Failure of the child to object, however,

# University of Massachusetts Medical Center
## Committee for the Protection of Human Subjects in Research
## Consent to Participate in a Research Project

Title: Patient Empowerment Program for People with Diabetes
Principle Investigator: James A. Fain, PhD, RN, BC-ADM, FAAN

Research Subject's Name _____ Date: _____

## PURPOSE
You are invited to volunteer for a research study. You have been chosen to take part in this study because you have diabetes. The main objective is to see if a program that helps develop skills and self-awareness in the areas of goal setting, problem solving, stress management, coping, and motivation would be beneficial to patients with diabetes. The purpose of this study is to try to find an effective way to prepare patients with diabetes to make decisions.

It is important for you to know that your participation is entirely voluntary. You may decide not to take part in or quit the study at any time, without any penalty. You will be told about any new information or changes in the study that might affect your participation.

To take part in this study you must agree to participate in an outpatient educational program. The program will take place weekly for 2 hours and last a total of six (6) weeks. Each session will involve a brief presentation of key concepts related to the topic; completion of self-assessment worksheets; and small group discussions.You will be encouraged to bring a spouse, family member, or friend to each session.

## PROCEDURES
If you agree to participate in this study, you will be invited to an orientation session where a discussion about the program along with sample worksheets will be presented. You will be asked to complete several questionnaires along with giving us permission to access your medical records to obtain the most recent glycosylated hemoglobin level which was performed as a routine procedure during your treatment at the diabetes clinic. In addition, at the end of 6 weeks, you will be asked to complete the questionnaires a second time along with giving us permission to access once again your glycosylated hemoglobin levels. Questions throughout the program will focus on exploring life satisfactions, coping with diabetes, addressing daily stresses, and setting priorities.

Not everyone in the study will initially participate in the program. You will either be assigned to attend the program (experimental group) or not attend (comparison group). At the conclusion of the program, all those individuals who did not attend the program will be asked to complete the questionnaires a second time. After that time, the program will be provided for all those individuals who did not initially participate in the program.

## RISKS
We can foresee few risks that might occur if you decide to participate in this study. A minor risk is the possibility that certain questions regarding anxiety, stress, and feelings toward diabetes may arouse psychologically distressing emotions. If this is the case, you will be able to speak to a member of the research team or staff within the clinic.

## BENEFITS
There is no promise or guarantee of any medical benefits to you resulting from your participation in this study. However, you might have a better insight into your own values, goals, and needs as they relate to living with diabetes. In addition, your participation may help others with diabetes in the future as a result of knowledge gained from this research.

## ALTERNATIVES
Your standard treatment will be the same whether or not you decide to be in the study. However, the educational program is not presently available off study.

## COSTS
There will be no additional cost to you from being in this research study. Patients will not be charged for any materials used in this research study.

## CONFIDENTIALITY
Your research records will be confidential. In all records of the study you will be identified by a code number and your name will be known only to the researchers. Your name will not be

*(continued)*

FIGURE 2.3 Example of an adult consent form.

**University of Massachusetts Medical Center
Committee for the Protection of Human Subjects in Research
Consent to Participate in a Research Project** (continued)

used in any reports or publications of this study. Once again, your participation in this study is entirely voluntary. You may withdraw from the study at any time.

Please feel free to ask any questions you may have about the study or about your rights as a research subject. If other questions occur to you later, you may contact James A. Fain, PhD, RN, BC-ADM, FAAN, the Principle Investigator, at (508) 856-5661. If at any time during or after the study, you would like to discuss the study or your research rights with someone who is not associated with the study, you may contact the Administrative Coordinator for the Committee for the Protection of Human Subjects in Research at UMMC, (508) 856-4261. Consent to Participate in the Research Project, H-2895 entitled "Patient Empowerment Program for People with Diabetes."

Subject's Name _____

P.I. Name _____
The purpose and procedures of this research project have been explained to me and I understand them. I have been told about all the predictable discomfort, risks, and benefits that might result, and I understand them. I agree to participate as a subject in this research project. I understand that I may end my participation at any time.

_____ Date: _____
　　　　　　　　Subject's Signature

NAME: (print) _____

Relationship to Subject: _____

Witness Signature: _____

Date: _____

NAME: (print) _____

FIGURE 2.3  Example of an adult consent form.

cannot be construed as assent. An example of a child's assent form is shown in Figure 2.4.

## Institutional Review Boards

In addition to ensuring that subjects give voluntary informed consent to participate in a study, most institutions and funding agencies have a mechanism for reviewing research proposals. As mentioned earlier, IRBs are review groups responsible for ensuring that researchers do not engage in unethical behavior or conduct poorly designed research studies.

The major responsibility of an IRB is to review research proposals at convened meetings to ensure that federal guidelines are followed. Proposals submitted to IRBs are reviewed in detail. The IRB ensures that the researcher is not violating the rights of human subjects. Lawyers, lay persons, and clergy often serve on IRBs to deal

**University of Massachusetts Medical Center
Committee for the Protection of Human Subjects in Research
Consent to Participate in a Research Project entitled:**

**Multidimensional Sense of Humor in School-Aged Children:
A Pilot Study**

---

Child's Name (print)                    Date

**Parent/Guardian Consent:** The purpose and procedures of this research project, the predictable risks, and the benefits that my child may experience have been explained to me. Alternatives to my child's participation in this study have also been discussed. I have read and understand this consent form. I voluntarily consent to my child's participation in this study I understand that my child and I may end our participation at any time.

---

Parent/Legal Guardian Signature          Date

---

Parent/Legal Guardian Signature (print)      Date

**Child Assent:** My parent/legal guardian has explained this study to me. We have Dr. Fain's telephone number and can call Dr. Fain at any time if we have any further questions. I have decided to do this study even though I know I do not have to.

---

Child's Signature

FIGURE 2.4  Example of a child's assent form.

with nonscientific issues. (Feasibility of conducting a study, however, is outside the realm of the IRB.) The IRB also reviews the procedures for selecting subjects, ensuring voluntary informed consent, clearly written descriptions, and confidentiality. The decision to approve, modify, or disapprove a proposal must be made by a majority of IRB members.

Some categories of research may qualify for an expedited review, such as when the use of noninvasive procedures is routine or if a study consists of surveys, interviews, or studies of existing records, provided that the data are collected in such a way that subjects cannot be identified and the study does not deal with sensitive issues. In the case of an expedited review, the chairperson and at least one other member of the IRB review the proposal. The advantage of an expedited review is that it is usually completed in less time than that required for a full IRB review.

### Evaluating Evidence for the Protection of Human Rights

Most research reports provide only a sentence or two concerning review by an appropriate committee. Excerpt 2.5 displays an example of what is usually written in research reports regarding protection of human rights. Without a detailed explanation of data collection procedures, a number of issues can be raised as to the ethical acceptability of a given study. The information presented in Table 2.3 can help the researcher evaluate the protection of human rights in research reports. Nurses at all levels typically find themselves involved in carrying out research activities. As patient advocates, nurses must make an effort to verify the nature of a study and whether the study has been reviewed by an IRB. When human rights are violated, the nurse must report the concern to both the researcher and the IRB. Similarly, the nurse should not assume that the rights of subjects have been adequately addressed unless the exact nature of protection has been specified. It is incorrect to assume that the rights of subjects and the process of informed consent have been handled adequately unless the procedures are clearly articulated.

## SUMMARY OF KEY IDEAS

1. The research process is a decision-making process.
2. The five general phases of the research process are selecting and defining the problem, selecting a research design, collecting data, analyzing data, and using research findings.
3. Research studies are classified based on the purpose of the study and degree of control.
4. Basic research refers to investigations conducted to develop, refine, or test theory.

---

**EXCERPT 2.5**

### EXAMPLE OF HUMAN SUBJECTS APPROVAL FROM THE HOSPITAL INSTITUTIONAL REVIEW BOARD (IRB)

The study was conducted in a 40-bed Level III NICU within a 500-bed regional referral hospital in a rural area of a Midwestern state. Permission was obtained from the hospital's Institutional Review Committee before the study was conducted. A total of 100 blood samples were obtained from a nonrandom sample of 38 infants who were admitted to the NICU over a 60-day period.

*Source: Martin, S, et al.: Comparison of two methods of bedside blood glucose screening in the NICU: Evaluation of accuracy and reliability. Neonatal Network 16:39, 1997.*

TABLE 2.3  GUIDELINES FOR EVALUATING THE PROTECTION OF HUMAN RIGHTS IN RESEARCH REPORTS

| Criteria for Evaluation | Comments |
| --- | --- |
| 1. Is the research problem a significant one for nursing? Is the design scientifically sound? | If an answer to the problem will not benefit subjects or contribute to nursing knowledge, it may not be eithical to involve subjects. |
| 2. Is the research designed to maximize benefit to human subjects and minimize risk? | If subjects are exposed to undue risk and the benefit or knowledge generated are minimal, ethical problems exist. |
| 3. Is the selection of subjects ethically appropriate to study the research problem? | It is ethically inappropriate to use captive subjects when they are not members of groups that would benefit from the results. |
| 4. Is there evidence of voluntary, informed consent? | Any evidence of subject coercion to participate and lack of information about the study purpose and subject participation violate human rights. |
| 5. Is there evidence of subject deception? | Deception should be avoided if at all possible. The researcher must inform subjects about any deception and the reason for that deception, prior to subjects' consent. Subjects must be debriefed about any deception at finish of study. |
| 6. Have subjects been invited to consent when under high stress? | Consent under stress should be avoided if possible. Invitations to participate should be timed so as to not add to periods of stress (e.g., immediately before surgery or other complex procedures). Timing invitations well in advance is preferred. |
| 7. Is informed consent given by a legal guardian or representative of a subject incapable of giving his or her own consent? | This type of consent must be done in the case of minors or subjects who are physically or mentally incapacitated. |
| 8. Is there evidence in the research report that individual subjects can be identified? | The researcher must take precautions that publication of the setting and data collection and analysis will protect the anonymity of subjects. |
| 9. Is there evidence of an independent ethics review by a board or committee? | An ethics review should be mentioned in the research report. |

5. Applied research refers to investigations conducted to generate knowledge that will have a direct impact on clinical practice.
6. Ethical principles relevant to nursing research were originally derived from the Nuremberg Code and Declaration of Helsinki.
7. The ANA has developed two documents that provide direction for nurses engaged in research activities: *Guidelines for the Investigative Function of Nurses* and *Human Rights Guidelines for Nurses in Clinical and Other Research.*
8. The basic rights of human subjects include the right to freedom from injury, the right to privacy and dignity, and the right to anonymity and confidentiality.

9. Informed consent includes the elements of adequate disclosure (providing subjects with enough information for them to make a voluntary decision), comprehension (ensuring that subjects understand the information provided), and freedom from coercion.
10. IRBs are responsible for reviewing research proposals and commenting on the rights of human subjects.

## LEARNING ACTIVITIES

1. Choose two research articles of interest to you.

   a. Does the researcher examine a problem that is relevant to nursing science?

   b. How would you classify the type of research conducted?

2. Choose a research article in which people were participants. Consider the issue of protecting human rights.

   a. How were human subject rights alluded to in the article?

   b. What information would you need to help you assess the adequacy of the protection of human rights?

   c. If you were to conduct a similar research study, what steps would you take to protect the rights and ensure the safety of the human subjects?

3. Identify several key points in the Tuskegee Syphilis Study, Willowbrook Study, and Crisis at John Hopkins University that raise ethical issues.

## References

1. Polit, DF, Beck, CT, and Hungler, BP: Essentials of Nursing Research: Methods, ed 5. Lippincott Williams & Wilkins, Philadelphia, 2001, pp 39–43.
2. Wilson, HK: Introducing Research in Nursing, ed 2. Addison-Wesley, New York, 1993.
3. Dellerfield, KS, and McDougall, GJ: Increasing metamemory in older adults. Nurs Res 45:284, 1996.
4. Hilton, JJ: Folic acid intake of young women. J Obstet Gynecol Neonatal Nurs 31:172, 2002.
5. Houldin, AD, Jacobsen, B, and Lowery, BJ: Self-blame and adjustment to cancer. Onc Nurs Forum 23:75, 1996.
6. Gennaro, S: Leave and employment in families of preterm low birthweight infants. Image J Nurs Sch 28:193, 1996.
7. Katz, J: Experimentation With Human Beings. Russell Sage Foundation, 1972, pp 289–290.
8. World Medical Association: Human experimentation code of ethics of the World Medical Association, Declaration of Helsinki. Br Med J 2:177, 1964.
9. Getz, K, and Borfitz, D: Informed Consent: The Consumer's Guide to the Risks and Benefits of Volunteering for Clinical Trials. Thomson Healthcare Inc, Boston, 2002, pp 70–121.
10. Brandt, AM: Racism and research: The case of the Tuskegee Study. Hastings Center Report 8:21, 1978.
11. Gillis, A, and Jackson, W: Research for Nurses: Methods and Interpretation. FA Davis, Philadelphia, 2002, pp 322–348.
12. Steinbrook, R: Protecting research subjects: The Crisis at John Hopkins. N Engl J Med 346:716, 2002.
13. Beecher, HK: Ethics and clinical research. N Engl J Med 274:1354, 1996.
14. Rothman, DJ: Were Tuskegee and Willowbrook studies in nature? Hastings Center Report 12:5, 1982.
15. American Nurses' Association Commission on Nursing Research: Guidelines for the Investigative Function of Nurses. American Nurses' Association, Kansas City, MO, 1981.
16. American Nurses' Association: Human Rights Guidelines for Nurses in Clinical and Other Research. American Nurses' Association, Kansas City, MO, 1985.

# part 2

# Planning a Research Study

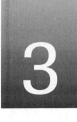

# Selecting and Defining the Problem

James A. Fain, PhD, RN, BC-ADM, FAAN

## LEARNING OBJECTIVES

*At the end of this chapter, you will be able to:*

1. Distinguish between a problem statement and the purpose of a study.
2. Identify several characteristics of a good problem statement.
3. Identify a problem statement in a journal article.
4. Cite different sources of ideas for selecting a research problem.
5. Describe the purposes of a literature review.
6. Identify the characteristics of a relevant literature review.
7. Differentiate between primary and secondary sources.
8. Compare advantages and disadvantages of print and computer database sources for searching the literature.

## GLOSSARY OF KEY TERMS

**Electronic databases.** Bibliographic files that can be accessed by the computer through an online search (i.e., directly communicating with a host computer over telephone lines or the Internet) or by CD-ROM (compact discs that store bibliographic information).

**Empirical literature.** Databased literature that presents reports of completed research; also called scientific literature.

**Literature review.** A critical summary of the most important scholarly literature on a particular topic. Scholarly literature can refer to research-based publications and conceptual or theoretical literature.

**Operational definitions.** Explanations of concepts or variables in terms of how they are defined for a particular study.

**Primary source.** Source reported by the person(s) who conducted the research or developed the theory; refers to original data or first-hand facts.

**Problem statement.** A statement of the topic under study, outlining all relevant variables within the study, providing justification for the choice of topic, and guiding the selection of the research design.

**Purpose statement.** A statement that describes why the study has been created.

43

**Refereed journals.** A journal that determines acceptance of manuscripts based on the recommendations of peer reviewers.

**Replication.** The duplication of research procedures in a second study to determine whether earlier results can be repeated.

**Scientific literature.** A database literature presenting reports of completed research.

**Secondary source.** Source reported by person(s) other than the individual(s) who conducted the research or developed the theory; usually represents a comment, summary, or critique of another's work.

**Theoretical literature.** Conceptual articles presenting reports of theories, some of which underlie research studies, and other nonresearch-related material.

Selecting and defining a research problem begins with identifying a potential problem and ends with at least one hypothesis or research question. The process is based on a thorough review and critical analysis of the literature. As the problem is identified, the researcher refines it until it is amenable to empirical investigation. This process entails much time and thought. This chapter focuses on the formulation and evaluation of problem statements and on how a researcher conducts a literature review.

## PROBLEM STATEMENT

Formulating and defining the problem is the first and most important step in the research process. The problem statement provides direction for the research design and is typically stated at the beginning of a research report or journal article. The opening sentences describe the problem and focus on what is being studied. The problem statement justifies the study by citing background information about the problem and its contributions to practice, theory, or both. In other words, the problem statement makes a case for conducting the study and provides the basis for generating a variety of research purposes. When the problem statement is effectively written, the remaining steps of the research process fall into place.

The **problem statement** is the foundation of the research design. Problem statements consist of several paragraphs identifying a significant researchable problem, citing significant literature sources to justify the research study, and stating the goals of the study. Complete problem statements are usually not found in most journal articles owing to a page limitation.

Excerpt 3.1 presents a problem statement that has been published in a journal article. Within the first few sentences, the author identifies an area of research (e.g., HIV infection and AIDS among women) and outlines pertinent variables.

### Characteristics

By definition, the problem statement describes a problem in need of investigation. A basic prerequisite of a research problem is that it must be researchable. A researchable problem is one that researchers can investigate by collecting and

## EXAMPLE OF A PROBLEM STATEMENT

AIDS is among the top five causes of death in women 15 to 44 years old. The rate of HIV infection in women is rising faster than that in men (Chu, Buehler, Berkelman, 1990; Centers for Disease Control [CDC], 1990). Although only 19 percent of all U.S. women are black or hispanic, these two minority groups constitute 72 percent of the AIDS cases in women. Low-socioeconomic women may be at increased risk for HIV infection from high-risk behavior, such as intravenous drug use or having multiple sexual partners who are infected with HIV (Chu, et al, 1990; McDonald & Jenssen, 1990). Because of their poverty, these women may have less access to health-care services and receive less health education. In other higher-risk groups such as bisexual and homosexual males (Becker & Joseph, 1988; CDC, 1985; Wickelstein, et al, 1987) and intravenous drug users (Stephens, Feucht, & Roman, 1991), educational programs have positively influenced their risk-taking behaviors. Less is known about the effect of educational intervention on other groups at risk for AIDS/HIV infection.

Participants in the WIC program for dietary supplementation form a unique group of women for AIDS prevention strategies. Although this population is potentially at risk for AIDS, it is also highly accessible to health-care providers. Based on the criteria of the WIC program, these mothers are economically poor, often have less than a high school education, and have few opportunities to change their socioeconomic situation (Williams, Lessler, Wheeless, & Wildfire, 1990). Research involving a similar population of participants at a family planning clinic indicates that many of the women who attend public health clinics are indeed engaging in activities that expose them to the AIDS virus (Weisman, et al, 1989; Valdiserri, Bonati, Proctor, & Glasser, 1988). Many of these women are from minority groups and have difficulty understanding or benefiting from traditional educational programs (Becker & Joseph, 1988; Hu, Keller, & Fleming, 1989).

The purpose of this study was to determine the level of knowledge, attitudes, and risk-taking behaviors concerning HIV infection among a low-socioeconomic population of women who are enrolled in a WIC program, and to evaluate the effect of two educational approaches on knowledge and behavioral intent.

*Source: Ashworth, CS, et al: An experimental evaluation of an AIDS educational intervention for WIC mothers. AIDS Education & Prevention 6:154, 1994, with permission.*

analyzing data. By using the scientific method, the researcher attempts to make conclusions based on data or information concerning key concepts in the problem. To collect these data, the researcher must create operational definitions.

**Operational definitions** are clear-cut statements of how variables are measured. These definitions are important if quantitative research is to be meaningful. For example, the concepts of knowledge, attitudes, and risk-taking behaviors are addressed in Excerpt 3.1. To render these concepts operational, the researcher provides measurable definitions that are valid reflections of the concepts. In most journal articles, the operational definitions are found in the "Methods" section under the subheading of "Instruments" or "Data Collection."

Ethical and philosophical problems are not researchable. These types of problems elicit a range of opinions with no right or wrong answers. For example, consider these problems: Should therapeutic abortions be legalized? Do nurses have the right to strike? Research can be used to assess how people feel about such problems but cannot resolve them. Debating these issues, however, may elicit further knowledge that might be useful.

Another characteristic of a problem statement concerns whether the problem is significant enough to warrant a study. The problem should have the potential for contributing to and extending the scientific body of nursing knowledge. Haber[1] has identified several criteria that serve as a guideline for selecting research problems (Table 3.1).

Once the problem has been identified, the feasibility of the study needs to be considered. Despite how researchable or significant a problem may be, the following variables must also be considered to determine whether a problem is appropriate for study: availability of subjects, time and money constraints, researchers' expertise, cooperation of others, available resources, and any ethical considerations. Access to faculty advisors or experienced researchers can help a beginning researcher decide a problem's feasibility.

## PURPOSE STATEMENT

The purpose of the study is a single statement that identifies why the problem is being studied. The **purpose statement** specifies the overall goal and intent of the research while clarifying the knowledge to be gained. The purpose of the study, seen more commonly in journal articles, is stated objectively and indicates the type of study to be conducted. The purpose statement is usually stated after the problem statement and under the subheading of "Introduction," "Literature Review," or "Background." Clearly, the purpose of the study is based on the problem statement, although the two are different.

In Excerpt 3.2, the purpose statement appears within the opening sentences of the journal article just before the review of the literature. The authors conducted this study using data collected from a larger study.

Brink and Wood[2] suggest that the purpose statement can be written in one of three ways: as a declarative statement, as a question, or as a hypothesis. Choosing which form to use depends on the researcher's knowledge of previous research findings.

---

TABLE 3.1 GUIDELINES FOR SELECTING RESEARCH PROBLEMS

- Clients, nurses, the medical community, and society will potentially benefit from the knowledge derived from the study.
- Results will be applicable to nursing practice, education, and/or administration.
- Results will be theoretically relevant.
- Findings will lend support to untested theoretical assumptions, challenge an existing theory, or clarify a conflict in the literature.
- Findings will potentially formulate or alter nursing practices or policies.

EXCERPT 3.2

## EXAMPLE OF A PURPOSE STATEMENT

Pregnant adolescents and young mothers are at a greater risk of contracting HIV than are the general population of youth because they often become sexually active at an early age, are likely to remain sexually active, and may have multiple partners over the course of their childbearing years. Furthermore, many of these young women have a history of having sexually transmitted diseases (STDs) or intravenous drug use, and may be sexual partners of individuals who practice high-risk behaviors (Amaro, Zuckerman, & Cabral, 1989; Pletsch, 1988). Use of other substances such as alcohol and marijuana during pregnancy and early parenthood may also indirectly contribute to young mothers' risk of acquiring HIV through increased sexual risk-taking.

The purpose of this investigation was to describe the relationship between sexual risk-taking and substance use and AIDS knowledge among a sample of pregnant adolescents and unpregnant young mothers. The data were collected as part of a larger survey designed to increase understanding about risk behaviors, AIDS knowledge, and attitudes of this vulnerable population.

*Source: Koniak-Griffin, D, and Brecht, ML: Linkages between sexual risk taking, substance use, and AIDS knowledge among pregnant adolescents and young mothers. Nurs Res 44:340, 1995, with permission.*

The purpose statement should include information about what the researcher intends to do (describe, identify, observe); information about the setting (where the researcher plans to collect data); and information about the subjects.

In Excerpt 3.1 the purpose statement was written as a declarative statement. The purpose of this study was to determine knowledge, attitudes, and risk-taking behaviors concerning HIV infections among a low socioeconomic population of women enrolled in the Women, Infants, and Children (WIC) program. This purpose statement contains information about what the researcher intends to do (describe), the setting of the study (WIC program), and the subjects of the study (women of low socioeconomic status).

## SOURCES AND SELECTION OF RESEARCH PROBLEMS

Selecting a problem can be a difficult step in the research process. Students may spend many hours or days asking themselves, "How am I going to identify a significant problem that is appropriate to study?" The problem is not a lack of problems; the possibilities are endless. Rather, the problem is learning how and where to find researchable problems, which can be an overwhelming task.

### Nursing Practice

Research problems come from a variety of sources. However, the most meaningful ones are usually those derived from nursing practice or the investigator's own experience. Burns and Grove[3] acknowledged that nursing practice offers an important source of clinically relevant research problems. Nurses can develop observational and analytical skills that maximize each opportunity for discovering important questions and problems.

As an example of research derived from nursing practice, Beyea and Nicoll[4] examined the practice of administering medications via the intramuscular (IM) route. A critical review of the literature revealed that the proper techniques for administering IM injections were non–research-based and reflected myths, tradition, and out-of-date recommendations. An integrated review of the literature dating from the 1920s was conducted, and pertinent research was reviewed and critiqued. A research-based protocol for the procedure was then developed and further areas of research were identified.

## Literature Review

Another source of research problems is the literature. Examining the literature can generate ideas for possible areas of research. Examples of many kinds of problems that have been observed by other researchers can be found in research studies reported in various nursing and related journals. Additional questions and problems identified from published studies can provide the opportunity to expand on the work of others.

Excerpt 3.3 highlights suggestions for further research, based on a study conducted by Beyea and Nicoll.[4] After completing a research-based protocol for the administration of IM injections, the researchers identified a number of studies worthy of further evaluation.

## Theory

Investigating problems derived from theory can provide meaningful contributions to nursing knowledge. Researchable problems based on theory are less likely to involve a clinical problem; they are usually concerned with more general and abstract explanations of phenomena.[3]

Reading theories developed in nursing and other disciplines can provide research problems through a deductive process. The researcher reads theoretical schemata and conceptual frameworks that have been published in existing literature and asks whether a particular theory, such as stress and coping, adaptation, or family theory, might explain certain patterns observed under specified conditions. As an example of generating research problems based on theories or conceptual models, Robinson[5] conducted a descriptive correlation study of widows during the second year of bereavement. The purpose of the study was to explore from a nursing perspective the grief response and the variables that had an impact on grief. The research was guided by Roy's adaptation model. Contextual stimuli (social support, social network, income/education, spiritual beliefs) were related to the cognator function (coping process), which was related to the adaptation outcome (grief response).

**EXCERPT 3.3**

## LITERATURE AS SOURCE OF RESEARCH PROBLEMS

There is sufficient research to support the protocol for the administration of IM injections. However, a variety of issues are evident and would be useful areas of further research, including the following:

1. What volume can be safely and comfortably injected? While there is consensus that 5 mL is the maximum volume, less information exists about the range of volumes for children and adults and for different muscles such as the deltoid.

2. What is the rate of absorption in the gluteus medius, the muscle of the ventrogluteal site? Evans, et al (1975) studied rates of absorption and found that the deltoid had the fastest absorption rate and the gluteus maximus the slowest, although the gluteus medius was not included in the study. In addition, what effect does the absorption rate have on the medication effect for the patient?

3. How does exercise affect the rate of absorption in the different muscle groups? For example, in ambulatory patients who receive an injection in the large gluteus muscles, does walking affect the rate of absorption? By what factors?

4. What specific nursing interventions would be appropriate for special complications of IM injections? Basic interventions are usually recommended. However, specific complications are usually identified such as tissue injury, abscesses, nerve injury, or bruising. What particular interventions are effective for each of these complications?

5. Can infants be given IM injections safely in the ventrogluteal site? A number of authors have suggested this site, but for the mainstay of pediatric practice the vastus lateralis remains the area of choice.

*Source: Beyea, SC, and Nicoll, LH: Administration of medications via the intramuscular route: An integrative review of the literature and research-based protocol for the procedure. Appl Nurs Res 8:23, 1995, with permission.*

Selecting a problem based on theory may be a bit complex for beginning researchers, which is not to say that a hunch based on experience will never lead to a theoretical problem. It is more probable, however, that such a problem will result in an applied research study.

## Replication

**Replication** is the duplication of research procedures in a second study to determine whether earlier results can be repeated. Beck[6] provided strong evidence that implementing research findings into nursing practice has been seriously hampered by the lack of replication studies. Some researchers believe replication to be less scholarly or less important than original research. Yet, replication of certain studies provides an excellent opportunity for researchers to discover results that conflict with previous research or disconfirm some aspect of an established theory.[7,8]

## Selecting a Research Problem

The first step in selecting a problem is to identify a general problem area related to your area of expertise. Examples of problem areas may include:

Factors that affect the duration of breast-feeding in adolescent mothers
Patients' psychosocial adjustment after a cardiac event
Perceived effect of illiteracy on patients receiving prenatal care
Roles of the family in post-traumatic stress syndrome
Communication patterns between health-care providers and child-care workers

A great deal of reading is required, and many hours must be devoted to planning and conducting the study. The next step is to narrow down the general problem area to a specific researchable problem. A problem that is too general would involve reviewing many unrelated articles. The literature review would inevitably be unnecessarily increased, resulting in many more hours spent in the library. This, in turn, would complicate the organization of the results and the subsequent hypothesis development. A problem that is too general leads to a study with too many variables that produces results that may be difficult to interpret.

# REVIEW OF RELATED LITERATURE

Having identified a researchable problem, the researcher is usually excited about moving ahead with the project. Too often, the literature review is considered a tedious and time-consuming process. This notion may be due to a lack of understanding of the purpose and importance of the literature review, along with a feeling of uneasiness by researchers who are not sure exactly how to proceed.

## Definition, Purpose, and Scope

The **literature review** involves identification and analysis of relevant publications that contain information pertaining to the research problem. The literature review serves several important functions that make it worth the time and effort. The major purpose of reviewing the literature is to discover what is already known about the problem. This knowledge not only helps the researcher avoid unintentional duplication but also provides the understanding and insight necessary to develop a logical framework. In other words, the literature review provides the researchers with important information concerning what has been done and what needs to be done. Krainovich-Miller[1] has summarized the overall purposes of a literature review (Table 3.2).

Beginning researchers seem to have difficulty determining the depth of a literature review. Although they understand that all literature directly related to their problem should be reviewed, they often do not know when to quit. They have trouble determining which articles are "related enough" to their problem to be included in the literature review. Deciding how much of a literature search is enough is based on the researcher's judgment. These decisions become easier after the researcher has conducted several literature reviews.

TABLE 3.2 PURPOSE OF A REVIEW OF LITERATURE

- Determines what is known and not known about a subject, concept, or problem.
- Determines gaps, consistencies, and inconsistencies in the literature about a subject, concept, or problem.
- Discovers unanswered questions about a subject, concept, or problem.
- Describes the strengths and weaknesses of designs/methods of inquiry and instruments used in earlier work.
- Discovers conceptual traditions used to examine problems.
- Generates useful research questions or problems for the discipline.
- Determines an appropriate research design/method (instruments, data collection, and data analysis methods) for answering the research question.
- Determines the need for replication of a well-designed study or refinement of a study.
- Promotes the development of protocols and policies related to nursing practice.
- Uncovers a new practice intervention or gains support for changing a practice intervention.

Several guidelines can help the beginning researcher determine what is appropriate for the literature review. First, the researcher must avoid the temptation to include everything. A well-defined literature review is preferred to one that contains many articles that are just somewhat related to the problem. Second, well-researched areas usually provide substantial amounts of literature directly related to the problem. Third, a common misconception is that the significance of a problem is related to how much literature is available. This is not so. In some areas of study, a lack of research-based articles increases the value of the study. However, researchers should not assume there is no further need of research when a topic reveals many already-published studies. Although topics are usually well developed, additional research may be needed and even specified in a published article.

## Searching for Relevant Literature

Once the problem has been identified, the search for appropriate literature can begin. Important considerations when beginning the literature search are as follows:

How many years back should you go?
What literature should you search?
How many articles and books do you need for an adequate literature search?
Do you go beyond the library resources for information?

To answer the foregoing questions, researchers need to acquaint themselves with the library and the process of searching through the literature. Deciding how much of the literature review is needed becomes a difficult task until part of the literature review has been accomplished. Locke, Spirduso, and Silverman[9] identified a retrieval system as the searching process by which researchers screen a variety of published literature (e.g., research reports, research reviews, theoretical speculation, and scholarly discourse). The retrieval systems in large health science libraries and smaller institutions may vary enormously. Each discipline also may have its own particular mechanisms for searching the literature. Locke, Spirduso, and Silverman[9] identified several rules that attempt to make any retrieval effort more efficient (Table 3.3).

---

**TABLE 3.3 RULES FOR SEARCHING THE LITERATURE**

1. Begin by planning how you will conduct your literature review. Do not just go to the library and start searching the literature. Instead, first talk with faculty and other colleagues who have some familiarity with the problem area, and find out what they think you should read. Gather the recommended articles, skim over them, and record full citations of those that seem appropriate. Review the reference list in each article to determine which citations are most directly related to the problem. Retrieving these citations should be your priority when you return to the library.
2. When you go back to the library, talk first with the reference librarian, who can identify the retrieval systems that are most likely to be appropriate for your research problem. Do not begin by starting to search for literature.
3. Plan to devote a considerable amount of time learning how each retrieval system works. Use computerized systems whenever they are available, but do not automatically assume that a manual search is without value.
4. Think of your retrieval efforts as consisting of a series of stages.
   a. *Identification.* Find and record citations that seem potentially relevant. This work is done with indexes, bibliographies, reference lists, and computers.
   b. *Confirmation.* Determine whether the items identified can be obtained. This is work done with library holdings of serials and books, reprint services, interlibrary loan, and microfiche files.
   c. *Skim and Screen.* Assess each item to confirm that it actually contains content to be reviewed. Much of this work can be accomplished without obtaining the actual resource item and by spending time in the stacks and at the microfiche reader. The most important retrieval skill is the ability to resist the temptation to stop skimming and screening and immerse yourself in reading.
   d. *Retrieval.* Acquire the literature by checking out books, copying articles from journals, ordering microfiche and reprints, and requesting interlibrary loans. Not everything must be (or should be) retrieved. There is a strong argument for not having every article at hand when you draft the literature review.
   e. *Review.* Read and study the literature.
5. Keep track of all words used to identify or describe what you have learned; these will become the key words used by indexing systems for accessing their holdings. Building a key word list is like acquiring a set of master keys to a large building.
6. Always take advantage of other people's work. Research reviews in your area should have the highest priority in your search plan, as should annotated bibliographies and the reference list at the back of every article and book you retrieve. What could be a better search strategy than reading the reviews of literature crafted by students who have worked on similar problems? *Dissertation Abstracts International* is the "Yellow Pages" of research retrieval.
7. Record a complete citation for every item you identify as being useful for your research problem. Keep a record of what you find by using index cards or a computer program that alphabetizes and sorts by key words. No frustration can match that of having to backtrack to the library for a missing volume or page number.
8. As you make notes during the skimming and screening stages, make sure that your notes are clearly your own and not those of another author. Write any quotes verbatim, and attach the proper page citation.

## Sources of Information

### Nursing Journals

Major sources of information for literature reviews are contained in nursing and social science journals that serve as available sources of the latest information on clinical topics. Because books usually take longer to publish, journals are the preferred mode for communicating the latest results of a research study. **Refereed journals** are important sources of scholarly literature. A refereed journal uses a panel of reviewers to review manuscripts for possible publication. Reviewers are chosen by the editor for their expertise as clinicians, researchers, and/or administrators. The reviews are usually performed blind, meaning that the reviewers do not know the name(s) of the author(s). A list of nursing journals that contain research and conceptual articles is found in Table 3.4. **Empirical literature,** sometimes referred to as **scientific literature,** is databased literature presenting reports of completed research. Conceptual articles refer to **theoretical literature** in which reports of theories, some of which underlie research studies, and other non–research-related material are presented.[1]

### Primary Versus Secondary Sources

Several sources of literature are available to help the researcher conduct a literature review. These sources are divided into two categories: primary sources and secondary sources. A **primary source** is written by the person(s) who developed the theory or conducted the research. An appropriate literature review mainly reflects the use of primary sources. In historical research, a primary source is an eyewitness or an original document. A **secondary source** is a brief description of a study, written by a person(s) other than the original researcher. Often a secondary source represents a response to, or a summary and critique of, the original researcher's work. Excerpt 3.4 provides an example of a secondary source of information.

---

TABLE 3.4  APPROPRIATE NURSING JOURNALS FOR LITERATURE REVIEWS

- *Advances in Nursing Science*
- *Applied Nursing Research*
- *Clinical Nursing Research*
- *Journal of Nursing Scholarship*
- *Journal of Professional Nursing*
- *Journal of Qualitative Research*
- *Nursing and Health Care*
- *Nursing Research*
- *Nursing Science Quarterly*
- *Research in Nursing and Health*
- *Scholarly Inquiry for Nursing Practice*
- *Western Journal of Nursing Research*

## Databases, Indexes, and Abstracts

Several strategies for locating research references are available. Most nursing students have access to college and university libraries with assistance from a reference librarian. **Electronic databases;** bibliographic files that can be accessed by the computer are available either through an online search (i.e., directly communicating with a host computer over telephone lines or the Internet) or by CD-ROM (compact disks that store bibliographic information).[10] Most electronic databases are available through computer searches and can be accessed using software programs such as OVID, PaperChase, and SilverPlatter. These programs are user-friendly and menu-

---

**EXCERPT 3.4**

## EXAMPLE OF A SECONDARY SOURCE

Morgan, W, Raskin, P, and Rosenstock, J: Comparison of fish oil or corn oil supplements in hyperlipidemic subjects with NIDDM. Diabetes Care 18:83, 1995.

**Commentary by James A. Fain, PhD, RN, BC-ADM, FAAN**

Advanced practice nurses need to interpret the results of this study with caution. Findings showed that subjects who used fish oil supplements had significantly lower total plasma triglycerides and plasma very–low-density lipoproteins (VLDL) compared with subjects who received corn oil supplements. A major lipid problem in patients with NIDDM is hypertriglyceridemia. Several studies have shown that hypertriglyceridemia in NIDDM is exaggerated by high-carbohydrate diets regardless of the carbohydrate source (e.g., simple or complex). Experimental and clinical studies further suggest that partial replacement of complex carbohydrates with monounsaturated fats may improve the hypertriglyceridemia of NIDDM without raising LDL cholesterol or compromising glycemic control.

Studies also have shown that polyunsaturated fatty acids (PUFAs) can lower plasma cholesterol levels, particularly LDL cholesterol. PUFAs are divided into two types: omega-6 and omega-3. These fatty acids may also have a beneficial effect for patients with NIDDM who have a greater risk of developing cardiovascular disease. The major source of omega-3 fatty acids may be beneficial to individuals with NIDDM because of the ability of fatty acids to reduce serum triglycerides. However, large doses of fish oils are needed to produce such an effect that, in turn, can elevate glucose levels and increase insulin requirements. More clinical trials with larger sample sizes are needed to confirm these findings of this study.

Advanced practitioners need to be aware that several capsule forms of omega-3 are available to the public and not regulated by the FDA. Dietary supplementation with fish oil capsules is generally not recommended. Instead, patients should be encouraged to eat 6 to 8 ounces of fish per week. Although salmon, mackerel, and herring are good sources of omega-3, consumption of all kinds of fish should be encouraged because of its low fat content and proportion of PUFAs.

Source: Fain, JA: A comparison of fish oil or corn oil supplements in hyperlipidemic subjects with NIDDM [Commentary]. APN SCAN 3:18, 1995, with permission.

driven and have onscreen support. With such advances in technology, the search for references on a particular topic is greatly enhanced.

Computer searches have traditionally been performed using centralized databases, such as Medical Literature On-Line (MEDLINE) (medicine, nursing, and hospital articles) offered by the National Library of Medicine. The Cumulative Index to Nursing and Allied Health Literature (CINAHL) is another useful database for nurses. CINAHL covers references to all Engligh-language and many foreign-language nursing journals as well as books, book chapters, nursing dissertations, and selected conference proceedings in nursing and allied health. The database covers materials dating from 1982 to the present.[10] PsycINFO (psychology on-line), AIDSLINE (AIDS information on-line), CancerLit (Cancer Literature), Health-STAR (Health Services, Technology, Adminisration, and Research), ERIC (Educational Resources Information Center), and CHID (Combined Health Information Database) are commonly used databases that have existed since the 1960s. Examples of commonly used databases along with Internet resources[11] relevant to nursing are shown in Table 3.5. A computer-assisted literature search is most effective when the topic has been well defined.

Knowing how to search the literature is an essential skill. Consulting with the reference librarian is well worth the time and effort. Among the most important

---

**TABLE 3.5 COMMON DATABASES AND INTERNET RESOURCES RELEVANT TO NURSING**

**Print Databases**

1. Cumulative Index to Nursing and Allied Health Literature (CINAHL) (formerly called Cumulative Index to Nursing Literature); known to many as "red books."
2. International Nursing Index (INI): published by the American Journal of Nursing Company in cooperation with the National Library of Medicine (NLM).
3. Nursing Studies Index: developed by Virginia Henderson; includes nursing literature from 1900 to 1959.
4. Index Medicus (IM); oldest health-related index.
5. Health and Psychosocial Instruments (HAPI).

**Electronic Databases**

1. CINAHL
2. MEDLINE
3. BIOETHICSLINE (Biomedical ethics coverage)
4. AIDSLINE (AIDS and HIV coverage)
5. PsychINFO
6. Social Sciences Citation Index

**Health-Related Internet Directories**

1. Health Web (http://www.healthweb.org)
2. Medscape (http://www.medscape.com)
3. National Library of Medicine (http://www.nlm.nih.gov)
4. Evidence-Based Nursing (http://www.bmjpg.com/dataebnpp.html)
5. National Center for Health Statistics (http://www.cdc.gov.nchswww)

approaches to finding relevant literature are manual searches of indexes. *Indexes* provide bibliographic citations, including names, titles, journals, dates, and pages. Indexes are used to find journal sources (periodicals) of data-based and conceptual articles on various topics. Depending on the topic, several indexes exist, including *Hospital Literature Index,* which covers nonclinical aspects of health care delivery such as health planning, financial management, cost containment, and utilization review. Each index contains several volumes. Another important index for nursing research is the *International Nursing Index,* published by the *American Journal of Nursing.* Examples of other frequently used indexes are shown in Table 3.5.

Abstracts are summaries of articles that appear in other journals. Because titles can be misleading, abstracts are especially useful for determining if a particular reference is relevant to an area of study, before searching for it on the shelves. Several abstract journals that are appropriate for nursing literature include *Nursing Abstracts, Psychological Abstracts, Sociological Abstracts, Child Development Abstracts,* and *Dissertation Abstracts.*

## Analyzing, Organizing, and Reporting

For beginning researchers, the hardest part of writing the literature review may be thinking about how difficult the task will be. More time may be spent worrying about the process than doing it. Analyzing, organizing, and reporting is made easier by following the steps outlined in Table 3.3. The researcher should begin by reading through the notes quickly, which refreshes the memory and may also reveal some references that no longer seem sufficiently relevant. The following steps are recommended for writing a literature review:

1. Identify the major ideas (usually two or three) that are related to the problem statement.
2. List the concepts either in descending order of importance or in terms of logical presentation. Determine whether one concept needs to be understood before another can be introduced.
3. Prepare an outline using the major concepts as major headings. The time put into the outline at this stage will save time later and increase the chances of having an organized literature review. The outline does not have to be extremely detailed to be useful (Table 3.6).
4. Divide each major heading into logical subheadings, if applicable. The need for further differentiation is determined by the problem. More complex problems require more subheadings (see Table 3.6).
5. In a sentence or two, summarize the major findings of each study. Include complete reference citations.
6. Write an introductory paragraph explaining the significance of the two or three major concepts.
7. At the end of each section, summarize the findings for each group of studies. Write a paragraph at the end of each major concept or topic that summarizes

TABLE 3.6 OUTLINING THE LITERATURE REVIEW

Research Question: What are the smoking behaviors of women after being diagnosed with lung cancer?
First-stage outline: Identify concepts that provide the rationale for the study.
Smoking is related to lung cancer.
Smoking behaviors are associated with sociodemographic variables.
Second-stage outline: Develop subheadings for each major concept.
   I. Smoking is related to lung cancer.
      A. Incidence of women who smoke.
      B. Gender-specific differences in smoking.
  II. Smoking behaviors are associated with sociodemographic variables.
      A. Relationship of smoking behaviors among women of color and ethnic background.
      B. Relationship of smoking behaviors of women in young, middle, and older adulthood.
Third-stage outline: Add most important references that support each subheading.
   I. Smoking is related to lung cancer.
      A. The percentage of women who smoke has decreased from 33% in 1974 to 23% in 1990. However, the rate of decline is slower in women than in men, and women are smoking at an increasingly earlier age (Centers for Disease Control, 1993; Grit, 1993; USDHHS, 1989). Even a family history of lung cancer does not deter some women from smoking (Horowit, Smaldone, & Viscoli, 1988).
      B. Investigations of gender-specific differences in smoking and quitting behavior suggest that women have more difficulty quitting (Blake, et al, 1989; Grit, 1982; Novotony, et al, 1990; Orlandi, 1987). Women are more likely than men to have tried to quit or to have actually quit after diagnosis of lung cancer (Grit, Nisenbaum, Elashoff, & Holmes, 1991).
  II. Smoking behaviors are associated with sociodemographic variables.
      A. In an analysis of smoking patterns of white, hispanic, and black men and women with cancer, white women were noted to have the highest smoking prevalence (29.6% of current smokers) (Spit, et al, 1990).
      B. Continued smoking was reported most frequently in women ages 20 to 34 years and less frequently in women ages 65 years and older. Middle-aged women (45 to 65 years), however, smoked the most cigarettes per day.

the key points, supports the cohesiveness of the subheadings, and establishes the relevance of the proposed problem.

8. Compile the entire literature review and scan it for coherence, continuity, and smoothness of transition from one topic to the next. Carefully check each citation for accuracy.

## QUESTIONS TO CONSIDER WHEN CRITIQUING REVIEWS OF LITERATURE

Identify a research study to critique. Read the study to see if you recognize any key terms discussed in this chapter. Remember that all studies may not contain all key terms. The following questions serve as a guide in critiquing literature reviews.

1. *Has the literature review been conducted in a thorough manner? Is the problem introduced within the first couple of paragraphs?* Within the first few paragraphs, the reader should be oriented quickly to the major areas of study. It is important that author(s) state the area of study concisely, what literature will be considered, and why some literature may be omitted.

2. *Can you identify the most relevant articles on the topic of interest? How far back (publication dates) were articles chosen to be included in the literature review?* Look over the reference list, and make an assessment that the literature chosen supports and explains the rationale for this particular study. Literature reviews can be somewhat misleading. The purpose is not to demonstrate a comprehensive understanding of the general area. Instead, author(s) should be placing the hypotheses and/or research questions in the context of previous work to support and explain knowledge that this study intends to fill.

3. *Have the author(s) used mostly primary rather than secondary sources?* In almost all instances, articles presented in nursing journals reflect original research written by those individuals who actually conducted the research (primary source). Use caution with secondary sources because the description of a study may not be entirely correct.

4. *Has evaluation of key articles been presented succinctly in terms of critical appraisal of methodology and interpetation of results?* Identify if the literature review is only a summary of past work, with a historical account of each study and important milestones that lead up to the present study. It is important to compare and contrast the contributions of key studies while discussing the strengths and weaknesses in existing research studies and identifying important gaps in the literature.

5. *Is there a summary statement or overall evaluation of the literature?* All good literature reviews end with a summary statement (or paragraphs) of the state of the science on the topic just discussed.

## SUMMARY OF KEY IDEAS

1. The problem statement presents the topic to be studied, along with a description of the background and rationale for its significance.

2. A good problem statement expresses a relationship between two or more variables and can be investigated by collecting and analyzing data.

3. The purpose of a study is expressed as a single statement or question that specifies the overall goal of the study.

4. Nursing practice and personal experiences are good sources of research problems. Ideas can also come from literature, nursing theory, and previous research.

5. A literature review involves identifying, obtaining, and analyzing literature that is related to the research problem.

## LEARNING ACTIVITIES

*Problem Statement 1*

Coronary heart disease (CHD) is the leading cause of death for women in the United States. Approximately 250,000 to 500,000 American women die of CHD annually (Cochrane, 1992; Rich-Edwards, Manson, Hennekens, & Buring, 1995; Steingart, et al, 1991; Wenger, 1985). However, most women are unaware of the risk associated with developing CHD relative to other diseases. For example, one of five women will die from CHD compared with one of nine women who will die from breast cancer (Rich-Edwards, et al, 1995; Steingart, et al, 1991). In fact, the mortality rate for women with CHD exceeds that for all neoplastic diseases combined.

Coronary heart disease has long been thought of as a man's disease (Rich-Edwards, et al, 1995). The fact that women have been underrepresented in nearly all randomized, controlled studies of CHD until recently both reflects and contributes to a mistaken belief that women are not significantly affected by CHD (Barry, 1992). Reasons for excluding women from such studies include fear of teratogenicity; increased variability caused by a woman's menstrual cycle, pregnancy, and menopause; increased cost; and the false belief that gender-specific effects are unlikely to significantly influence treatment outcomes (Annual Report/Women's Health Research, 1991).

Consequently, little is known about gender differences in the presentation, pathophysiology, and treatment outcomes for CHD. Research involving women with CHD is in its infancy; the scientific basis for care offered to women with CHD is based largely on data extrapolated from clinical trials in which most of the subjects were men (Cochrane, 1992). The lack of data about women with CHD raises yet more questions regarding gender differences.

Of particular concern is the poorer survival rate for women compared with men following a myocardial infarction (MI). This finding is based on data from landmark studies such as the Framingham Heart Study and the Multicenter Investigation of the Limitation of Infarct Size or MILIS Trial (Tofler, et al, 1987; Wingate, 1993). The increased incidence of mortality among women who experience an MI may reflect their older age and more coexisting illness at onset, suboptimal or delayed treatment, or both (Wenger, Speroff, & Packard, 1993).

A delay in treatment of MI has extensive consequences because myocardial cell death with irreversible loss of cellular function begins to occur 20 to 40 minutes after the onset of myocardial ischemia. Early intervention and treatment can dramatically reduce the irreversible loss of myocardial tissue (Ayanian & Epstein, 1991; Maynard, 1992). Therefore, early intervention for MI is paramount.

Yet several studies show that women undergo less intensive or less invasive evaluations than men, despite equal or more severe symptoms (Wenger, et al, 1993). Tobin and colleagues (1987) found that 4 percent of women, compared with 40 percent of men, with abnormal radionuclide scan during exercise were referred for cardiac catheterization. Data from the Multicenter Survival and Ventricular Enlargement (SAVE) Trial showed that women with a confirmed MI were less likely than their male counterparts to undergo cardiac catheterization (Mark, Shaw,

DeLong, Califf, & Pryor, 1994; Steingart, et al, 1991). Using data from Massachusetts and Maryland state insurance claims (11,865 discharge summaries from Massachusetts and 6894 from Maryland), the overall rate for coronary angiography referrals among patients hospitalized for known CHD was 15 percent to 28 percent higher for men than for women (Ayanian & Epstein, 1991).

Maynard and Weaver (1992) suggested that there is something about the characteristics of chest pain at the time of emergency room evaluation and during the first few days of hospitalization that make it difficult to arrive at the diagnosis of acute MI in women. In fact, the clinical presentation of women with ischemic-type sensations may differ from that of males; women may actually have a different constellation of symptoms associated with MI. Data from the Myocardial Infarction Triage and Intervention (MITI) Registry revealed differing associated symptoms. Women complained more often of fatigue, nausea, and upper abdominal pain than men, and more men than women experienced diaphoresis (Maynard, 1992). In addition, data from the Framingham Heart Study showed that more women than men experience silent ischemia (the absence of chest pain)—34 percent versus 27 percent, respectively.

The current practice of differentiating between typical versus atypical symptoms of MI based on data extrapolated from clinical trials in which most of the subjects were male could be problematic. The purpose of this study is to determine whether a relationship exists between the gender differences in the presenting symptoms of acute MI and the typical evaluation of women with CHD.

### Problem Statement 2

Osteoporosis is an age-related skeletal disorder with multiple etiologies, characterized by decreasing bone mass and increasing bone fragility when there are no other identified diseases (Ockene, 1994; Lappe, 1994). Fifty percent of all American women older than 45 years develop osteoporosis; 75 percent are affected by age 90 years (McMahon, Peterson, & Schilke, 1992). One in four white women will have at least one fracture by age 65, resulting in 1.5 million fractures/year (Erickson & Jones, 1992). The current health-care cost of $7 to $10 billion/year related to fractures resulting from postmenopausal osteoporosis is expected to reach $31 to $62 billion/year by the year 2020 (Lappe, 1994).

The primary treatment of postmenopausal osteoporosis is building and maintaining peak bone density during the years of skeletal maturation. Peak bone mass is reached by age 30 years. The goal of early intervention in young women is to maximize the bone mass by affecting the risk factors for osteoporosis. Lappe (1994) identified the major risk factors for development of postmenopausal osteoporosis as genetic influences; metabolic and endocrine status; dietary factors; exercise patterns; and exposure to drugs, alcohol, and cigarettes.

Dietary intake of calcium and protein affects the body's ability to achieve peak bone mass by age 30 years. At birth the total skeleton contains 25 g of calcium and increases to 1000 g at maturity, all from dietary intake (El-Choufli, Nelson, & Kleerekoper, 1994). One study recommended that young women monitor dietary intake of calcium and use calcium supplements to achieve the recommended calcium intake of 1200 to 1500 mg/day for adolescents and young women (Erickson & Jones, 1992).

Physical activity and weight-bearing exercises influence bone density in the maturing skeleton through the process of mechanical loading on bones. This longitudinal force stimulates osteoblasts to increase production, thereby maximizing and strengthening bone mass. Decreased activity levels have resulted in increased urinary excretion of calcium, with resultant decreases in bone mass and skeletal growth (Rutherford, 1990). A study of gender and developmental differences in exercise beliefs and performance compared boys and girls in grades six, seven, and eight in two school districts (Garcia, et al, 1995). Findings showed that girls continue to be a high-risk group for inactivity and could develop lifelong sedentary habits, with increased risk for skeletal deterioration.

Several studies have been published related to osteoporosis and behaviors aimed at its prevention in perimenopausal and postmenopausal women. However, no data are available about younger women and osteoporosis. A study of 91 postmenopausal women revealed that these women did not perform adequate osteoporosis prevention behaviors (Ali & Bennet, 1992). This study investigated the relationship between knowledge of osteoporosis and osteoporosis prevention behaviors, perceptions of barriers and benefits to milk intake, and health-promoting behaviors such as exercise. Higher levels of knowledge were associated with more consistent health practices and greater milk intake. Older postmenopausal women generally had less knowledge about osteoporosis than did younger postmenopausal women.

The lack of published research about osteoporosis knowledge, beliefs, and prevention behaviors in women who are still young enough to affect their peak bone mass reflects a significant problem. This information is critical to the development of appropriate educational and health-maintenance programs for younger women. The purpose of this descriptive study is to assess the knowledge of osteoporosis risk factors and preventive behaviors among women between the ages of 16 and 22 years.

*Activity*

1. Evaluate problem statements 1 and 2 by identifying:
   a. What is being studied
   b. The justification for the study
   c. The focus of the study (statement of purpose)
   d. The population being studied
2. Rank each problem statement on a scale of 1 to 5 (5 = Excellent, 4 = Very Good, 3 = Good, 2 = Fair, 1 = Poor) as to the:
   a. Clarity
   b. Importance to nursing
   c. Comprehensiveness
   d. Logical presentation
3. Select a topic of interest. Identify four articles related to one of the concepts within the topic, and complete an outline similar to the one in Table 3.6.

## References

1. Haber, J: Research problems and hypotheses. In LoBiondo-Wood, G, and Haber, J (eds): Nursing Research: Critical Appraisal and Utilization. Mosby, St. Louis, 1998, pp 65, 95, 102.
2. Brink, PJ, and Wood, ME: Basic Steps in Planning Nursing Research: From Question to Proposal, ed 5. Jones & Bartlett, Boston, 2001, pp 69–82.
3. Burns, N, and Grove, SK: The Practice of Nursing Research: Conduct, Critique, & Utilization, ed 4. WB Saunders, Philadelphia, 2001, pp 87, 90.
4. Beyea, SC, and Nicoll, LH: Administration of medications via the intramuscular route: An integrative review of the literature and research-based protocol for procedure. Appl Nurs Res 8:23, 1995.
5. Robinson, JH: Grief responses, coping processes, and social support of widows: Research with Roy's model. Nurs Sci Q 8:158, 1995.
6. Beck, CT: Replication strategies for nursing research. Image J Nurs Sch 26:191, 1994.
7. Martin, PA: More replication studies needed. Appl Nurs Res 8:102, 1995.
8. Taunton, R: Replication: Key to research application. Dimens Crit Care Nurs 8:156, 1989.
9. Locke, LF, Spirduso, WW, and Silverman, SJ: Proposals That Work, ed 3. Sage Publications, Newbury Park, CA, 1995, pp 66–95.
10. Polit, DF, Beck, CT, and Hungler, BP: Essentials of Nursing Research: Methods, Appraisal, and Utilization, ed 5. Lippincott Williams and Wilkins, Philadelphia, 2002, pp 122–127.
11. Gillis, A, and Jackson, W: Research for Nurses: Methods and Interpretation. FA Davis, Philadelphia, 2002, pp 79–84.

# Applying Appropriate Theories and Conceptual Models

James A. Fain, PhD, RN, BC-ADM, FAAN

## LEARNING OBJECTIVES

*At the end of this chapter, you will be able to:*
1. Discuss the relationship between research and theory.
2. Describe the processes of inductive and deductive reasoning.
3. Differentiate among the three types of theories (i.e., grand, middle-range, and practice).
4. Discuss the importance of borrowed theories.
5. Distinguish between a concept and a construct.
6. Suggest a theory or conceptual model for a topic of inquiry.

## GLOSSARY OF KEY TERMS

**Borrowed theories.** Theories taken from other disciplines and applied to nursing questions and research problems.

**Concepts.** Symbolic statements describing a phenomenon or a class of phenomena.

**Conceptual model.** A set of abstract and general concepts that are assembled to address a phenomenon of interest.

**Constructs.** Higher-level concepts that are derived from theories and that represent nonobservable behaviors.

**Deductive approach.** An approach to reasoning that generates theory by beginning with known facts, moving from the general to the specific. It is an approach used to test predictions and validate existing relationships.

**Grand theories.** Theories that are complex and broad in scope. Grand theories attempt to explain broad areas and include numerous concepts that are not well defined and that have ambiguous and unclear relationships.

**Inductive approach.** An approach to reasoning that involves collecting observations that lead to conclusions or hypotheses. This approach moves from specific observations to general statements that can be tested through research.

**Metaparadigm.** Refers to the primary or central phenomena that are of interest to a particular discipline.

**Middle-range theories.** Theories that look at a piece of reality and that contain clearly defined variables in which the nature and direction of relationships are specified.

**Nursing theory.** A specific and concrete set of concepts and propositions that accounts for or characterizes phenomena of interest to the discipline of nursing.

**Practice theories.** Theories that are more specific than middle-range theories and that produce specific directions or guidelines for practice.

**Theory.** An organized and systematic set of interrelated statements (concepts) that specify the nature of relationships between two or more variables, with the purpose of understanding a problem or nature of things.

Research is not conducted just to answer research questions or to test hypotheses; rather, it is conducted to develop through generating or testing of theory a body of knowledge unique to nursing. To build this knowledge effectively, the research process should be developed within some theoretical structure that faciliates analysis and interpretation of findings. When a study is placed within a theoretical context, it is theory that lets us speculate on the questions of why and how treatment works and what variables are related to one another. Thus, theory provides the structure for a research study, allowing the researcher to generalize beyond a specific situation and make predictions about what should happen in other, similar situations.[1] Research without theory results in disconnected information or data, which does not add up to an accumulated knowledge of nursing. This chapter provides a basic overview of theory as it relates to research and presents common terminology associated with the elements of theory. Criteria for evaluating theories and conceptual models will be described. Students interested in learning more about theories and conceptual models should pursue additional readings to acquire an in-depth understanding of the topic.

## OVERVIEW OF THEORY

As researchers begin to explain and predict phenomena as a way of gaining knowledge, facts are collected through empirical investigations. As these facts accumulate, there is need for integration, organization, and classification in order to make the isolated facts meaningful. Researchers bring empirical findings into meaningful patterns that take the form of theories.

Defining theory is not an easy task because of the many fields of inquiry that contribute to the development of nursing knowledge.[2] At a basic level, **theory** is an organized and systematic set of interrelated statements (concepts) that specify the nature of relationships between two or more variables with the purpose of understanding a problem or nature of things.[3] Theories are organized and provide meaning to a complex collection of individual facts and observations. Theories pull together the results of observations, allowing researchers to make general statements about variables and the relationships among variables.

Theories serve several purposes in the development of science and clincal practice, depending on how we choose to use them. Theories summarize existing knowledge, giving meaning to isolated empirical findings. Theory provides a structure or framework that describes, explains, and predicts. It offers organization of nursing knowledge and provides a systematic means of collecting data to describe, explain, and predict nursing practice.[1]

The term *framework* refers to the conceptual underpinnings of a study. In a study based on a theory, the framework is usually referred to as the *theoretical framework*. In a study that has its roots in a specified conceptual model, the framework is often called the *conceptual framework*. These terms—*theoretical framework, conceptual framework,* and *conceptual model*—are often used interchangeably throughout the literature.[4]

## Inductive Versus Deductive Approach to Discovering New Knowledge

The role that theory plays in clinical practice and research is best described by examining the relationship between theory and data. Figure 4.1 identifies the integration of inductive and deductive reasoning, starting from observations and moving up to concepts and theories. Researchers agree that the role of theory and data collection are essential features of the scientific method. There are two approaches to discovering or testing new knowledge. The researcher may move from observations to an idea (inductive approach) or from an idea to observations (deductive approach). Researchers who stress theory versus those who emphasize observations reflect a deductive theory-testing approach versus an inductive inquiry that is oriented toward discovery.

The **inductive approach** involves collecting observations that lead to conclusions or hypotheses. This approach begins with specific observations and moves to general statements that can be tested through research. Inductive reasoning underlies qualitative approaches to inquiry. In situations where conclusions are arrived at using very specific or limited data, generalizations of results can be erroneous.[5] Thus, study results can only be generalized to the sample in which data were collected.

The **deductive approach** generates theory by beginning with known facts moving from the general to the specific. It is an approach used to test predictions and validate existing relationships. Specific hypotheses can be deduced from a theory that serves as a more general statement of interrelated phenomena. Deductive reasoning helps to unveil existing relationships. As with inductive reasoning, inherent problems may exist using the deductive approach. Not all deductions can be verified, particularly when the methods of measurement are poor or undeveloped.

The validity of nursing knowledge generated through inductive and deductive reasoning depends on the accuracy of information or premises with which one is working. Conclusions are valid if the premises (statements) on which they are based are valid. Research is used to confirm or refute premises so nurses in practice may use them.[6]

## Classification of Theories in Nursing

Theories unique to nursing help define how nursing is different from other disciplines. Fawcett[7] defines **nursing theory** as a specific and concrete set of concepts

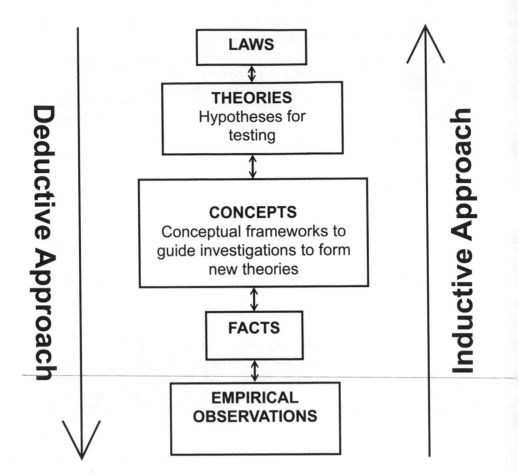

**FIGURE 4.1** Integration of inductive and deductive reasoning.

and propositions that claims to account for or characterize phenomena of interest to the discipline of nursing.

The term **metaparadigm** refers to the primary phenomena that are of interest to a particular discipline. The primary or central phenomena within nursing revolve around the concepts of *person, environment, health,* and *nursing.*[7] The first nurse scholar to disseminate writings on the central phenomena was Fawcett. The four concepts were not formalized as the metaparadigm of nursing until 1984. Definitions of each metaparadigm concept are displayed in Table 4.1.

Theories that deal with these four metaparadigm concepts are referred to as nursing theories. Nursing theories are classified according to the complexity and amount of abstraction in addressing person, environment, health, and nursing. *Grand theory* (macrotheory) describes a comprehensive conceptual framework; *middle-range*

TABLE 4.1 NURSING'S FOUR METAPARADIGM CONCEPTS

1. The metaparadigm concept **person** refers to the individuals, families, communities, and other groups who are participants in nursing.
2. The metaparadigm concept **environment** refers to the person's significant others and physical surroundings, as well as to the setting in which nursing occurs, which ranges from the person's home to clinical agencies to society as a whole. The metaparadigm also refers to all the local, regional, national, and worldwide cultural, social, political, and economic conditions that are associated with the person's health.
3. The metaparadigm concept **health** refers to the person's state of well-being at the time that nursing occurs, which can range from high-level wellness to terminal illness.
4. The metaparadigm concept **nursing** refers to the definition of nursing, the action taken by nurses on behalf of or in conjunction with the person, and the goals or outcomes of nursing actions. Nursing actions are typically viewed as a systematic process of assessment, labeling, planning, intervention, and evaluation.

*theory* describes a framework that is relatively focused; and *practice or prescriptive theory* is smallest in scope.

## Grand Theories

**Grand theories** are complex and broad in scope. They attempt to explain broad areas and include numerous concepts that are not well defined and that have ambiguous and unclear relationships. Because these theories are not grounded in empirical data, they are usually not useful as guides for nursing practice. In most instances, grand theories require further specification and partitioning of theoretical statements for them to be empirically tested and theoretically verified.

Use of a systems approach that focuses on the human needs of protection or relief of stress is central to the discipline of nursing. Gerstle, All, and Wallace[8] conducted an exploratory correlational study guided by the Neuman Systems Model to explore the impact of stressors on the quality of life of adult patients with chronic pain. Patients' perceptions of their health, functional status, and socioeconomic status as well as psychological, spiritual, and familial aspects of life were examined. The Neuman model views an individual as a system containing five components (i.e., physiological, psychological, developmental, sociocultural, and spiritual). Stability of the system is determined by its ability to cope with stressors. Based on Neuman's model, results revealed that a higher quality of life was associated with participants who were older, female, and employed, whereas a lower quality of life was associated with participants with a low income, higher treatment costs, and a lack of workers' compensation insurance. Other examples of grand theories developed by nurse theorists are presented in Table 4.2.

## Middle-Range Theories

Middle-range theories were first introduced in the field of sociology[9] during the late 1960s. By the mid-1970s, middle-range theories were recognized as the latest step

TABLE 4.2 EXAMPLE OF GRAND THEORIES

- Faye G. Abdellah: Patient-Centered Approaches to Nursing
- Virginia Henderson: The Principles and Practice of Nursing
- Dorothea E. Orem: The Self-Care Deficit Nursing Theory
- Dorothy Johnson: The Behavioral System Model
- Betty Neuman: The Neuman Systems Model
- Imogene King: King's Systems Framework and Theory of Goal Attainment
- Myra E. Levine: The Conservation Model
- Sister Callista Roy: The Roy Adaptation Model
- Jean Watson: Nursing—Human Science and Human Caring: A Theory of Nursing
- Martha Rogers: The Science of Unitary and Irreducible Human Beings
- Margaret Newman: Health as Expanding Consciousness
- Rosemarie Parse: The Theory of Human Becoming

in knowledge development. Merton[9] describes **middle-range theories** as those that look at a piece of reality and contain clearly defined variables in which the nature and direction of relationships are specified.

Over the past 10 years, middle-range nursing theories have gained more popularity than grand theories because they are more specific and contain fewer concepts that are concrete and operationally defined. Nursing has recognized middle-range nursing theories as appropriate for defining or refining the substantive component of nursing science and practice. The purpose of middle-range theories is to describe, explain, and predict phenomena; unlike grand theories, they are explicit and testable.

Health-promoting behaviors directed toward health enhancement is important for people of all ages. Kerr, Lusk, and Ronis[10] used Pender's Health Promotion Model (HPM) to identify factors that influenced Mexican American workers' use or nonuse of hearing protection devices (HPDs). Derived from social cognitive theory, the HPM is a useful middle-range theory. The HPM contains three major components: modifying factors, cognitive-perceptual factors, and health-related behavior use of HPDs. Modifying factors such as demographic characteristics and interpersonal

TABLE 4.3 EXAMPLE OF MIDDLE-RANGE THEORIES

- Patricia Benner: Benner's Model of Skills Acquisition in Nursing
- Madeline Leininger: Cultural Care Diversity and Universality Theory
- Nola Pender: Health Promotion Model
- Merle Mishel: Uncertainty of Illness Theory
- Pamela Reed: Self-Transcendence Theory
- Joan Eakes: Theory of Chronic Sorrow
- Mary Burke and Margaret Hainsworth: Chronic Sorrow
- Elizabeth Lenz: Theory of Unpleasant Symptoms
- Cheryl Cox: Motivation in Health Behavior (Health Self-Determinism)
- Cheryl Beck: Postpartum Depression Theory
- Ramona Mercer: Maternal Role Attainment

influences are proposed as indirect influences on health-related behavior, exerting their influence through the cognitive-perceptual factors that directly affect behavior. Other examples of middle-range theories used in nursing are presented in Table 4.3.

### Practice Theories

Practice theories, sometimes referred to as prescriptive theories, are important in developing a science of nursing practice.[3] **Practice theories** are more specific than middle-range theories and produce specific directions or guidelines for practice. These theories are aimed at providing knowledge about what nurses do in their practice, how they get to do what they do in practice, and what is affected (outcomes).[3] Practice theories can cover a particular element of a specialty, such as oncology nursing, obstetric nursing, or operating room nursing, or they may relate to another aspect of nursing, such as nursing administration or nursing education. Such theories typically describe elements of nursing care, such as cancer pain relief, or a specific experience such as dying and end-of-life care.[1] Practice theories contain few concepts and are easily understandable. They are usually narrow in scope, limited to specific populations, and explain a small aspect of reality.[1] Some examples of practice theories are presented in Table 4.4.

### Borrowed Theories

As a practice profession, nursing often deals with phenomena that are not unique to nursing. A significant number of theories used as frameworks in nursing are based on theoretical work from other disciplines, such as sociology (e.g., sick-role theory), psychology (e.g., social-cognitive theory), or physiology (e.g., theory of pain perception). **Borrowed theories** are taken from other disciplines and applied to nursing questions and research problems. Knowledge gained from borrowed theories is useful provided the fit and relevance to nursing is clarified. Some examples of borrowed theories are presented in Table 4.5.

## CONCEPTS

Concepts are the building blocks of a theory. They are defined and understood within the theory of which they are part. **Concepts** are symbolic statements describing a phenomenon or a class of phenomena.[3] From birth, we begin to structure empirical impressions of the world around us in the form of concepts, such as "play," "food," or "mother," each of which implies a complex set of recognitions and expectations. Concepts vary in level of abstraction, from highly abstract (e.g., hope,

---

TABLE 4.4  EXAMPLE OF PRACTICE THEORIES

- Theories of Caring, Empowerment, and Communication
- Theories of Clinical Inference and Clinical Decision Making
- Theories of Suctioning, Wound Care, Rest, and Learning
- Theory of End-of-Life Decision Making

TABLE 4.5 EXAMPLE OF BORROWED THEORIES

- Theories from Sociology
- General Systems Theory
- Role Theory
- Feminist Theory
- Critical Social Theory
- Theories from the Behavioral Sciences
- Psychoanalytic Theory
- Interpersonal Theory
- Operant Conditioning
- Human Needs Theory
- Person-Centered Theory
- Stress, Coping, Adaptation Theory
- Theories from the Medical Sciences
- Germ Theory and Principles of Infection
- Homeostasis
- Theories of Immunity and Immune Function
- Genetic Principles and Theories
- Pain Management: Gate Control Theory

love, empowerment, grief) to relatively concrete (e.g., pain, blood loss, temperature). Concepts are formulated in words that enable people to communicate their meanings about realities in the world.[3] Concepts develop within the context of experience and feelings so that they meet with our perception of reality. We supply labels to sets of behaviors, objects, and processes, which allow us to identify and discuss them. A concept may be a single word (e.g., grief,) or a phrase (e.g., maternal role attachment, health-promoting behaviors). Concepts may likewise have a theoretical or operational definition. In a *theoretical definition*, the concept is defined in relation to other concepts. A theoretical definition provides meaning to a term in the context of a theory. The *operational definition* identifies empirical indicators of the concept, which permits observation and measurement. An example of a theoretically and operationally defined concept is presented in Excerpt 4.1. Note how a theoretical definition of resilience is provided under the subheading Resilience (within the literature review), and the operational definition of resilience is provided under the subheading Methods (Measures).

Higher level concepts that are dervied from theories and that represent nonobservable behaviors are called **constructs.** Examples of constructs are motivation, intelligence, anxiety, self-concept, achievement, aptitude. What is observable is the behavior presumed to be a consequence of the hypothesized construct.

## Conceptual Models

The term conceptual model is synonymous with such terms as *conceptual framework* and *conceptual system*. A **conceptual model** is defined as a set of abstract and general concepts that are assembled to address a phenomenon of central interest.[4,7] Conceptual models represent ideas or notions that have been put together in a

EXCERPT 4.1

EXAMPLE OF THEORETICALLY AND OPERATIONALLY
DEFINED CONCEPT: RESILIENCE

## Resilience

Stewart and colleagues (1997) define resilience as the capacity of individuals to cope successfully with significant change, adversity or risk; that capacity changes over time and is enhanced by protective factors within the person and the environment.

## Methods

## Measure

*Resilience Scale (RS).* Resilience, defined as beliefs in one's personal competence and acceptance of self and life that enhances individual adaptation, was measured by the Resilience Scale (RS). The RS is a 25-item self-report scale with a 7-point Likert response format. Possible scores ranged from 25 to 175 with higher scores indicating more resilience.

*Source: Rew, L, Taylor-Seehafer, M, Thomas, NY, and Yockey, RD: Correlates of resilience in homeless adolescents. J Nurs Scholarship 33:33, 2001.*

unique way to describe a particular area of concern. The process may be likened to experiencing the world by "looking through someone else's glasses" or "walking in someone else's shoes." Because each person has different life experiences, wearing another's shoes changes the experience of events. Similarly, conceptual models put specific ideas or notions into a meaningful framework for viewing the world.[9] Conceptual models are loosely structured, as compared with theories, but provide a framework for communicating a particular perception of the world. In addition, conceptual models, like theories, can help facilitate the generation of hypotheses to be tested.

## Conceptual Models of Nursing

Conceptual models of nursing not only provide direction for a study but also present nursing in relation to the four central metaparadigm concepts (i.e., person, environment, health, nursing). Although some nurse researchers have used conceptual models of nursing that do not reflect all four concepts, the advantage of utilizing a nursing model is that the researcher views a study from a nursing perspective from the beginning. Within the nursing framework, each nursing model defines and relates the concepts in a unique manner. In essence, conceptual nursing models frame the way in which nursing will be viewed and the direction a research study will take.

## QUESTIONS FOR CRITIQUING THEORIES AND CONCEPTUAL MODELS

Identify a research study to critique. Read the study to see if you recognize any key terms discussed in this chapter. Remember that all studies may not contain all key

terms. The following questions[11] serve as a guide in critiquing theories and conceptual models.

1. *Was a theoretical framework clearly identified?* Discussion of the theoretical framework should be incorporated into several sections of the research report. First, the theoretical framework should be introduced and briefly described in the problem statement. Second, the framework should be described in more detail under its own heading, usually at the end of the literature review. Description of the theory should be from primary sources. Also, because theoretical frameworks are unfamiliar to many nurses, it is very important to read over the particular theory and become familiar with the concepts, relationships, and usefulness of the theory in extending nursing science. It will be difficult to determine if the theory was clearly stated, not knowing what the theory is all about.

2. *What type of theory (i.e., grand, middle-range, practice) was discussed? Was the theory from nursing or another discipline?* Look over the types of theories cited in Tables 4.2 to 4.5, and identify the theory stated in the research article. It is likewise important to examine the depth and extent of the literature review conducted. Has the author provided a sufficient amount of information to demonstrate the problem? Does the research contribute to the understanding of the phenomenon of interest? Is there a discussion related to the four metaparadigm concepts of nursing?

3. *Are concepts clearly and operationally defined in the study?* Concepts are selected for a theoretical framework based on their relevance to the phenomenon of interest. Thus, the problem statement, which describes the phenomenon of concern, will be a rich source of concepts for the framework. Each concept included in the framework needs to be defined conceptually and operationally in the methods section of the research report. This will explain how the framework influences or is reflected in the study's design, data collection strategies, and data analysis methods.

4. *Are study findings related to the theoretical rationale?* Findings of the study need to be discussed in terms of how they illustrate, support, challenge, or contradict the theoretical framework.

## SUMMARY OF KEY IDEAS

1. A theory is a set of interrelated concepts that provide a view of reality for the purpose of describing, explaining, or predicting the phenomena of interest.
2. Nursing knowledge can be acquired through inductive and deductive reasoning.
3. The three types of theories (grand, middle-range, practice) are classified according to their level of abstraction.
4. Grand theories are global and attempt to describe and explain everything about a subject. Middle-range theories focus on a particular area of study,

have clear propositions from which hypotheses can be derived. Practice theories are more specific and produce specific directions or guidelines for practice.
5. Knowledge gained from borrowed theories is useful, provided the fit and relevance to nursing are clarified. Concepts are the building blocks of theory.
6. A conceptual model is a set of abstract and general concepts that are assembled to address a phenomenon of interest.
7. Conceptual nursing models deal with the central phenomena of concern to nursing (i.e., person, environment, health, and nursing).

## LEARNING ACTIVITIES

1. Select one of the theories cited in Table 4.1, and read one primary source of the theorist's original work. Review several research articles that cite the work of the particular theory, and answer the following questions:

   a. Do the research articles appear to use the theory appropriately?

   b. Are the studies consistent in their use of the theory?

   c. Did the studies contribute to the knowledge base of the theory? How?

2. Select one of the middle-range theories cited in Table 4.2, and read one primary source of the theorist's original work. Review several research articles that cite the work of the particular theory, and answer the following questions.

   a. Do the research articles appear to use the theory appropriately?

    b. Are the studies consistent in their use of the theory?

    c. Did the studies contribute to the knowledge base of the theory? How?

## *References*

1. McEwen, M, and Wills, EM: Theoretical Basis for Nursing. Lippincott Williams & Wilkins, Philadelphia, 2002, pp 23–68.
2. Chinn, PL, and Kramer, MK: Theory and Nursing: Integrated Knowledge Development, ed 5. Mosby-Year Book, St. Louis, 1999, pp 50.
3. Kim, HS: The Nature of Theoretical Thinking in Nursing, ed 2. Springer Publishing Company, New York, 2000, pp 1–30.
4. Polit, DF, Beck, CT, and Hungler, BP: Essentials of Nursing Research: Methods, Appraisal, and Utilization, ed 5. Lippincott Williams & Wilkins, Philadelphia, 2001, pp 143–161.
5. Feldman, HR: Theoretical Framework. In LoBiondo-Wood, G, and Haber, J (eds): Nursing Research: Methods, Critical Appraisal, and Utilization, ed 4. Mosby-Year Book, St. Louis, 1998, pp 133–153.
6. Gillis, A, and Jackson, W: Research for Nurses: Methods and Interpretation. FA Davis Company, Philadelphia, 2002, pp 10, 37–67.
7. Fawcett, J: Analysis and Evaluation of Contemporary Nursing Knowledge: Nursing Models and Theories. FA Davis Company, Philadelphia, 2000, pp 3–33.
8. Gerstle, DS, All, AC, and Wallace DC: Quality of life and chronic nonmalignant pain. Pain Mgmt Nurs 2:98, 2001.
9. Merton, RK: Social Theory and Social Structure. The Free Press, New York, 1968.
10. Kerr, MJ, Lusk, SL, and Ronis, DL: Explaining Mexican American workers' hearing protection use with the health promotion model. Nurs Res 51:100, 2002.
11. Brockopp, DY, and Hastings-Tolsma, MT: Fundamentals of Nursing Research, ed 3. Jones and Bartlett Publishers, Boston, 2003, pp 81–135.

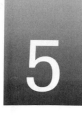

# Understanding Evidence-Based Practice

James A. Fain, PhD, RN, BC-ADM, FAAN

LEARNING OBJECTIVES

*At the end of this chapter, you will be able to:*
1. Define evidence-based practice (EBP).
2. Distinguish between evidence-based medicine (EBM) and evidence-based nursing (EBN).
3. Define meta-analysis.
4. Identify several reasons for the delay in using research findings in nursing practice.
5. List some limitations associated with EBP.
6. Describe some of the more commonly used electronic database in EBM.
7. Discuss the level of evidence associated with appraising research studies.

GLOSSARY OF KEY TERMS

**ACP Journal Club.** The ACP Journal Club summarizes and interprets the best evidence of one recent study or review article from traditional journals, based on the criteria provided by the practitioner.

**Agency for Healthcare Research and Quality (AHRQ).** The AHRQ has promoted EBP through the establishment of 12 Evidence-Based Practice Centers (EPCs). These EPCs are responsible for developing evidence guidelines and technology assessments on various clinical topics.

**The Cochrane Database of Systematic Reviews.** One of the most popular databases is The Cochrane Library, which reviews and summarizes individual clinical trials and systematic reviews from more than 100 medical journals.

**Evidence-based medicine (EBM).** The conscientious, explicit, and judicious use of current best evidence in making decisions about the care of individual patients. The practice of EBM means integrating individual clinical expertise with the best available external clinical evidence from systematic research.

**Evidence-based practice (EBP).** The conscientious, explicit, and judicious use of theory-derived, research-based information in making decisions about care delivery to individuals or groups of patients and in consideration of individual needs and preferences.

**InfoPOEMS.** Info-POEMS (Patient-

Oriented Evidence that Matters) is a database similar to the ACP Journal Club and it reviews and provides commentary on recent articles.

**MD consult.** A database that provides full-text access to textbooks, journal articles, practice guidelines, patient education handouts, and drug awareness.

**Meta-analysis.** A statistical method that takes the results of many studies in a specific area and synthesizes their findings to draw conclusions regarding the state of the science in the area of focus.

**National Guideline Clearinghouse.** The Clearinghouse provides a collection of evidence-based clinical practice guidelines.

Nurses use a variety of sources of information in making care decisions around certain treatments, therapies, and interventions. Unfortunately, many of these sources of information may have been derived from a textbook or journal article or perhaps from a conversation with a respected colleague or professor. To a lesser extent, information may have come from scientific research findings. Although nurses have advocated research-based practice for years, this goal has been difficult to achieve. During the past decade, there has been a renewed call for health-care professionals to base their care on the best research evidence available. The EBP movement is consistent with nursing's goal of providing research-based care to patients. This chapter provides an overview of EBP along with a discussion of an assortment of evidence-based tools.

## EVIDENCE-BASED PRACTICE: WHAT IS IT?

**Evidence-based practice (EBP)** was derived from the principle that health-care professionals should not center their practice on tradition or experience but on scientific research findings. The concept of EBP originated within the field of medicine; it was initially termed **evidence-based medicine (EBM).** EBM was originally defined by Sackett and colleagues[1] as the conscientious, explicit, and judicious use of current best evidence in making decisions about the care of individual patients. EBM means integrating individual clinical expertise with the best available external clinical evidence from systematic research.

The concept of EBM has been expanded and applied across all health-care areas under the term evidence-based health care (EBH) or evidence-based practice (EBP). Both terms refer to the critical appraisal of research findings and decisions regarding whether and how to use findings in the care of patients.

Ingersoll[2] differentiated evidence-based nursing (EBN) from EBM by suggesting that EBN is the conscientious, explicit, and judicious use of theory-derived, research-based information in making decisions about care delivery to individuals or groups of patients and in consideration of individual needs and preferences. EBN de-emphasizes ritual, isolated, and unsystematic clinical experiences, ungrounded opinions, and tradition as a basis for practice; instead, it stresses the use of research findings.[3]

## Characteristics of EBP

Important features or characteristics of EBP exist. First, EBP is a problem-solving approach that considers the context of the nurse's current clinical experience.[3] Clinical experience refers to the nurse's ability to use his or her clinical skills and past experience to identify each patient's unique health state and diagnosis, the individual risks, and benefits of potential interventions.[4]

Second, EBP brings together the best available research evidence by combining research with knowledge and theory.[3] Use of the best evidence from patient-centered clinical research allows for accuracy and precision of diagnostic tests; the power of prognosis markers; and the efficacy and safety of therapeutic and preventive regimens.[4] Finally, EBP allows patient values to be heard. If they are to serve the patient, the unique preferences, concerns, and expectations each patient brings to a clinical encounter are integrated into clinical decisions.

## THE RESEARCH-PRACTICE GAP

The research-practice gap refers to that period from when knowledge is produced to when it is practiced by health-care professionals.[5] Although the concept and movement of EBP continue to gain popularity, there is still a delay in using nursing research findings in practice. Several reasons[3,5] for this delay are listed in Table 5.1.

## LIMITATIONS OF EBP

Several limitations associated with the science and practices of EBM have been identified. Three limitations that are universal to science include a shortage of coherent, consistent scientific evidence; difficulties in applying any evidence to care of individual patients; and barriers to any practice of high-quality medicine.[4] Limitations unique to the practice of EBM include a need for developing skills in

TABLE 5.1 REASONS FOR THE DELAY IN USING RESEARCH FINDINGS IN NURSING PRACTICE

1. Nurses in practice do not know about research findings.
2. Nurses in practice are often not clear about who will benefit from the research findings or about the risks involved.
3. Nurses in practice do not usually associate with those individuals (i.e., scientists, academic researchers) who produce knowledge. There is often a lack of dialogue between researchers and clinicians.
4. Nurse researchers and nurse clinicians use different languages.
5. Nurses in practice lack the skills of locating and reading research reports.
6. Research is often reported in language of statistics instead of being reported in clinically meaningful terms.
7. Nurses and nurse managers do not develop opportunities for acceptance and introduction of innovation.

researching and appraising the research; the limited amount of time in practice to master such skills; and scarce resources to access the evidence.[4]

## HOW IS EBM ACTUALLY PRACTICED?

The practice of EBM consists of the following five steps[4]:

Step 1. Converting the need for information (about prevention, diagnosis, prognosis, and therapy) into an answerable question

Step 2. Tracking down the best evidence with which to answer that question

Step 3. Critically appraising the evidence for its validity (closeness to truth), impact (extent of effect), and applicability (usefulness in clinical practice)

Step 4. Integrating the critical appraisal with clinical expertise and patient's unique values and circumstances

Step 5. Evaluating the effectiveness and efficiency of steps 1 to 4

### Asking Clinical Questions

Questions in practice usually crop up from central issues involved in caring for patients. A list of issues related to writing clinical questions are presented in Table 5.2.[4] This listing is neither exhaustive nor mutually exclusive.

---

TABLE 5.2 ISSUES TO CONSIDER WHEN WRITING CLINICAL QUESTIONS

1. **Clinical findings:** How to properly gather and interpret findings from the history and physical examination.
2. **Etiology**: How to identify causes for disease.
3. **Clinical manifestations**: Knowing how often and when a disease causes clinical manifestations and how to use this knowledge in classifying patients' illnesses.
4. **Differential diagnosis**: When considering the possible causes of patients' clinical problem, how to select those that are likely, serious, and responsive to treatment.
5. **Diagnostic test**: How to select and interpret diagnostic tests in order to confirm or exclude a diagnosis, based on considering their precision, accuracy, acceptability, safety, etc.
6. **Prognosis:** How to estimate your patient's likely clinical course over time.
7. **Therapy:** How to select treatments to offer your patients that do more good than harm and that are worth the efforts and costs of using them.
8. **Prevention:** How to reduce the chance of disease by identifying and modifying risk factors and how to diagnose disease early in screening.
9. **Experience and meaning:** How to empathize with your patients' situations, appreciate the meaning they find in the experience, and understand how this meaning influences their healing.
10. **Self-improvement:** How to keep up to date, improve your clinical and other skills, and run a better, more efficient clinical practice.

---

*Source: Sackett, DL, et al: Evidence-Based Medicine: How to Practice and Teach EBM, ed 2. Churchill Livingstone, Edinburgh, 2000, pp 1–35.[4]*

## Tracking Down the Best Evidence

As you begin to track down the best evidence, it is a good idea to start searching broadly rather than beginning specifically. Identify the indexes, journals, databases, and other sources of which you are aware, and spend some time persuing them. Textbooks will not be helpful; although you may find some useful information about the pathophysiology of a disease, textbooks are not appropriate for establishing the cause, diagnosis, prognosis, prevention, or treatment of the disorder.

As you begin to launch your search, you might consider working with the librarian at your institution. Share your clinical questions with the librarian. He or she will be able to point you in the right direction and provide some consultation. It is important for you to work with the librarian and participate in the computerized searching that needs to be conducted. Your understanding of the topic and your clinical experience are extremely valuable when working with the librarian.

## EVIDENCE DATABASES

Current best evidence from specific research studies can be found in a number of electronic databases. The best of these is Evidence-Based Medicine Reviews (EBMR) from OVID Technologies (www.ovid.com). EBMR combines several electronic databases including MEDLINE, HealthSTAR, CANCERLIT, AIDSLINE, Best Evidence (BE), and The Cochrane Database of Systematic Reviews. Several of these databases are also available as separate databases on CD-ROM and the Internet.

## MEDLINE

MEDLINE is the largest biomedical research literature database and is available on CD-ROM and the Internet. MEDLINE comprises information from several print indexes, including Index Medicus, Index to Dental Literature, and International Nursing Index. MEDLINE indexes published research in allied health, biological sciences, information sciences, physical sciences, and the humanities. Because of its large size (over 10 million references), it is challenging to get exactly what you want. More specialized clinical research databases are available and easier to use (i.e, the Cochrane Database of Systematic Reviews).

## HEALTHSTAR

HealthSTAR indexes published literature on health services, technology, administration, and research. The focus in this database is on both clinical and nonclinical aspects of health-care delivery. In addition to journals, HealthSTAR indexes material from books, book chapters, government documents, newspaper articles, and technical reports.

## CANCERLIT

CANCERLIT indexes cancer literature including journal articles, government reports, technical reports, meeting abstracts and papers, and monographs.

## AIDSLINE

AIDSLINE indexes published literature on HIV infections and AIDS. It focuses on the biomedical, epidemiological, oncological, health-care administration, social, and behavioral sciences literature. AIDSLINE indexes literature from journal articles, monographs, meeting abstracts and papers, newsletters, and government reports.

### The Cochrane Library

The Cochrane Library is an electronic library designed to make available the evidence needed to make informed health-care decisions. The program presents the growing body of work of the Cochrane Collaboration and others interested in EBM. Currently, the library maintains four databases:

1. The Cochrane Database of Systematic Reviews
2. The Database of Abstracts of Reviews of Effectiveness
3. The Cochrane Controlled Trials Register
4. The Cochrane Review of Methodology Database

The **Cochrane Database of Systematic Reviews** is one of the most popular databases in The Cochrane Library; the database reviews individual clinical trials and summarizes systematic reviews from over 100 medical journals. When searching the Cochrane Review of Methodology Database, explicit selection criteria are needed. Each review includes the same predefined sections (i.e., Description of study; Methodological qualities of included studies; Results; Discussion; Implications for practice). The Cochrane Review of Methodology Database provides an efficient method of interpreting the results of many studies.

There are several ways a researcher pulls together the accumulated information on a topic. Results of many studies are synthesized to produce new knowledge by a statistical method called meta-analysis. **Meta-analysis,** sometimes referred to as quantitative synthesis, is not a research design; rather, it is a method that takes the results of many studies in a specific area and synthesizes their findings to draw conclusions regarding the state of the science in the area of focus.[6] Instead of individual subjects being the unit of analysis, individual studies are the unit of analysis. Information is extracted about the strength of the relationship of the independent and dependent variables of each study. This information is quantified and an average score is computed across all studies.[7]

### Other Resources on Evidence-Based Health Care

**ACP Journal Club.** The ACP Journal Club is published by the American College of Physicians—American Society of Internal Medicine (http://www.

acponline.com). The ACP Journal Club summarizes and interprets the best evidence of one recent study or review article from traditional journals based on the criteria provided by the practitioner. Use of the ACP Journal Club is important when you need to know quickly about one study or review. Such a resource provides the best evidence from high-quality studies selected from a variety of journals.

**InfoPOEMS.** InfoPOEMS (Patient-Oriented Evidence that Matters) is published by the Journal of Family Practice (http://www.infopoems.com). InfoPOEMS is a database similar to the ACP Journal Club in that it reviews and provides commentary on one recent article.

**National Guideline Clearinghouse.** The National Guideline Clearinghouse (http://www.guideline.gov) provides a collection of evidence-based clinical practice guidelines, without providing an integrative review. The Clearinghouse provides recommendations on a given topic from more than one organization, often several (e.g., American Medical Association, Agency for Healthcare Research and Quality). These guidelines may reflect the bias of the particular author.

**MD Consult.** MD Consult (http://www.mdconsult.com) provides full text access to textbooks, journal articles, practice guidelines, patient education handouts, and drug awareness. Use MD Consult when you need to find some quick background information on a particular topic in a variety of formats. MD Consult provides current information, such as medical news, what patients are reading, clinical topics, and weekly updates from several journals.

**Agency for Healthcare Research and Quality (AHRQ).** AHRQ (http://www.ahcpr.gov) was formerly known as the Agency for Health Care Policy and Research (AHCPR). AHRQ has promoted EBP through the establishment of 12 Evidence-Based Practice Centers (EPCs). These centers are responsible for developing evidence guidelines and technology assessments on various clinical topics. These guidelines include Diagnosis of Sleep Apnea; Depression: Newer Pharmacotherapeutics; Acute Sinusitis in Children; and Treatment of Attention-Deficit/Hyperactivity Disorder.

Many computerized databases are user-friendly and have a great deal of help incorporated into their programs to help you with what you are looking for while teaching you to be a better searcher. Basic tips associated with searching some of databases listed above are provided in Table 5.3.

## Appraising the Evidence Critically

After completing the search on a particular topic, it is important to critically appraise or "rank" the resulting evidence. Different sources of evidence are needed to address varied clinical questions. A hierarchy of research evidence is presented in Figure 5.1. Refer to Sackett et al[4] for a detailed discussion of levels of evidence and grades of recommendation.

## ETHICAL CONCERNS AROUND EBP

In practicing EBM it is important for all health-care professionals to share research findings and research evidence with patients and their families as part of the

- Meta-analysis of randomized clinical trials
- Individual randomized clinical trials
- Individual cohort study
- Outcomes research
- Individual case-control study
- Case studies
- Expert opinion

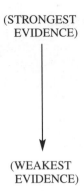

(STRONGEST EVIDENCE)

(WEAKEST EVIDENCE)

FIGURE 5.1 Hierarchy of research evidence.

decision-making process regarding care and treatment.[5] Information must be shared in ways that invite patients to participate in these decisions. Presentation of information should include whether there is a great deal of evidence in support of a certain treatment and/or therapy; what benefits are likely to be realized and which ones are more in doubt; and a separation of likely adverse outcomes from uncommon ones. You need not feel obligated to present findings and evidence independent of your appraisal of them; you should feel free to express your views regarding the meaning of findings, particularly as they apply to the patient with whom you are talking.[5]

TABLE 5.3 TIPS ON SEARCHING DATABASES

1. Basic/Background Information
   MD Consult
   National guidelines
   MEDLINE/reviews
2. Short critiques or recent studies/reviews
   MEDLINE/abstracts
   InfoPOEMS
   Best Evidence
3. Common well studies topics
   MEDLINE/reviews
   InfoPOEMS
   Best Evidence
   Cochrane
4. Guidelines/Algorithms
   National guidelines
   Cochrane
   MD Consult
   MEDLINE/guidelines
5. Uncommon/specific/current topic
   MEDLINE

**SUMMARY** OF KEY IDEAS

1. Evidence-based medicine (EBM) is a movement that has developed to assist health-care professionals to base their care on the best research evidence possible.
2. Evidence-based nursing (EBN) eliminates the attention to the type of research design, incorporating the use of theory-derived and research-based information.
3. A delay in using nursing research findings in clinical practice still exists today.
4. The practice of EBM is focused on several steps, including asking the right clinical question, tracking down the best evidence, appraising the evidence critically, and integrating the critical appraisal with the patient's unique values and circumstances.
5. Best evidence from research studies is found in a number of electronic databases. The best of these is Evidence-Based Medicine Reviews (EBMR) from OVID Technologies, which includes The Cochrane Database of Systematic Reviews.
6. Meta-analysis is a statistical technique that takes the results of many studies in a specific area and synthesizes their findings to draw conclusions regarding the state of the science in the area of focus.
7. It is important for health-care professionals to share research evidence and findings with patients and their families.

**LEARNING** ACTIVITIES

1. Obtain a copy of a research-based practice guideline developed by one of the Evidence-Based Practice Centers through the Agency for Healthcare Research and Quality (AHRQ).

   Complete the Appraisal of Evidence Form for Practice Guidelines listed below.

   *Synopsis*

   What does the guideline address?

   What population of patients is the guideline intended for?

What are the key decision points addressed by the guideline?

What process was used to develop the guideline?

*Credibility Profile*

Is the guideline based on a comprehensive meta-analysis or integrative review?

Is the scientific basis for each recommendation provided?

Are the key decision points addressed?

At each decision point, was the full range of actions evaluated?

Is the discussion of the way the panel reached decisions convincing that all evidence was considered in an impartial manner?

Are the guidelines current?

Was the panel that developed the guidelines made up of people with the necessary skills, expertise, and backgrounds?

Are the recommendations credible?

*Applicability Profile*

Does the guideline address a problem, decision, or situation seen in practice?

Is the guideline being used in whole or in part?

Are the recommended courses of action acceptable and feasible to you and your patients?

To follow the guideline, what will you have to do differently?

Do you have the resources, skills, and equipment to implement this guideline accurately and safely?

Should you adopt this guideline in its entirety?

Should you adopt parts of it?

How will you know if your patients are benefiting from your use of the guideline?

## References

1. Sackett, DL, et al: Evidence-based medicine: What it is and what it isn't. Br Med J 312:71, 1996.
2. Ingersoll, GL: Evidence-based nursing: What it is and what it isn't. Nurs Outlook 48:151, 2000.
3. McEwen, M, and Wills, EM: Theoretical Basis for Nursing. Lippincott Williams & Wilkins, Philadelphia, 2002, pp 356–358.
4. Sackett, DL, et al: Evidence-Based Medicine: How to Practice and Teach EBM, ed 2. Churchill Livingstone, Edinburgh, 2000, pp 1–35.
5. Brown, SJ: Knowledge for Health Care Practice: A Guide to Using Research Evidence. WB Saunders, Philadelphia, 1999, pp 15–19, 188–196, 241.
6. LoBiondo-Wood, G, and Haber, J: Nonexperimental designs. In LoBiondo-Wood, G, and Haber, J (eds). Nursing Research: Methods, Critical Appraisal, and Utilization, ed 4. Mosby-Year Book, St. Louis, 1998, pp 207–210.
7. Polit, DF, Beck, CT, and Hungler, BP: Essentials of Nursing Research: Methods, Appraisal, and Utilization, ed 5. Lippincott Williams & Wilkins, Philadelphia, 2001, p 134.

# 6

# Formulating Hypotheses and Research Questions

James A. Fain, PhD, RN, BC-ADM, FAAN

## LEARNING OBJECTIVES

*At the end of this chapter, you will be able to:*

1. Define a hypothesis.
2. Identify characteristics of a hypothesis.
3. Write different types of hypotheses.
4. Compare and contrast inductive versus deductive hypotheses, directional versus nondirectional hypotheses, simple versus complex hypotheses, and statistical (null) versus research hypotheses.
5. Describe the appropriate use of research questions.
6. Define independent, dependent, and extraneous variables.

## GLOSSARY OF KEY TERMS

**Dependent variable.** A variable that is observed for changes or to assess the possible effect of a treatment or manipulation; may be the effect or outcome of an experimental procedure; also referred to as a criterion variable. Usually symbolized by the letter Y.

**Directional hypothesis.** A hypothesis that makes a specific prediction about the direction of the relationship between two variables.

**Extraneous variable.** A variable that is not controlled for in a study, threatening the internal validity of the study.

**Hypothesis.** A statement about the relationship between the variables that are being investigated.

**Independent variable.** A variable that is manipulated and controlled by the

researcher; also called a predictor variable. Usually symbolized by the letter X.

**Nondirectional hypothesis.** A hypothesis that does not stipulate in advance the direction and nature of the relationship between two variables.

**Null hypothesis ($H_o$).** A hypothesis stating that no relationship or difference exists between two variables. Also called statistical hypothesis.

**Research hypothesis ($H_1$ or $H_a$).** A hypothesis stating a relationship or difference between two variables. Also called an alternative, declarative, or scientific hypothesis.

**Variable.** A measurable characteristic that varies among the subjects being studied.

Hypotheses and research questions are formulated after the review of literature has been completed. The literature review identifies prior findings and provides a basis for understanding how the proposed study relates to previous knowledge. Hypotheses and research questions influence the study design, sampling techniques, and plans for data collection and analysis. Stating hypotheses and research questions requires the researcher to identify variables that are pertinent to the study. Determining how these variables are defined is important for purposes of measurement. This chapter focuses on the formulation of hypotheses and research questions; various types of variables are introduced and described.

## HYPOTHESES

A **hypothesis** is a statement that explains or predicts the relationship or differences between two or more variables in terms of expected results or outcomes of a study. The researcher does not set out to prove hypotheses but rather to collect data that either support or refute the hypotheses. A common misconception is that data must support the hypotheses for a study to be successful. Research studies do not have to prove anything to be considered worthwhile. Some of the most important findings have come from research in which the data did *not* support the hypotheses. A lack of support in research data forces the researcher to reevaluate the hypotheses.

Hypotheses serve several purposes.[1] One purpose is to guide scientific inquiry for the advancement of knowledge. Researchers must go beyond mere gathering of isolated data and seek relationships and generalizations about the data. Another purpose is to provide direction for the research design and the collection, analysis, and interpretation of data. Hypotheses provide a basis for selecting the sample, the statistical analyses needed, and the relationships to be tested. For example, when the aim of a study is to explain certain relationships, the major emphasis is on linking the variables. Finally, hypotheses can also provide a framework for reporting the conclusions of a study; each hypothesis can be tested separately, and conclusions relevant to each can be stated. This section of the research report can be organized around each hypothesis to make a more meaningful and readable presentation.

Hypotheses are not needed for research that is classified as descriptive (describing rather than explaining phenomena). Descriptive research is important for laying the foundation for further study.

### Characteristics of Hypotheses

Nurses must know what constitutes good hypotheses to be able to read and critique research effectively. Good hypotheses state clearly and concisely the expected relationship (or difference) between two or more variables. Regardless of the specific format used to state a hypothesis, the statement includes the variables being studied, the population being studied, and the predicted outcomes. A general model for stating hypotheses is as follows: Subjects who receive X are more likely to have Y than subjects who do not receive X.

In the following examples, X represents the treatment (independent variable) or variable manipulated by the researcher and Y the observed outcome (dependent variable). Words and phrases such as "greater than," "less than," "positively," "negatively," and "difference" denote the direction of the proposed hypotheses.

Children ages 5 to 10 years old who are provided with prior information about their tonsillectomy will experience less postoperative anxiety than children of the same age who do not receive information.

> Subjects = Children ages 5 to 10 years old
> X = Provided with prior information
> Y = Less postoperative anxiety

Nursing home residents exposed to 10 minutes of calming music experience less agitation than those who receive no such intervention.

> Subjects = Nursing home residents
> X = 10 minutes of calming music
> Y = Less agitation

Children with a high sense of humor adjust better to having cancer than do those children with a low sense of humor.

> Subjects = Children
> X = Sense of humor (high versus low)
> Y = Better adjustment to cancer

Patients who have had internal mammary artery grafting following coronary artery bypass surgery will experience greater chest pain or discomfort than patients who have had saphenous vein grafting.

> Subjects = Patients
> X = Internal mammary artery grafting following coronary artery bypass surgery
> Y = Greater chest pain or discomfort

Excerpt 6.1 provides an example of two hypotheses from one study. In both examples, the population being studied (chemically-dependent women), the treatment (subjects who participated in experiential and cognitive therapy groups versus those who did not), and the outcomes (higher levels of general and social self-efficacy) were presented.

All nouns in hypotheses or research questions should be defined first conceptually and then operationally. What if the characteristics of the subjects were not further defined in the article? How would you interpret the term "subjects"? People older than age 50 years? 60 years and older? 70 years and older? In applying research findings to practice, it is important to know how subjects are defined, to be able to make a judgment about the applicability of the findings to a particular population. Similarly, a definition of "increased memory self-efficacy" should also be provided in this example. Later in this research report, an explanation of the

---

**EXCERPT 6.1**

## EXAMPLE OF TWO HYPOTHESES

To explore self-efficacy further with chemically dependent women, the following hypotheses were examined:

1. Chemically dependent women who have participated in experiential or cognitive therapy groups will have higher levels of general self-efficacy than will women who are chemically dependent but who have not participated in either therapy group.
2. Chemically dependent women who have participated in experiential and cognitive therapy groups will have higher levels of social self-efficacy than will women who are chemically dependent but who have not participated in either therapy group.

*Source: Washington, OGM: Effects of group therapy on chemically dependent women's self-efficacy. Image J Nurs Schol 32:347, 2000, with permission.*

---

intervention and memory self-efficacy is given, along with a description of the population being studied.

Variables identified in hypotheses must be operationally defined. This means specifying how the variables will be measured in terms of the instruments, scales, or both, that will be used. Research studies have been criticized for lack of a clear definition of the concepts and variables being studied. Concepts and variables need to be logically defined according to their relationship to the problem. The hypotheses presented in Excerpt 6.2 include a definition of the instruments that measure the dependent variables. In the first hypothesis, depression is measured by a score on the Center for Epidemiologic Studies Depression Scale (CES-D), with fatigue being measured by a score on the Piper Fatigue Scale (PFS). In the second hypothesis, transformational coping is measured by utilizing two subscales of the Jalowiec Coping Scale. Both examples illustrate the collection of data using quantitative instruments. Many statistical techniques can then be applied to measure interval and ratio variables.

A hypothesis must state an expected relationship between two variables. In the example, "If adults with chronic non-malignant pain (CNP) differ from one another, they will differ from one another in quality of life (QOL)," there is no proposed relationship to test. An expected relationship could be stated as: There is a higher perception of QOL in a group of adults with CNP who completed a pain management program compared with adults with CNP who have not completed a program.

A hypothesis that states several relationships among variables can be difficult to decipher. Limiting hypotheses to a single relationship between two variables adds clarity in terms of understanding the intended relationship and the conclusions that follow data analysis.

A well-stated hypothesis must be testable. Hypotheses are never proved right or wrong through hypothesis testing. Hypotheses are either supported or not supported, based on the collection and analysis of data. Variables included in the hypothesis lend themselves to observation, measurement, and analysis. The predicted outcomes

## EXCERPT 6.2

### OPERATIONAL DEFINITION OF VARIABLES WITHIN HYPOTHESES

The purpose of this study was to examine the relationship between individual hardiness and caregiver strain, as measured by depression and fatigue in persons caring for functionally impaired older adults (high stress conditions), and to determine if use of transformational coping strategies mediates the relationship between hardiness and caregiver outcomes.

**Hypotheses**

1. Caregivers with higher individual hardiness will experience lower strain as measured by depression (Center for Epidemiological Studies Depression Scale—CES-D) and fatigue (Piper Fatigue Scale—PFS).
2. Caregivers with higher individual hardiness will use more transformational coping strategies (as measured by two subscales of the Jalowiec Coping Scale—Confrontive and Optimistic Scales) than caregivers with lower individual hardiness.

*Source: Clark, PC: Effects of individual and family hardiness on caregiver depression and fatigue. Res Nurs Health 25:37, 2002, with permission.*

proposed in the hypothesis either will or will not be congruent with the actual outcome when the hypothesis is tested. Hypotheses advance scientific knowledge by confirming or not confirming relationships. Some studies may require more than one hypothesis.

## TYPES OF HYPOTHESES

Hypotheses are classified as simple versus complex, nondirectional versus directional, and statistical versus research.

### Simple Versus Complex

A simple hypothesis states the relationship between two variables. Using a simple but clearly stated format makes it easier for readers to understand and formulate conclusions following data analysis. A complex hypothesis states the relationship between two or more independent variables and two or more dependent variables. Simple hypotheses are easier to test, measure, and analyze because nursing research involves human beings, who are complex. Many hypotheses in nursing research may be complex; however, the most important considerations for researchers to think about are the following:

What type of hypothesis is best for your study?
Is the study you are planning feasible?

If, for example, a complex hypothesis is appropriate but you cannot collect the data to test it, then a simple hypothesis should be used instead. Several examples of simple and complex hypotheses are presented in Table 6.1.

---

TABLE 6.1  SIMPLE AND COMPLEX HYPOTHESES

---

**Simple Hypotheses**

1. Subjects will have less discomfort following administration of the two-track intramuscular injection compared with administration by standard injection.
   *Independent variable = Type of injection administered (two-track versus standard)*
   *Dependent variable = Discomfort*
2. Patients with greater knowledge of diabetes will have significantly higher rates of adherence to the treatment regimen than will patients who have less knowledge about diabetes.
   *Independent variable = Amount of knowledge (greater versus lesser)*
   *Dependent variable = Compliance adherence*
3. Healthy young adults who consume 720 cc of ice water within 10 minutes will have a significant increase in systolic blood pressure as compared with healthy young adults who consume 720 cc of room-temperature water within 10 minutes.
   *Independent variable = Temperature of water (ice water versus room temperature)*
   *Dependent variable = Systolic blood pressure*

**Complex Hypotheses**

1. Newborns fed at 1, 2, and 3 hours of life (HOL) produce stool earlier, have lower serum indirect bilirubin levels, less observed jaundice at 48 HOL, and a lower percentage of weight loss than do infants initially fed at 4 HOL.
   *Independent variable = Time of feeding (1, 2, and 3 HOL versus 4 HOL)*
   *Dependent variables = Time of stool, level of indirect bilirubin, presence/absence of jaundice at 48 HOL, percentage of weight loss*
2. Abdominal surgery patients who received preoperative teaching will have a decreased perception of pain and request fewer analgesics than patients undergoing abdominal surgery who receive structured postoperative teaching.
   *Independent variable = Timing of teaching (preoperative versus postoperative)*
   *Dependent variables = Perception of pain, request for analgesics*
3. Nurses who deliver nursing care using a primary nursing model will have an increase in patient satisfaction with nursing care, a decrease in absenteeism, and an improvement in their perception of the work environment as compared with nurses who deliver nursing care by the conventional method of team nursing.
   *Independent variable = Delivery of nursing care (primary versus team nursing)*
   *Dependent variables = Patient satisfaction, absenteeism, perception of work environment*

---

## Nondirectional Versus Directional

A **nondirectional hypothesis** states a relationship between variables, but it has no specific direction. Nondirectional hypotheses are used when past research provides conflicting results or when the direction of the relationship is unknown. Instead of writing nondirectional hypotheses, researchers may instead ask, "What is the relationship between X and Y?" A **directional hypothesis** states the direction of the relationship between variables. Such hypotheses are usually derived from conceptual models or findings from previous research. Directional hypotheses are clearer and more logical than nondirectional hypotheses. Using directional hypotheses, researchers are better able to indicate a direction of the relationship between the

EXCERPT 6.3

## EXAMPLE OF TWO DIRECTIONAL HYPOTHESES

The purpose of this study was to investigate a conceptual model in which depression was proposed to have direct negative effects on positive health practices as well as indirect negative effects through maternal-fetal attachment.

Based on this framework, the following hypotheses were examined:
1. Women who have higher levels of depressive symptoms will have lower levels of maternal-fetal attachment.
2. Women who have higher levels of depressive symptoms will report fewer positive health practices.

*Source: Lindgren, K: Relationship among maternal-fetal attachment, prenatal depression, and health practices in pregnancy. Res Nurs Health 24:203, 2001, with permission.*

variables being studied, as knowledge about that particular topic increases. Two examples of directional hypotheses are shown in Excerpt 6.3.

### Statistical Versus Research

A statistical hypothesis, also referred to as a **null hypothesis ($H_o$),** states that no relationship (or difference) exists between two variables. Statistical hypotheses are usually used because they suit the statistical techniques that determine whether an observed relationship is probably a chance relationship or probably a true relationship. Excerpt 6.4 provides an illustration of a null hypothesis.

Because null hypotheses do not reflect the researcher's true expectations of a study's results, two hypotheses are often stated. This is done in various ways. A declarative research hypothesis may be used to communicate the researcher's true expectations, along with a statistical hypothesis to permit statistical testing. Another strategy is to state a research hypothesis, analyze the data (assuming a null hypothesis), and make inferences based on the target population identified in the research hypothesis. Given that few studies are really designed to verify the nonexistence of a relationship, it seems logical that most studies should be based on research hypotheses.

EXCERPT 6.4

## EXAMPLE OF NULL HYPOTHESIS

**Hypothesis**

There will be no significant difference in the weights of children obtained while being held by an adult on adult scales compared with the weights of children obtained using infant scales.

*Source: Vessey, JA, and Stueve, DL: A comparison of two techniques for weighing young children. Pediatr Nurs 22:327, 1996, with permission.*

A **research hypothesis,** also referred to as an alternative ($H_1$ or $H_a$), declarative, or scientific hypothesis, states that a relationship or difference exists between variables. Such hypotheses indicate what the researcher expects to find as a result of conducting a study. Research hypotheses can be simple or complex, directional or nondirectional. In each of the four hypotheses illustrated in Excerpt 6.5, the authors state that a difference exists between variables. The four hypotheses are nondirectional because no clear indication of the nature of the relationships has been previously confirmed in the literature. Guidelines for measuring heart rate (pulse-counting techniques) have conflicting results throughout the literature.

Another way to categorize hypotheses is according to how they are derived. Hypotheses can be derived inductively or deductively. Inductive reasoning moves from specific observations to general. For example, after working many years with people who have type 2 diabetes, you notice that specific observations or patterns emerge every time you talk about blood glucose monitoring. Inductive reasoning is used when these specific observations begin to generate a way to care for this population of people. From these observations, you are able to propose a model or framework on how to incorporate the importance of blood glucose monitoring in working with people who have type 2 diabetes that could possibly be tested through formal research. Certain variables are noted to be related in most situations, which warrants development of a tentative explanation, or hypothesis. Related literature is then reviewed, and a formal hypothesis is formulated. Deductive hypotheses are derived from theory and contribute to the science of nursing by providing evidence that supports, expands, or contradicts a given theory. A deductive hypothesis that is based on a theoretical framework is illustrated in Excerpt 6.6.

---

## EXCERPT 6.5

### EXAMPLE OF RESEARCH (ALTERNATIVE) HYPOTHESES

Based on recommendations from Jones, our study was designed to test the following hypotheses:

1. The accuracy of radial pulse-rate assessments taken by nursing personnel with different levels of status and education will be different.
2. The accuracy of 1-minute resting radial pulse rates per minute taken by nursing personnel for 15 seconds multiplied by 4, 30 seconds multiplied by 2, and for 60 seconds will be different compared with rates shown in simultaneous electrocardiographic (ECG) tracings.
3. The accuracy of radial pulse-rate assessments per minute taken by nursing personnel will differ on the basis of number of years of experience.
4. The accuracy of radial pulse-rate assessments obtained by nursing personnel palpating the right radial artery will differ compared with assessments obtained by those palpating the left radial artery.

*Source: Hollerbach, AD, and Sneed, NV: Accuracy of radial pulse assessment by length of counting interval. Heart Lung 19:258, 1990, with permission.*

**EXCERPT 6.6**

EXAMPLE OF DEDUCTIVE HYPOTHESES

In addition, two hypotheses based on Rubin's propositions were tested:

1. High-risk women (HRW) will report lower maternal role competence than low-risk women (LRW) during postpartum hospitalization and at 1, 4, and 8 months post-partum.
2. There is a significant relationship between maternal competence and maternal attachment from postpartum hospitalization through 8 months postpartum.

*Source: Mercer, RT, and Ferketich, SL: Predictors of maternal role competence by risk status. Nurs Res 43:38, 1994, with permission.*

## TESTING HYPOTHESES

Hypothesis testing is what scientific research is all about. To test a hypothesis, the researcher determines the sample, measuring instruments, design, and procedure for collecting data. A testable hypothesis is one that contains variables that are measurable, with a relationship that can be either supported or not supported based on the data collected.

Hypotheses are evaluated by statistical analyses. The choice of an appropriate statistical measure depends not only on the nature of the data but also on the level of measurement appropriate for those data. Correlational analyses are conducted to determine the existence, type, and strength of the relationship between the variables being studied. Inferential statistics (e.g., t-test, analysis of variance) is used to evaluate hypotheses that examine differences between and among categories or levels of variables. Results obtained from testing a hypothesis are described using certain research terminology. When a study is completed and a significant relationship exists between two variables or there is a difference between groups, the null hypothesis is "rejected." Rejection of the null or statistical hypothesis is similar to acceptance of the research hypothesis. This indicates the possibility that a relationship or difference does exist. Failure to reject the null of statistical hypothesis implies there is insufficient evidence to support the idea of a real difference.

## RESEARCH QUESTIONS

Research studies do not always contain hypotheses but may instead be organized around research questions. A research question is a concise, interrogative statement written in the present tense and including one or more variables (or concepts). Research questions focus on describing variable(s), examining relationships among variables, and determining differences between two or more groups regarding the selected variable(s).[2]

Researchers specify the type of research and the purpose of the study by using phrases such as "to identify" and "to describe." Research questions are used when prior knowledge of the phenomenon is limited and the research seeks to identify or describe the phenomenon (as in exploratory or descriptive studies), or both. A general model for writing research questions is:

1. How is X described? *(describing variables)*
2. What is the perception of X? *(describing variables)*
3. Is X related to Y? *(examining relationships)*
4. What is the relationship between X and Y? *(examining relationships)*
5. Is there a difference between groups 1 and 2 with respect to Y? *(determining differences)*

The three research questions presented in Excerpt 6.7 focus on *describing* the recovery of patients undergoing laparoscopic cholecystectomy. The purpose of the study was to describe and understand what patients experience after outpatient laparoscopic cholecystectomy procedures. In Excerpt 6.8 the focus of the study is *examining* relationships—identifying the relationship between a woman's age and social support while experiencing the stress of undergoing a breast biopsy. Excerpt 6.9 illustrates the third type of research question, *determining* differences between groups.

Research questions are written as interrogative statements. The interrogative form seeks an answer. All research variables and the population to be studied are included in the interrogative statement. In contrast to the problem statement, research questions are more precise and specific. The research question flows naturally from the purpose statement, narrowing the focus of the study.

## CLASSIFICATION OF VARIABLES

A **variable** is a measurable characteristic that varies among the subjects being studied. As the definition implies, the characteristic or phenomenon under study varies in some way. Research variables are classified as either independent or dependent.

---

**EXCERPT 6.7**

## FOCUS OF RESEARCH QUESTIONS: DESCRIBING VARIABLE(S)

**Purpose of Study**

After reviewing the results of these previous studies, we believed that additional research was indicated to evaluate and describe the recovery course of short-stay patients undergoing laparoscopic cholecystectomy procedures, comparing their experiences with those reported in the literature. We addressed these specific research questions in our study:

- What is the pattern of occurrence of symptoms (e.g., pain, vomiting, nausea, fatigue, loss of appetite) and how do these symptoms change during the perioperative and recovery periods?
- How many patients require analgesic medications and for how long after surgery?
- How quickly after surgery do patients resume normal eating and living patterns?

*Source: Cason, CL, Seidel, SL, and Bushmaier, M: Recovery from laparoscopic cholecystectomy procedures. AORN J 63:1099, 1996, with permission.*

## EXCERPT 6.8

### FOCUS OF RESEARCH QUESTIONS: EXAMINING RELATIONSHIPS

**Review of the Literature**

There is a scarcity of research studying how a woman's age may influence the strength and size of her social support. An awareness of the age-related needs of women experiencing stress is important. The literature espouses the importance of social support in maintaining and promoting health but does little to specify gender- and age-related differences in seeking and utilizing social support. That definitive knowledge may assist health professionals in helping women cope with stress by anticipating social support deficits.

**The Problem**

The purpose of this study was to identify the relationship between a woman's age and social support while experiencing the stress of undergoing a breast biopsy. The study was designed to answer the following research questions: (1) Do social support network size and social support affect a woman's stress at the time of breast biopsy? (2) Is the age of the woman related to her social support network size or strength?

*Source: Seckel, MM, and Birney, MH: Social support, stress, and age in women undergoing breast biopsies. Clin Nurse Specialist 10:137, 1996, with permission.*

An **independent variable** is a variable that is observed, introduced, or manipulated to determine the effect it has on another variable. Depending on the research approach, the independent variable may be classified as an experimental, treatment, intervention, or predictor variable. The terms "experimental" and "treatment" are not to be confused with experimental treatment that is associated with therapeutic care. "Treatment" means manipulation, not necessarily therapeutic procedures.

## EXCERPT 6.9

### FOCUS OF RESEARCH QUESTIONS: DETERMINING DIFFERENCES

The purpose of this study was to compare African Americans and Caucasians in a diabetes education weight control program and describe the differences between the two groups regarding health beliefs about diabetes. A second purpose was to learn more about attrition from the program by examining the differences in sociodemographic characteristics and beliefs about diabetes treatment between African Americans who dropped out and those who completed the program. Therefore, the research questions are:

1. What are the differences in health beliefs about diabetes between Caucasians and African Americans in the program?
2. What are the differences in sociodemographic characteristics of Caucasian and African-American participants in a diabetes education research program for persons with NIDDM?

*Source: Wierenga, ME, and Wuethrich, KL: Diabetes program attrition: Differences between two groups. Health Values 19:12, 1995, with permission.*

Consider the following hypothesis:

> Children ages 5 to 10 years old who are provided with prior information about their tonsillectomy will experience less postoperative anxiety than children of the same age who do not receive prior information.

Providing prior information about tonsillectomies, in this case, is the independent variable and is considered the treatment (manipulation) used to discover its effect on postoperative anxiety. "Postoperative anxiety" is the dependent variable, or focus, of the study.

The **dependent variable,** also called the criterion or outcome variable, is the variable that is observed for change or reaction after the treatment is applied. The dependent variable is that which is under investigation; it is this variable that the researcher determines to be a result of conducting the study. The researcher can manipulate conditions that affect the variability in the dependent variable. The researcher intends to understand, explain, or predict the dependent variables; they constitute what the researcher measures about subjects after subjects have experienced or been exposed to the independent variable. Consider the following hypothesis:

> Men ages 25 to 50 years old, who experience migraine headaches and perform biofeedback therapy, report fewer headaches than do men in the same age range who do not perform biofeedback therapy.

In this hypothesis, the independent variable or intervention (treatment) is biofeedback therapy. This therapy is designed to control the number of migraine headaches among men ages 25 to 50 years old. Another group of men ages 25 to 50 years old does not receive the intervention. The number of headaches is the dependent variable and represents the area of interest under investigation. The number of headaches reflects the effect of and/or the response to the treatment of biofeedback (independent variable). Several independent or dependent variables, or both, can be used in one study.

**Extraneous variables** are characteristics that are not under investigation but that may, or may not, be relevant to the study. These variables exist in all studies and are primarily of concern in quantitative research. Extraneous variables are classified as controlled or uncontrolled and as recognized or unrecognized. If these extraneous variables are not taken into account, they can confuse the interpretation of the results and confound the effects of the independent variable. Therefore, extraneous variables are sometimes called confounding variables. Attempts should be made to identify and control extraneous variables. Quasiexperimental and experimental designs have been developed to control the influence of extraneous variables.

## QUESTIONS TO CONSIDER WHEN CRITIQUING HYPOTHESES AND/OR RESEARCH QUESTIONS

Identify a research study to critique. Read the study to see if you recognize any key terms discussed in this chapter. Remember that all studies may not contain all key

terms. The following questions[1,3] serve as a guide in critiquing hypotheses and/or research questions:

1. *Can you identify the hypotheses and/or research questions in the study? Were the hypotheses directional or nondirectional?* Phrases such as "the study tested the following hypotheses" or "it was hypothesized that" help locate hypotheses in a research study. Research questions are easy to identify; they focus on describing variables, examining relationships, and/or determining differences. When research questions are used, the purpose of the study tends to be descriptive or exploratory.
2. *If the study contains hypotheses, are they worded so that there is an expected relationship between two or more variables?* Remember that all hypotheses may not be explicitly stated as described in this chapter.
3. *Is the absence of hypotheses in a research study justifiable?* Consider the research problem and design of the study. Descriptive studies attempt to describe what exists, with no intention to explain relationships, test hypotheses, or make predictions. Results of descriptive studies often lead to the formation of hypotheses that can then be tested.
4. *If the study contains research questions, are they stated clearly and concisely?* Look to see if the research question(s) begin(s) with "why." These research questions are difficult to answer. Such questions may reflect personal values or judgments and are not based on research evidence.
5. *Can you identify how study variables were defined?* Once a problem has been formulated, variables must be defined operationally. Look to see if the study explains how variables are measured, including the instruments and/or procedures used to obtain those measurements. The operational definitions should be sufficiently detailed so that the procedures can be replicated.

## SUMMARY OF KEY IDEAS

1. The hypothesis is the researcher's prediction about the outcome of a study.
2. Hypotheses provide direction for the researcher's efforts and determine the research method and type of data to be collected.
3. A good hypothesis states clearly and concisely the expected relationship (or difference) between two or more variables in measurable terms.
4. Hypotheses can be classified as (1) simple versus complex, (2) nondirectional versus directional, and (3) statistical versus research.
5. A research question is a clear, concise, interrogative statement that is stated in the present tense and includes one or more variables.
6. Research questions are used when prior knowledge of the phenomenon is limited and the research seeks to identify or describe a phenomenon (exploratory or descriptive studies), or both.
7. A variable is a measurable characteristic that varies in a population.
8. Independent variables, sometimes referred to as experimental or treatment variables, are used to explain or predict a result or outcome. Dependent

variables reflect the effects of or response to the independent variables; dependent variables are sometimes called outcome variables.

## LEARNING ACTIVITIES

1. Identify whether the hypotheses listed here are simple or complex, directional or nondirectional, or statistical (null) or research (alternative).

    a. There is a relationship between self-efficacy and uncertainty among patients with sickle-cell disease.

    b. With the use of an imagery protocol for asthmatic children, lower levels of dyspnea and use of fewer pharmacological agents are reported as compared with asthmatic children who do not receive imagery protocol.

    c. Cancer patients receiving chemotherapy who are enrolled in the nursing telephone intervention group have higher hope scores as compared with cancer patients in the control group who receive the standard nursing care.

    d. There is no difference in attitude among junior and senior baccalaureate nursing students toward caring for patients with AIDS.

    e. High levels of perceived stress are significantly related to elevated blood glucose levels in elderly people with type 2 diabetes.

2. Identify the independent and dependent variables in each of the following hypotheses:

   a. Children with cancer who have a high sense of humor have greater immune function and less incidence of infections as compared with children with a low sense of humor.

   b. Attitude and perceived control significantly predict the intention of newly diagnosed patients with type 1 diabetes to enroll in a diabetes education program.

   c. Spinal cord–injured patients treated on the Kinetic Treatment Table have a decreased length of stay in the neurointensive-care unit as compared with spinal cord–injured patients who are immobilized on the Stryker Frame/Wedge turning device.

   d. There is a difference in the intensity, quality, and location of chest pain in patients who have had internal mammary artery grafting following coronary artery bypass surgery as compared with patients who have had only saphenous vein grafting.

   e. There is a relationship between various health-related, physiological, and balloon-related factors and the development of lower-limb ischemia in patients treated with the intraaortic balloon pump.

3. Read the article cited as the source of Excerpt 6.8. Within the limits of the information provided in the article, describe how the terms "stress" and "social support" were operationally defined.

## References

1. Polit, DF, Beck, CT, and Hungler, BP: Essentials of Nursing Research: Methods, Appraisal, and Utilization, ed 5. Lippincott Williams & Wilkins, Philadelphia, 2001, pp 95–117.
2. Burns, N, and Grove, SK: The Practice of Nursing Research: Conduct, Critique, and Utilization, ed 4. WB Saunders, Philadelphia, 2001, p 171.
3. Langford, RW: Navigating the Maze of Nursing Research. Mosby, St. Louis, 2001, pp 92–135.

# 7

# Selecting the Sample and Setting

James A. Fain, PhD, RN, BC-ADM, FAAN

## LEARNING OBJECTIVES

*At the end of this chapter, you will be able to:*
1. Define a sample and a population.
2. List the characteristics, uses, and limitations of each kind of probability and nonprobability sampling.
3. Distinguish between random selection and random assignment.
4. Discuss the importance of a representative sample.
5. Define external validity.

## GLOSSARY OF KEY TERMS

**Accessible population.** Population that is readily available to the researcher and that represents the target population as closely as possible.

**Cluster sampling.** Type of sampling in which the researcher selects groups of subjects rather than individual subjects; also called multistage sampling.

**Convenience sampling.** Type of nonprobability sampling in which the researcher selects subjects or elements readily available; also called accidental sampling.

**External validity.** Extent to which results of a study can be generalized from the study sample to other populations and settings.

**Network sampling.** Type of nonprobability sampling that takes advantage of social networks.

**Nonprobability sampling.** Type of sampling in which the sample is not selected using random selection.

**Population.** Entire set of subjects, objects, events, or elements being studied; also called the target population.

**Probability sampling.** Type of sampling in which every subject, object, or element in the population has an equal chance or probability of being chosen.

**Purposive sampling.** Type of nonprobability sampling in which the researcher selects only subjects that satisfy prespecified characteristics; also called judgmental or theoretical sampling.

**Quota sampling.** Type of nonprobability sampling in which quotas are filled.

**Random assignment.** Allocation of subjects to either an experimental or a control group.

**Random selection.** Type of selection in which each subject has an equal, independent chance of being selected.

**Sample.** A subset of a population.

**Sampling.** The process of selecting a subset from a larger population.

**Sampling frame.** A list of all elements in a population.

**Simple random sampling.** Method of selecting subjects for a sample, in which every subject has an equal chance of being chosen.

**Snowball sampling.** Type of nonprobability sampling that relies on subjects identifying other subjects with similar characteristics.

**Stratified random sampling.** Type of random sampling in which the population is divided into subpopulations, or strata, on the basis of one or more variables, and a simple random sample is drawn from each stratum.

**Systematic sampling.** Type of sampling in which every $k^{th}$ (where "k" is some convenient number) member of the population is selected into the sample.

**Target population.** Population for which study outcomes are intended. Although the intended (target) population is usually evident, having access to members of this population (accessible) can be difficult.

The purpose of selecting a sample is to gain information from a small group so that findings can be generalized to a larger group. Because generalizations concerning a population are based on characteristics of a sample, the sample must represent the larger population. Matching sampling techniques to the purpose and design of the study determines the meaningfulness of study findings. A clear rationale for sampling techniques helps to ensure correct selection of subjects. This chapter focuses on basic concepts of sampling as they relate to research design, type of sampling, and sample size.

## SAMPLING CONCEPTS

### Sample and Population

Regardless of the technique used in selecting a sample, the first step is to define the population. A **population** is an entire set of subjects, objects, events, or elements being studied.[1,2] It is a well-defined group whose members possess specific attributes. Populations may consist of individuals or elements, such as medical records, patient falls, diagnoses, episodes of care, or any other units of interest. For example, researchers may be interested in describing the characteristics of private versus public institutions in different geographic locations. Type of institution and geographic areas would be the units that define this population.

Because it is not feasible to study everybody in a particular population, a small subset of the population, called a **sample,** is selected.[1,2] When the sample represents the total population, the researcher may conclude that the study results can be generalized to include the entire population and settings being studied.

The population for a study is often called the **target population** (i.e., the entire set of elements about which the researcher would like to make generalizations). If a researcher studies people with type 2 diabetes, the target population is all people with type 2 diabetes. Finding and contacting all people with type 2 diabetes is impossible. Instead, researchers will identify some portions of the target population that have a chance of being selected. The sample will come from an **accessible population** that is readily available to the researcher and that represents the target population as closely as possible. Perhaps the researcher has access to a large academic health science center, several community hospitals, or home care services, all of which provide care for people with type 2 diabetes. Individuals with type 2 diabetes from any or all of these institutions constitute an accessible population.

## Sampling

**Sampling** is the process of selecting individuals for a study in such a way that individuals represent the larger group from which they were selected. As mentioned earlier, it is not possible to examine each and every element in a population. When sampling is conducted properly, it allows the researcher to draw inferences and make generalizations about the population without examining every element in the population. Sampling procedures ensure that the characteristics of the phenomena of interest will be, or are likely to be, present in all of the units being studied. With a representative sample, researchers are in a stronger position to draw conclusions from the sample findings that are generalizable to the population.

### Types of Sampling

Sampling is classified under two major categories: probability sampling and nonprobability sampling.[1,2] Table 7.1 identifies the most common types of probability and nonprobability sampling. **Probability sampling** occurs when every subject, object, or element in the population has an equal chance, or probability, of being chosen. In **nonprobability sampling,** the sample is not selected randomly. The probability of inclusion and the extent to which the sample represents the population are unknown. Probability and nonprobability sampling strive to represent the population under study, but they employ different methods.

---

TABLE 7.1 TYPES OF SAMPLES

---

**Probability Sampling**
- Simple random sample
- Stratified random sample
  Proportional
  Disproportional
- Cluster (multistage) sample
- Systematic sample

**Nonprobability Sampling**
- Convenience (accidental)
  Snowball
  Network
- Quota sample
- Purposive sample

---

Both types of sampling have advantages and disadvantages. In probability sampling, the researcher chooses a random sample considered to be representative of the population from which it is drawn. In nonprobability sampling, the researcher has no way of estimating the probability of each subject's being included in the sample.

There is a misconception about probability versus nonprobability sampling. The assertion that probability sampling is preferred over nonprobability sampling is incorrect. Such a statement can lead to conceptual errors in planning a study. The critical issue in defining a population is the ability to generalize from sample findings back to the population from which the sample was drawn. Probability and nonprobability methods of sampling are both appropriate, based on how the problem is conceptualized and according to the method used to achieve representation.

## PROBABILITY SAMPLING

### Simple Random Sample

In **simple random sampling,** every subject has an equal and independent chance of being chosen. Selection of one individual in no way affects selection of another. Random samples are only *considered* to represent the target population; however, it is possible that they do not do so. No sampling technique guarantees a representative sample.

Excerpt 7.1 illustrates simple random sampling. Notice that "simple" does not occur in the excerpt. The authors state that a sample of 40 patients experiencing supraventricular tachycardia were randomly selected from a list obtained from the medical records department. Whenever researchers use the phrase "randomly selected," the samples being described are simple random samples.

True random sampling involves defining the population and identifying a sampling frame. A **sampling frame** is a list of all subjects, objects, events, or units

---

EXCERPT 7.1

## EXAMPLE OF SIMPLE RANDOM SAMPLING

### Sample

The target sample included patients aged 20 to 80 years experiencing CABG for the first time. Patients with current valve replacements or valve repairs were not included. A sample of 40 patients experiencing SVT and 40 patients not experiencing SVT was randomly selected from a list obtained from the medical records department with use of the International Classification of Disease code to identify patients undergoing CABG for the first time during the calendar year 1991. The obtained list was not in any systematic chronologic or alphabetic order.

*Source: Nally, BR, et al: Supraventricular tachycardia after coronary artery bypass grafting surgery and fluid and electrolyte variables. Heart Lung 25:31, 1996, with permission.*

in the population. After the sampling frame has been identified, there are several ways to conduct random selection. One method is to write each individual's name, or other elements of the population, on separate pieces of paper, put the names into a container, shake the contents, and blindly select names until the desired number of individuals is chosen. This procedure is not always satisfactory or possible. A more appropriate method is to use a table of random numbers, which can be generated by a computer; it contains thousands of digits with no systematic order or relationship. Tables of random numbers, also located in the appendix of most statistics books, usually consist of three or five digits. An example of a five-digit table of random numbers appears as Table 7.2. To select a random sample using a table of random numbers, follow these steps:

1. Identify the population.
2. Determine the desired sample size.
3. List all members of the accessible population.
4. Assign all individuals on the list a consecutive number from one up to the required number.
5. Select an arbitrary number in the table of random numbers (just close your eyes and point to one). From that number, read consecutive numbers in some direction (horizontally, vertically).
6. If you chose a table of random numbers with five digits and your population has 800 members, you need to use only the first three digits of the number. If your population has 75 members, you need to use only the first two digits.
7. If the number chosen corresponds to that assigned to any of the individuals in the population, then that individual is in the sample. For example, if a population had 800 members and the number selected was 375, the individual assigned number 375 would be in the sample. If the population had only 300 members, however, in this case individual number 375 would be ignored.
8. Go to the next number in the column and repeat step 7. Continue this process until the desired number of individuals have been selected for the sample.

Simple random sampling is time-consuming. It may also be impossible to obtain an accurate or complete listing (sampling frame) of every element in the accessible population. When random selection is performed appropriately, sample representation in relation to the population is maximized.

## Random Selection Versus Random Assignment

**Random selection** is often confused with random assignment. Random selection—the equal, independent chance of being selected—refers to how individuals may be chosen to participate in a study. Random selection is not a prerequisite for random assignment. **Random assignment** is the random allocation of subjects to either an experimental or a control group. Random assignment is often used to provide at least some degree of randomness when random selection is impossible. Figure 7.1

TABLE 7.2 TABLE OF RANDOM NUMBERS

| 23795 | 97005 | 43923 | 81292 | 39907 | 67758 | 10202 |
| 57096 | 70158 | 36006 | 25106 | 92601 | 54650 | 27591 |
| 52750 | 69765 | 42110 | 38252 | 80201 | 21099 | 70577 |
| 90591 | 58216 | 04931 | 78274 | 10943 | 27273 | 28333 |
| 20809 | 23068 | 84638 | 99566 | 41598 | 25664 | 02400 |
| 57292 | 76721 | 75277 | 37751 | 79009 | 75957 | 22333 |
| 02266 | 97120 | 05055 | 34236 | 42475 | 80604 | 02227 |
| 61795 | 15534 | \ 45465 | 68798 | 02943 | 90934 | 63729 |
| 18021 | 45643 | 82756 | 50833 | 16365 | 87969 | 78079 |
| 52404 | 24573 | 72667 | 17693 | 04332 | 43579 | 24459 |
| 53104 | 80180 | 30612 | 24735 | 63414 | 67892 | 37053 |
| 78245 | 43321 | 64458 | 95647 | 57757 | 82849 | 15238 |
| 96198 | 06398 | 76790 | 63703 | 85749 | 07026 | 46901 |
| 64823 | 65665 | 43284 | 84972 | 92214 | 97669 | 62556 |
| 65083 | 67708 | 58513 | 18046 | 88476 | 13211 | 11675 |
| 30047 | 05312 | 47866 | 90067 | 41508 | 44709 | 70493 |
| 27052 | 80915 | 10914 | 62544 | 01246 | 59280 | 95348 |
| 84438 | 29174 | 15154 | 97010 | 53558 | 58741 | 53713 |
| 09083 | 21005 | 15203 | 76311 | 39195 | 62019 | 29929 |
| 96548 | 06390 | 56577 | 99863 | 58951 | 08673 | 26284 |
| 68927 | 37828 | 17069 | 73928 | 26582 | 08496 | 19678 |
| 07519 | 29067 | 53047 | 49285 | 05174 | 86393 | 19820 |
| 15246 | 16092 | 88491 | 46453 | 01504 | 61322 | 55766 |
| 97306 | 47296 | 94565 | 29597 | 34592 | 67680 | 33930 |
| 72590 | 71948 | 34123 | 04318 | 55899 | 96852 | 90471 |
| 89228 | 75728 | 32272 | 24197 | 71581 | 14731 | 42090 |
| 35188 | 64410 | 86923 | 25630 | 91336 | 05930 | 16148 |
| 79344 | 21677 | 43388 | 36013 | 37128 | 48252 | 36783 |
| 92450 | 37916 | 46903 | 53061 | 38117 | 65493 | 06579 |
| 42567 | 05694 | 82727 | 39689 | 77779 | 53564 | 49126 |
| 88541 | 53575 | 41679 | 00275 | 42844 | 21185 | 56025 |
| 48490 | 44531 | 58369 | 05146 | 29999 | 49853 | 70192 |
| 48498 | 60958 | 77913 | 74738 | 27821 | 56080 | 46295 |
| 66570 | 93573 | 73521 | 99191 | 90791 | 94440 | 83853 |
| 14134 | 59770 | 58818 | 47782 | 14536 | 08728 | 26317 |

illustrates random selection and random assignment. After researchers choose a target population, the sample is selected to participate.

## Stratified Random Sampling

**Stratified random sampling** is the process of selecting a sample to identify subgroups in the population that are represented in the sample. This process reduces the possibility that the sample might be unrepresentative of the population. Stratified random sampling achieves a greater degree of representativeness with each subgroup, or stratum, of the population. An example of a stratified random

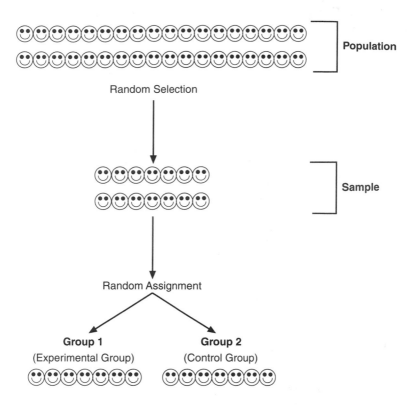

FIGURE 7.1 Random selection versus random assignment.

sample is seen in Excerpt 7.2. A sampling frame was obtained of 462 female employees in clerical and lower administrative positions at a large public university in southern Brazil. Using stratified random sampling, 60 women were selected. In particular, proportional stratification was used to represent accurately the three clerical categories (strata) of administrative technicians, typists, and clerical staff. Disproportional stratified sampling is sometimes useful if comparisons among strata are needed and strata are very different sizes.

Another example of stratification is seen in Excerpt 7.3. In this study, using purposive nonprobability sampling of 25 Polish immigrants, the sample was stratified according to three historically distinct waves of Polish immigration, yielding three subgroups (strata): post–World War II; mid- to late-1970s; and 1980 to 1988. Regardless of the type of sampling reported (purposive, more commonly seen with qualitative approaches to research), stratification was appropriate to ensure adequate representation. Populations can also be stratified according to age, gender, ethnicity, socioeconomic status, diagnosis, type of care, type of institution, geographical location, and so on.

**EXCERPT 7.2**

## EXAMPLE OF PROPORTIONAL STRATIFIED SAMPLING

**Sample**

This study was part of a larger international research project which incorporated both qualitative and quantitative data analysis in the study design. As a result, the sampling strategy was primarily a function of the quantitative analysis. From a master computer list of the 462 female employees in clerical and lower administrative positions at a large public university in southern Brazil, a stratified random sample of 60 women was obtained. The process of proportional stratification ensured a sample representation of each of the three clerical categories of administrative technician (53%), typist (26%), and clerical staff (21%).

*Source: Meleis, AI, et al: Women's work environment and health: Clerical workers in Brazil. Res Nurs Health 19:53, 1996, with permission.*

## Cluster Sampling

In **cluster sampling** (multistage sampling), groups, not individuals, are randomly selected. Cluster sampling is used for convenience when the population is very large or spread over a wide geographic area. Sometimes it may be the only feasible method of selecting an adequately large sample. Selection of individuals from within clusters may be performed by random or stratified random sampling. However, it may be impossible to obtain a complete list of all members of the population (sampling frame) to perform a true random selection.

An example of cluster sampling is displayed in Excerpt 7.4. Los Angeles and North Carolina were the identified clusters, representing sites of the Epidemiologic Catchment Area (ECA) study. The ECA was a five-site program initiated by the

**EXCERPT 7.3**

## STRATIFICATION: PURPOSIVE SAMPLE (NONPROBABILITY SAMPLING)

**Sample**

A purposive sample of 25 Polish immigrants, who resided in the Seattle area and had been in the United States ranging from 4 months to 39 years, was obtained for this study. Purposive sampling involved stratifying waves of Polish migration (Szulc, 1988), yielding three comparison groups of subsamples. Breakdown of the sample by wave of migration was as follows: subsample 1 (post–World War II era) (n = 6), subsample 2 (mid- to late-1970s) (n = 5), and subsample 3 (1980 to 1988) (n = 14). The mean length of time in the USA in years was 30.83 (range: 23 to 29), 14.20 (range: 8 to 22), 3.86 (range: 0.4 to 7) for subsamples 1, 2, and 3, respectively. The sample included 15 males and 10 females and the mean age was 43.92 (range: 26 to 77).

*Source: Aronia, KJ: A model of psychological adaptation to migration and resettlement. Nurs Res 39:5, 1990, with permission.*

**EXCERPT 7.4**

## EXAMPLE OF CLUSTER (MULTISTAGE) SAMPLING

**Sample**

Respondents were selected using multistage area probability sampling from household residents 18 years of age and older at each site. The Los Angeles sample was selected to represent adults in two mental health catchment areas in Los Angeles County, one of which was 83% Latino and the other, 21% Latino. The Latino residents were largely of Mexican cultural or ethnic origin. The interview was translated into Spanish (Karo, Burnman, Escobar, Hough, & Eaton, 1983), and the Spanish version validated before use with ECA respondents (Burnam, Karo, Hough, Escobar, & Forsythe, 1983). The North Carolina sample was selected to represent adults in two mental health areas in North Carolina, one consisting of Durham County, which is primarily urban, and the other of four contiguous rural counties.

*Source: Golding, JM: Sexual assault history and limitations in physical functioning in two general population samples. Res Nurs Health 19:33, 1996, with permission.*

National Institute of Mental Health, whose primary goals were to estimate the prevalence of specific psychiatric disorders and examine patterns of health and mental health services. Respondents at the Los Angeles and North Carolina sites were selected using multistage probability sampling and were asked questions regarding lifetime sexual assault and current physical functioning.

### Systematic Sampling

In **systematic sampling,** individuals or elements of the population are selected from a list by taking every $k^{th}$ individual. The "k," which refers to a sampling interval, depends on the size of the list and desired sample size. Systematic sampling is not strictly probability sampling, but pragmatically it may be just as good. A major difference between systematic sampling and other types of sampling is the fact that all members of the population do not have an independent chance of being selected for the sample. After the first individual is selected, the rest of the individuals to be included are automatically determined. For example, to select 250 patients from a population list of 1000 patients, you might divide 1000 by 250 to determine the size of the sampling interval. If $k = 4$, selection involves taking every fourth name. Even though selection is not independent, some researchers consider systematic sampling a type of probability sampling if the population list is randomly ordered. A major advantage of systematic sampling is that data are collected more conveniently and efficiently.

Excerpt 7.5 illustrates the use of systematic sampling without the researchers specifying a sampling interval. Between 1984 and 1986, 4000 mothers of toddlers who were born full-term and who were delivered vaginally or by cesarean section (sampling frame) were identified. To select 146 mothers from the list of 4000, every 27th subject was selected.

EXCERPT 7.5

## EXAMPLE OF SYSTEMATIC SAMPLING

**Sample**

Mothers of toddlers were defined as the biological mothers of children between 12 months and 36 months of postnatal age, inclusive. Full-terms were defined as infants born at greater than 36 weeks gestation and who weighed greater than 2500 grams at birth. The full-term population consisted of 4000 mothers of toddlers born at a large northeastern metropolitan hospital between 1984 and 1986, who were full-terms delivered vaginally or by C-section, and products of single births with no congenital anomalies. Systematic random sampling of hospital chart codes was used to identify a target population of 146 mothers to contact for participation. The preterm population consisted of 116 mothers of preterm infants born at the same hospital during the same time period, who had birth weights less than 2500 grams, were less than 36 weeks gestation at birth, and who were products of a single birth with no known congenital anomalies.

*Source: Gross, D, et al: Maternal confidence during toddlerhood: Comparing preterm and fullterm groups. Res Nurs Health 12:1, 1989, with permission.*

## NONPROBABILITY SAMPLING

In nonprobability sampling, chance plays no role in determination of the sample. In many studies, the researcher does not begin with a sampling frame in which each member has an independent chance of being included. Many nursing research studies use nonprobability sampling because of the difficulties in obtaining random access to populations. Although these samples are more feasible for the researcher to obtain, the ability to make generalizations about the findings is in jeopardy. The sample chosen may not represent the larger population.

### Convenience Sampling

**Convenience sampling,** sometimes called accidental or nonrandom sampling, is the collection of data from subjects or objects readily available or easily accessible to the researcher. This type of sample does not use random selection. Sample subjects are not selected from a larger group of subjects (population). Instead, the researcher collects data from whomever is available and meets the study criteria. The advantage of using a convenience sample is the ease in carrying out the research and savings in time and money. The disadvantages are the potential for sampling bias, the use of a sample that may not represent the population, and limited ability for results to be generalized. Excerpts 7.6 and 7.7 illustrate the use of the terms "convenience" and "nonrandom" sampling. In Excerpt 7.6, a convenience sample was used within a longitudinal research design. Assessment of mood state was completed on hospital admission, every 2 weeks until antepartum hospital discharge or delivery, and every 2 through 6 weeks postpartum.

EXCERPT 7.6

## EXAMPLE OF CONVENIENCE SAMPLING

The purpose of this study was to describe dysphoria, a composite of symptoms of negative affect for women admitted to the hospital on antepartum bed rest.

**Methods**

The convenience sample for this longitudinal repeated measures study consisted of 63 pregnant women admitted to the hospital on antepartum bed rest. Women were admited to one of three university-affiliated hospitals with tertiary obstetric services located in two cities in the Midwest. After study approval by the Institutional Review Boards, informed consent was obtained for all subjects by the research staff. Data collection took place in one of four sites: in one of three hospital inpatient units or subjects' home after hospital discharge. Data was collected on all subjects upon hospital admission through 6 weeks postpartum.

*Source: Maloni, JA, et al: Dysphoria among high-risk pregnant hospitalized women on bed rest. Nurs Res 51:92, 2002, with permission.*

**Snowball sampling** is a useful technique in situations where one cannot get a list of individuals who share a particular characteristic. It is useful for studies in which the criteria for inclusion specify a certain trait that is ordinarily difficult to find. Snowball sampling relies on previously identified members of a group to identify other members of a population. As newly identified members name others, the sample "snowballs." This technique is used when limiting a population is not possible. Excerpt 7.8 illustrates a combination of convenience and snowball sampling. Women who were at least 18 years of age and who experienced fatigue as they carried out daily activities at home, school, or work were asked to serve as informants to help identify other women who experienced similar fatigue. The researcher had no listing of women who shared similar experiences of fatigue. As one woman was identified, she gave the names of others to contact.

EXCERPT 7.7

## USE OF THE PHRASE NONRANDOM SAMPLE

**Sample**

This nonrandom sample consisted of 85 spouses of patients awaiting HT at three sites: Loyola University of Chicago Medical Center (LUMC), Hines Veterans Affairs Hospital (HVAH), and the University of Alabama Birmingham Medical Center (UABMC). LUMC and HVAH are adjacent medical centers and had a combined HT program. UABMC was chosen because LUMC and UABMC were collaborating already on an ongoing National Institutes of Health grant.

*Source: Collins, EG, et al: Spouse stressors while awaiting heart transplantation. Heart Lung 25:4, 1996, with permission.*

### EXCERPT 7.8

## CONVENIENCE AND SNOWBALL SAMPLING

**Sample and Setting**

The study was conducted in a rural setting in the Pacific Northwest area of the United States, with a convenience sample of generally healthy, nonpregnancy, premenopausal women who were at least 18 years of age. Regular participation in daily activites at school, work, or home was the first component of the operational definition of "generally healthy." The second component was normal (±5%) results on laboratory tests that included a complete blood count (CBC), nonfasting blood sugar, blood urea nitrogen (BUN), serum creatinine, and serum iron. All study participants were premenopausal, as indicated by an established pattern of regular menstrual periods. Forty women participated in the study. Sample size was chosen in anticipation of a large effect size with alpha set at .05. The researchers used "snowball" techniques to recruit women for the study. The process began with women known to the investigators and was extended as participants introduced other women to the investigators for participation.

*Source: Dzurec, LC, et al: Acknowledging unexplained fatigue of tired women. J Nurs Schol 34:41, 2001, with permission.*

Network sampling is another useful technique in situations where there are limited formal lists or ways of reaching potential subjects. Network sampling procedures also take advantage of social networks and the fact that friends tend to have characteristics in common. When the researcher has found a few subjects with the needed criteria, these individuals are asked to help the researcher get in touch with others having similar characteristics. Obvious biases with network sampling exist because subjects are not independent of each other and because they volunteer to participate. Excerpt 7.9 illustrates use of convenience and network sampling. Elderly parents and adult children caregivers were recruited through network sampling procedures. Networking with other elders and their adult children caregivers was employed to identify other potential elders and caregivers for the sample. Excerpt 7.10 demonstrates the use of a networked sample in the context of a qualitative study. Nurses volunteered to participate in a study to discuss the knowledge and expertise inexperienced nurses need to help patients and families through the process of making decisions about consent for a do-not-resuscitate status. Some nurses participated after hearing about the study through colleagues (network sampling).

### Quota Sampling

Quota sampling is similar to stratified random sampling. A quota sample identifies the strata of the population based on specific characteristics. Quota sampling differs from stratified random sampling in that subjects are not randomly selected for each stratum. The quota is computed proportionally or disproportionally to the popula-

EXCERPT 7.9

## CONVENIENCE AND NETWORKING SAMPLING

The purpose of the study was to explore factors that affect health and social service use among elderly Russian immigrants from the perspectives of the elders, their adult caregiving children, and the health and social service professionals who serve them.

**Sample**

The sample for this study included 17 elderly immigrants from the former Soviet Union, 8 adult children who were caregivers for elderly parents, and 15 health professionals who served this immigrant group. Elders and adult children were recruited from the primary author's larger study on immigrant adjustment or through network sampling procedures. Providers were identified by key informants and were recruited to include various disciplines and practice areas.

*Source: Aroian, KJ, et al: Health and social service utilization among elderly immigrants from the former Soviet Union. J Nurs Schol 33:265, 2001, with permission.*

tion under study. Once the quota for each stratum is determined, subjects are solicited via convenience sampling. Researchers who want to sample proportionally need to know the specific composition of the population. Disproportional quota sampling occurs when the number of elements in each stratum is not proportional to the number in the target population. Excerpt 7.11 illustrates an example of quota sampling that was used to ensure equal numbers of families expecting a first baby and families expecting a second baby. In this investigation, researchers filled their quota of families expecting a first baby from one site (e.g., public health prenatal clinic) and moved on to another site to find additional subjects (e.g., community Lamaze classes). This process was followed for families expecting a second baby.

EXCERPT 7.10

## NETWORKED SAMPLE: QUALITATIVE STUDY

**Sample**

To be included in the study, nurses practiced in their present setting for at least one year and had multiple self-reported experiences with patients and families signing DNR consents. Volunteer participants were obtained through local chapters of professional organizations (Oncology Nurses Society and American Association of Critical Care Nurses) and by a networked sample. I addressed the local chapters of these organizations to explain the study and the nurses' role in the study if they chose to participate. Eleven critical care nurses and 10 oncology nurses volunteered to participate. The remainder of participants volunteered after hearing about the study through colleagues.

*Source: Jezewski, MA: Obtaining consent for do-not-resuscitate status: Advice from experienced nurses. Nurs Outlook 44:114, 1996.*

EXCERPT 7.11

## EXAMPLE OF QUOTA SAMPLING

**Sample**

Subjects were 160 women (and their partners when available) selected by a quota sampling technique. This was to ensure equal numbers of families expecting a first baby and families expecting a second baby. Both the woman and her partner were interviewed in 65 of the 160 families. A family was defined as a psychosocial unit composed of two or more adults who have a commitment to each other and who live together. Subjects were drawn from a county public health prenatal clinic (n = 96) and Lamaze classes (n = 64) in a community in the southeastern United States. Families were included in the study if the woman was (1) in the third trimester of pregnancy; (2) anticipating a normal infant; (3) having her first or second child; and (4) living in a family that included at least one other adult (partner, parent, friend, or relative).

*Source: Tomlinson, B, et al: Family dynamics during pregnancy. J Adv Nurs 15:683, 1990.*

## Purposive Sampling

**Purposive sampling,** also known as judgmental or theoretical sampling, is commonly used in qualitative research. It is a type of nonprobability sampling in which the researcher "hand-picks" or selects certain cases to be in the study. Those chosen are thought to best represent the phenomenon being studied and to be typical of the population. In purposive sampling, the researcher makes a judgment regarding the type of subjects needed to provide the most useful information.

An advantage of purposive sampling is its allowance for the researcher to hand-pick the sample, based on his or her knowledge of the phenomenon under study. However, as with any nonprobability sample, sampling bias remains a constant threat. Excerpt 7.12 illustrates purposive sampling and how important it was to sample the lives of women who were directly at risk for AIDS. Study findings were aimed at developing a curriculum for women's AIDS education programs and at providing a foundation for future research projects on women and AIDS.

## ADEQUACY OF THE SAMPLE

### Sample Size

The most frequently asked question by researchers is "How many subjects do I need?" or "How large a sample should I be worrying about?" The answer is usually, "Large enough!" Although this is not a good answer, there are no hard and fast rules about sample size. In qualitative studies, the purpose is to explore meanings and phenomena; an adequate sample size in these types of studies is one that is large enough to accomplish this goal. Excerpt 7.3 illustrates a qualitative approach to

EXCERPT 7.12

## EXAMPLE OF PURPOSIVE SAMPLING

**Subjects and Site**

Subjects or their significant others were clients of an outpatient methadone treatment program for opiate addicts in a medium-sized northeastern city where a majority of reported AIDS cases are associated with injection drug use and where a quarter of the cases are women. Subjects had either used illegal injection drugs themselves, or were the sexual partner of men who did.

Purposive sampling was used to capture the richness of a wide range of perspectives. Subjects were selected on the basis of race or ethnicity, personal history of drug abuse and treatment, and personal experience with AIDS. All subjects spoke English and were approached individually by the researcher. Informed consent was obtained verbally and each participant was given a copy of the consent form.

*Source: Williams, AB: Women at risk: An AIDS educational needs assessment. Image J Nurs Schol 23:208, 1991, with permission.*

research by using an example of grounded theory methodology (see Chapter 14). In this study, the researcher investigated the implications of migration on emotional status over time among 25 Polish immigrants. The sample was stratified according to the three distinct waves of immigration described earlier. In another study (see Excerpt 7.12), 21 women were interviewed who were at risk for AIDS because of injection drug use or because they were heterosexual partners of injection drug users. In both examples, the exact number of subjects was not determined in advance. The researchers continued sampling subjects until the phenomenon under study was clear.

In quantitative studies, sample size is linked to data collection and the type of analysis. Unfortunately, there is a tendency to believe that results from studies with large sample sizes are more valid than studies with smaller sample sizes. Although this is not true, researchers need to consider the following criteria when evaluating the adequacy of the sample: purpose of the study, research design, sampling method, and data analysis. It is also possible to calculate an exact number of subjects needed by using a statistical procedure called power analysis. A discussion of power analysis is too complicated to be included in this book. Refer to Burns and Grove,[1] Polit, Beck, and Hungler[2], or Cohen[3] for specific information on power analysis formulas and tables.

Two critical questions for determining adequacy of a sample include:

1. How representative is the sample relative to the target population?
2. To whom does the researcher wish to generalize the results of the study?

The object of sampling is to have a sample as representative as possible with as little sampling error as possible. Every study will contain some error; results will never be 100-percent representative of the population. Samples that are biased or too small, however, threaten the external validity of the design.

## External Validity

**External validity** is the extent to which study results can be generalized from the study sample to other subjects, populations, measuring instruments, and settings. Researchers need to assess how well the sample they studied represents the larger population to which results are to be generalized. Threats to the ability to generalize findings (external validity), in terms of study design, are discussed in the following sections.

### Interaction of Selection and Treatment

For subjects who are sampled and selected according to specific characteristics (e.g., diagnosis, age range, race, socioeconomic status), those characteristics define the target population. When samples are confined to certain types of subjects, it is not reasonable to generalize results to those who do not have these characteristics. In addition, selecting subjects who are willing to participate in a study can be difficult and time-consuming. If a large number of subjects approached to participate in a study decline to participate, the sample selected tends to be limited in ways that might not be evident at first glance. The number of subjects who were invited to participate and refused should be reported in order to ascertain threats to external validity.

### Interaction of Setting and Treatment

Bias exists when members of different settings agree to participate in studies. For example, if a researcher demonstrates a relationship between the use of an exercise program and functional improvement using patients in a rehabilitation hospital, can these results be generalized to nursing homes? These two types of institutions (rehabilitation hospital and nursing home) may be different in important ways, leading to an interaction of setting and treatment that limits generalizability. This question can be answered only by replicating effects in different settings.

### Interaction of History and Treatment

This threat to external validity concerns the ability to generalize results to different periods in the past or future. For example, researchers examining the results of nutritional studies on reducing cholesterol in the diet would find results today that differ from those obtained 20 years ago. The effects of diet and exercise on cardiovascular fitness were less well known then, as was society's role in promoting health and fitness. This type of generalization is supported when results are replicated in future studies and when previous research corroborates an established relationship. In critiquing a study, researchers need to consider the period of history during which the study was conducted and the effect of the reported findings on nursing practice and societal events during that time.

## QUESTIONS TO CONSIDER WHEN CRITIQUING THE SAMPLE AND SETTING

Identify a research study to critique. Read the study to see if you recognize any key terms discussed in this chapter. Remember that all studies may not contain all key terms. The following questions[2,4] serve as a guide in critiquing sampling plans:

1. *Can you identify the sample? Were terms like "target" and "accessible populations" used? Can you determine what the population was?* Because populations tend to be inferred rather than directly stated, determining the population to whom results are generalized may be a bit more difficult.
2. *Can you determine whether a probability or nonprobability sampling technique was used?* Look for key words such as "random" for probability samples and "convenience" for nonprobability. If the technique is not specified, chances are great that the sampling technique is nonprobability.
3. *Could you determine any inclusion criteria for study participation?* This is usually discussed under the Methods/Sample section of a research report. In some instances, you might read about reasons why subjects were excluded from the study.
4. *Could you identify the sample size? Was the sample size adequate enough to yield a representative sample?* This may be difficult to answer based on information presented in this chapter. Refer to texts in the reference list for a more detailed discussion of techniques for weighing results to get a better reflection of the population whose characteristics one is trying to estimate. A more appropriate question is around the idea of response rate or impact of refusals.
5. *Can you tell the response rate associated with returned questionnaires or surveys and/or what percentage of participants elected not to participate in the study and for what reasons?* Response rates are reported as a percentage of returned questionnaires/surveys. However, it is not clear what conclusions one can legitimately draw if the response rate is 30 percent.
6. *Was the setting described?* There should be an adequate description of the setting in which data were gathered, particularly when aspects of the environment may have been crucial to the study. For example, in nonexperimental research designs, lack of environmental control may be viewed as an uncontrolled extraneous variable. For these reasons, possible ways in which the setting may have influenced the results should be considered.

## SUMMARY OF KEY IDEAS

1. Sampling is the process of selecting elements or individuals for a study so as to represent the larger group from which the sample group is selected.
2. There are two major types of sampling procedures: probability and nonprobability.

3. Probability samples (every member of a population has an equal chance of being chosen) are representative samples. Types of probability sampling include simple random, stratified random, cluster, and systematic.

4. Nonprobability samples (members of a population do not have an equal chance of being chosen) are not representative. Types of nonprobability sampling include convenience (snowball and networking), quota, and purposive.

5. Sampling methods must be evaluated to determine if the sample represents the population.

6. Probability and nonprobability sampling are rendered appropriate based on how the study is conceptualized, along with the method used to achieve representation.

7. Sample size, regardless of the type of sampling, affects generalizability.

8. External validity is the extent to which results of a study can be generalized from the study sample to other populations and settings.

9. Power analysis is a statistical method of calculating a needed sample size.

## LEARNING ACTIVITIES

1. In each of the studies listed, (1) identify the sample and sample selection procedure used and (2) indicate whether the sample and sample selection procedures are described adequately.

   a. Allen, JK: Coronary risk factor modification in women after coronary artery bypass surgery. Nurs Res 45:260, 1996.

   b. Hughes, LC, et al: Describing an episode of home nursing care for elderly postsurgical cancer patients. Nurs Res 51:110, 2002.

   c. Bolton, LB, et al: A response to California's mandated nursing ratios. Image J Nurs Schol 33:179, 2001.

d. Gaberson, KB: The effect of humorous and musical distraction on preoperative anxiety. AORN J 62:784, 1995.

e. Peden, AR, et al: Reducing negative thinking and depressive symptoms in college women. Image J Nurs Schol 32:145, 2000.

f. Knobf, MT: Carrying on: The experience of premature menopause in women with early-stage breast cancer. Nurs Res 51:9, 2002.

## References

1. Burns, N, and Grove, SK: The Practice of Nursing Research: Conduct, Critique, and Utilization, ed 4. WB Saunders, Philadelphia, 2001, pp 365–384.
2. Polit, DF, Beck, CT, and Hungler, BP: Essentials of Nursing Research: Methods, Appraisal, and Utilization, ed 5. Philadelphia, Lippincott Williams & Wilkins, 2001, pp 231–256.
3. Cohen, J: Statistical Power Analysis for the Behavioral Sciences, ed 2. Academic Press, Hillsdale, NJ, 1988.
4. Langford, RW: Navigating the Maze of Nursing Research. St. Louis, Mosby, 2001, p 121.

# Principles of Measurement

James A. Fain, PhD, RN, BC-ADM, FAAN

## LEARNING OBJECTIVES

*At the end of this chapter, you will be able to:*
1. Compare and contrast the four types of scales of measurement.
2. Discuss the issue of reliability and distinguish among the various types.
3. Discuss the issue of validity and distinguish among the various types.
4. Discuss the relationship between reliability and validity.

## GLOSSARY OF KEY TERMS

**Continuous variable.** Variable that takes on an infinite number of different values presented on a continuum.

**Cronbach's alpha (coefficient alpha).** Widely used index of the extent to which a measuring instrument is internally stable.

**Dichotomous variable.** A nominal variable that consists of two categories.

**Instrument.** A device, piece of equipment, or paper-and-pencil test that measures a concept or variable of interest.

**Interval level of measurement.** Level of measurement characterized by a constant unit of measurement or equal distances between points on a scale.

**Measurement.** The assignment of numerical values to concepts, according to well-defined rules.

**Nominal level of measurement.** Lowest level of measurement, which consists of assigning numbers as labels for categories. These numbers have no numerical interpretation.

**Operational definition.** A definition that assigns meaning to a variable and the terms or procedures by which the variable is to be measured.

**Ordinal level of measurement.** Level of measurement that yields rank-ordered data.

**Psychometric evaluation.** Evaluating properties of reliability and validity in relation to instruments being used to measure a particular concept or construct.

**Ratio level of measurement.** Highest level of measurement, characterized by equal distances between scores having an absolute zero point.

**Reliability.** Value that refers to the consistency with which an instrument or test measures a particular concept. Different ways of assessing reliability include test-retest, internal consistency, and interrater.

**Validity.** Value that refers to the accurac with which an instrument or test measures what it is supposed to measure. Different types of validity include content, criterion, and construct.

In order to make sense out of data collected, each variable must be defined operationally using a variety of measurement techniques. The specific technique chosen depends on the particular research question and the availability of instruments. One measurement technique is not necessarily better than another. Depending on how each variable is measured, different kinds of data are produced, which represent different scales or levels of measurement. Each level of measurement is classified in relation to certain characteristics. In addition, whether a researcher is testing hypotheses or answering research questions, some characteristics of the instrument are important in terms of determining the accuracy and meaning of results. Two major characteristics that are essential to the meaning and accuracy produced by an instrument are reliability and validity. This chapter focuses on the four levels of measurement and examines the issues of reliability and validity.

## MEASUREMENT

**Measurement** is the systemic assignment of numerical values to concepts to reflect properties of those concepts.[1] Whether the data are collected through observation, self-report, or some other method, the researcher must specify under what conditions and according to what criteria the numerical values are to be assigned. Researchers establish the level of measurement for variables under study and decide which statistical analyses are appropriate. The four levels of measurement, in order of increasing sophistication, are nominal, ordinal, interval, and ratio.

### Nominal

**Nominal level of measurement** represents the lowest level of measurement; numbers classify subjects or objects into two or more categories. Questions of "more" or "less" have no meaning in nominal measurement; data simply show the frequency of subjects or objects in each category.

Many variables in nursing research are measured on a nominal scale. Expressions commonly used to denote this level of measurement include nominal scale, nominal data, nominal measurement, and categorical data. Common examples of nominal data include gender (1 for males, 2 for females) and religion (1 for Catholic, 2 for Protestant, and 3 for Jewish). In each case, subjects are put into categories. No one category has "more" gender or "less" religion. The category names are simply labels, arranged in random order, without disturbing their meaning.

Numbers are assigned as category names when entering data into a computer. However, these numbers do not represent amounts. Numbers in nominal measurement cannot be manipulated mathematically; the results mean nothing. For example, a person's blood type can be entered into the computer by assigning 1 for type AB, 2 for type A, 3 for type B, and 4 for type O. The numbers have no numerical importance other than to serve as labels for each category. A label of "average blood type," for example, has absolutely no meaning.

Excerpt 8.1 illustrates seven different variables (age, gender, race, marital status, education, employment status, and household income). Each variable is defined as a characteristic that can be measured quantitatively using numbers. An important question in any study is how the variables are measured and defined. When nominal data have just two categories, as in the variable of gender (male or female), they are termed **dichotomous variables.**

## Ordinal

**Ordinal level of measurement** specifies the order of items being measured, without specifying how far apart they are. Ordinal scales classify categories incrementally and rank-order the specific characteristics of each category. Rank-ordered data are measured on an ordinal scale and rank subjects from highest to lowest and from most to least. For example, a researcher interested in patient satisfaction may classify 20 subjects as "1" (very satisfied); another 15 as "2" (somewhat satisfied), and another 25 as "3" (not satisfied). Although ordinal scales show which subjects reported a higher level of patient satisfaction, they do not indicate *how* much higher. In other words, intervals between ranks are not equal; the difference between "very satisfied" and "somewhat satisfied" is not measurably the same as between "somewhat satisfied" and "not satisfied." Expressions commonly used to denote this level of measurement include ordinal scale, ordinal data, ordinal variables, and ordinal measurement.

Ordinal data are common in nursing research. Many instruments and scales used to measure psychosocial variables yield ordinal data. Although an ordinal scale results in more precise measurement than a nominal scale, it still does not allow the precision usually warranted in a research study. In addition, ordinal scales do not lend themselves well to other statistical analyses. Knapp[2,3] provides an overview of the ongoing debate among researchers regarding the use of ordinal and interval scales.

In Excerpt 8.1, education and household income are measured and operationally defined by the research on an ordinal scale. An **operational definition** assigns meaning to a variable and the terms or procedures by which it is to be measured. In this example, numbers are assigned to each category and arranged in a natural order (e.g., lowest to highest). Like nominal data, ordinal data are not manipulated mathematically. Ordinal data are simply ranks, specifying which term was first, second, third, and so forth. The variable household income is defined as 1 = $0 to $4999, 2 = $5000 to $9999, 3 = $10,000 to $19,999, 4 = $20,000 to $29,999, and 5 = $30,000 to $49,999.

## Interval

**Interval level of measurement** possesses all characteristics of a nominal and ordinal scale, in addition to having an equal interval size based on an actual unit of measurement. Many instruments and scales used in nursing research report "scores" and are usually referred to as interval data or interval variables. When scores have equal intervals, the difference between a score of 20 to 30 is essentially the same as a score of 100 to 110. Because the difference between intervals is the same, it is meaningful to add and subtract these numbers and to compute averages.

**EXCERPT 8.1**

## ILLUSTRATION OF NOMINAL, ORDINAL, AND INTERVAL/RATIO VARIABLES

**Demographics of the Pretest Sample**

| | |
|---|---|
| Age, y | |
| Mean | 51 |
| Range | 25–77 |
| Gender | |
| Female | 73% |
| Male | 27% |
| Race | |
| African-American | 100% |
| Marital Status | |
| Single, living alone | 9% |
| Single, with children | 13% |
| Married | 12% |
| Widowed | 17% |
| Divorced | 4% |
| Other | 4% |
| Education, y | |
| ≤6 | 24% |
| 8 | 10% |
| 11–12 | 52% |
| 13–16 | 14% |
| Employment Status | |
| Employed, full-time | 43% |
| Employed, part-time | 18% |
| Unemployed | 13% |
| Disabled | 4% |
| Retired | 18% |
| Other | 4% |
| Household Income | |
| $0–$4999 | 40% |
| $5000–$9999 | 20% |
| $10,000–$19,999 | 40% |
| $20,000–$29,999 | 5% |
| $30,000–$49,999 | 5% |

Source: Anderson, W, et al: Culturally competent dietary education for Southern rural African Americans with diabetes. Diabetes Educ 28:245, 2002, with permission.

Interval scales, however, do not have a true zero point. Temperature is a good example of an interval scale in that a temperature of zero changes, depending on whether the researcher uses a Fahrenheit (F) or Celsius (C) scale. It makes no sense to say that a temperature of 10°F is twice as hot as a temperature of 5°F. Likewise, a temperature of zero is not absolute. Days that are 0°F do not have an absence of temperature.

Many highly reliable psychosocial instruments or scales yield interval data. There are, however, many nurse researchers who interpret ordinal data as if they were interval data and have even shown empirically that it matters little if an ordinal scale is treated as an interval scale. Knapp[2,3] attempts to resolve the controversy by insisting that researchers look to an instrument's "appropriateness" and "meaningfulness." That is, what descriptive statistics are appropriate for ordinal and interval scales? What meaning does a score associated with each scale have? Does the raw score on a given scale resemble an actual unit of measurement? Does the scale have a true zero point?

## Ratio

**Ratio level of measurement** is the highest level of measurement. The categories in ratio scales are different, ordered, and separated by a constant unit of measurement; ratio scales also have an absolute zero point. A zero point indicates absolutely none of the property. Temperature on the Fahrenheit scale is not a ratio measurement because a temperature of 0°F does not represent absolutely no heat. Ratio data can be manipulated using any arithmetic operation. Ratio levels of measurement include time, weight, and length. From a statistical standpoint, interval and ratio measurements are treated the same. More advanced statistical analyses are used to analyze data collected on an interval and ratio scale. The result of having an increased number of options for data analysis is that the description of what has actually happened in the study is more precise.

Age and education (years) in Excerpt 8.1 were defined operationally by researchers on an interval/ratio scale. Calculating a mean and standard deviation is appropriate for both these variables. Both variables are defined as continuous. A **continuous variable** is one that takes on an infinite number of different values presented on a continuum.

## Errors Associated with Measurement

Whenever data are collected, some amount of error is encountered. Researchers attempt to reduce error so data provide a more accurate reflection of the truth. Measurement error refers to how well or how poorly a particular instrument performs in a given population. No instrument is perfect. For a more thorough discussion of measurement error, refer to Burns and Grove.[4]

## Measurement Scales

In defining or quantifying concepts or variables within a study, a researcher may use various types of instruments to obtain a score. An **instrument** is a device, piece of equipment, or paper-and-pencil test that measures a concept or variable of interest. Many instruments used in nursing include questionnaires, surveys, and rating scales. (see Chapter 9). Psychosocial measures are by far the most commonly used data collection methods in nursing research. Some instruments make sense, whereas others may be difficult to follow, irrelevant, or poorly developed. The most important issues to consider when examining the worth of any instrument used to measure variables in a study are reliability and validity.

## RELIABILITY

**Reliability** refers to the consistency with which an instrument or test measures whatever it is supposed to measure.[1,4] The more reliable a test or instrument, the more a researcher can rely on the scores obtained to be essentially the same scores that would be obtained if the test were readministered. Reliability can be conceptualized by researchers in three ways.[5] In some studies, researchers ask, "To what extent does a subject's measured performance remain consistent across repeated testings?" In other studies, the question of interest takes a slightly different form: "To what extent do individual items that go together to make up an instrument or test consistently measure the same underlying characteristic?" In still other studies, the concern over reliability is expressed in the question, "How much consistency exists among the ratings provided by a group of raters?" Despite the differences among these three questions, the notion of consistency is central.

Reliability is expressed as a reliability coefficient (r). A high reliability coefficient indicates high reliability. Reliability coefficients range from 0.00 to 1.00: a completely reliable test has a reliability coefficient of 1.00, and a completely unreliable test has a reliability coefficient of 0.00.

Reliability testing focuses on three aspects: stability, equivalence, and homogeneity. Within each of these areas, several different types of reliability exist, each dealing with a different kind of consistency. Test-retest reliability (stability), internal consistency (homogeneity), and interrater reliability (equivalence) are measures of reliability and are determined by use of correlations.

### Test-Retest Reliability

Stability is concerned with the consistency of repeated measurements. This is usually called test-retest reliability or coefficient of stability. It is the extent to which scores are consistent over time. It indicates a score variation that occurs from time 1 to time 2. In many studies, a researcher measures a group of subjects twice with the same measuring instrument or test, the two testings being separated by a time interval. A concern with this type of reliability is how to determine the amount of time that should elapse between the two testings. Knapp and Brown[6] argue that there is no methodological justification for greater than a 2-week time interval. However, the time interval may actually be as brief as 1 day or as long as 1 year. Test-retest reliabilities are generally higher when the time lapse between the testing is short, usually no longer than 4 weeks. If the interval is too short, however, mem-

---

EXCERPT 8.2

## REPORTING TEST-RETEST RELIABILITIES

Independent categories, physical dimension, and overall (total) scores are expressed in percentages, with higher scores indicating greater functional difficulties. Test-retest reliability coefficients across categories ranged from 0.80 to 0.88, and internal consistency levels (Cronbach's alpha) for the total score were 0.97 and 0.94 in 1976 field trials, respectively.

*Source: Leidy, NL: Functional performance in people with chronic obstructive pulmonary disease. Image J Nurs Schol 27:23, 1995, with permission.*

---

ory of the responses given during the first session may influence responses during the second session.

In Excerpt 8.2, the researcher reports test-retest reliability coefficients, ranging from $r = 0.80$ to 0.88. However, the researcher does not mention the time interval associated with retesting. Caution is advised when reading research reports, regarding how stable the measurement is when researchers do not indicate the length of time between the two testings. In Excerpt 8.3, note how the authors report the coefficient of stability (test-retest reliability) at 2 weeks and 1 month (0.87 and 0.81, respectively).

### Internal Consistency Reliability

Researchers sometimes assess the extent to which a measuring instrument possesses internal consistency. From this perspective, reliability is defined as consistency

---

EXCERPT 8.3

## REPORTING TEST-RETEST RELIABILITY WITH TIME INTERVAL

**Measurement**

The QOL Index (Ferrans & Powers, 1985) was developed to measure the quality of life as perceived by healthy or ill individuals. It consists of 64 items that are rated by using a 6-point Likert-type scale. A total score as well as subscale scores are derived from the instrument. The possible range for each subscale and for overall scores is 0 to 30 (Ferrans, 1990; Ferrans & Powers, 1985; Ferrans & Powers, 1992; Mellors, Riley, & Erlen, 1997; Oleson, 1990). The subscales measure the perception of the individual's health and functioning, socioeconomic, psychological/spiritual, and family-related QOL. Test-retest correlations were performed at 2 weeks and 1 month and were adequate (0.87 and 0.81 respectively). Internal consistency reliability was established through Cronbach's alpha calculations at 0.95 for the total instrument, 0.90 for the health and functioning scale, 0.84 for the socioeconomic scale, 0.93 for the psychological/spiritual scale, and 0.66 for the family scale (Ferrans & Powers, 1985).

*Source: Gerstle, D, et al: Quality of life and chronic nonmalignant pain. Pain Management Nurs 2:98, 2001, with permission.*

across items of an instrument, with individual items being individual questions. To the extent that certain items "hang together" and measure the same thing, an instrument is said to possess high internal consistency reliability.

To assess internal consistency, a researcher administers a measuring instrument to a group of individuals. After all responses are scored, one of several statistical procedures is applied. The procedure examines the extent to which all the items in the instrument measure the same concept. One of the more popular statistical procedures used to assess internal consistency is **Cronbach's alpha (coefficient alpha).** This statistical procedure is more versatile than others because it can be used with instruments composed of items that can be scored with three or more possible values. An example is a Likert-type scale (see Chapter 9) in which the response option for each statement is scored from 1 (strongly agree) to 5 (strongly disagree). Another statistical procedure used to assess internal consistency is called Kuder-Richardson #20, or simply KR-20. This procedure is used when the items of an instrument are scored dichotomously (e.g., 1 = yes and 0 = no; or 1 = true and 0 = false).

Use of assessing internal consistencies by Cronbach's alpha is illustrated in Excerpt 8.3, in which the researcher reports the range of internal consistency reliabilities for three subscales associated with the Quality of Life (QOL) Index: 0.90 for the health and functioning scale, 0.84 for the socioeconomic scale, and 0.66 for the family scale. An acceptable level of reliability is an alpha coefficient of 0.80 for a well-developed psychosocial measurement instrument. For newly developed instruments, an alpha coefficient of 0.70 is considered acceptable.[4] Excerpt 8.4 illustrates an example of a researcher reporting the results of KR-20. Subjects responded either "yes" or "no" to the 10-item Family Stressors Index (FSI). A moderate reliability coefficient ($r = 0.64$) was reported.

The reliability of instruments can be affected by several factors, including the characteristics of the sample, the number of items or questions, how closely connected the items or questions are, and the response format. Researchers who develop instruments need to understand that these areas potentially affect the reliability of instruments. Gable and Wolf[7] provide a more thorough discussion of developing an instrument and issues of reliability.

### Interrater Reliability

In some studies, researchers collect data by having raters evaluate a particular situation. To quantify the amount of consistency among raters, the researcher computes an index of interrater reliability. One popular statistical procedure that quantifies the degree of consistency among raters is called Cohen's kappa. This statistical procedure is used with nominal data and is designed for situations in which raters classify the items being rated according to discrete categories. If all raters agree that a particular item belongs in a given category and there is total agreement for all items being evaluated, then Cohen's kappa assumes the value of +1.0. To the extent that raters disagree, Cohen's kappa value becomes smaller. Knapp and Brown[6] report that Cohen's kappa statistic of 0.75 or greater indicates good agreement.

**EXCERPT 8.4**

## USE OF KUDER-RICHARDSON 20 RELIABILITY

Family life changes and transitions were measured with the Family Stressors Index (FSI). The FSI, a 10-item self-report instrument that records developmental and situational changes experienced by the families in the past year, is designed for use with families across the life span. Items have a dichotomous yes or no response scale. The reliability coefficient (Kuder-Richardson 20) for the total study sample was 0.64. Both respondents were asked to complete the instrument, and any item to which either person responded positively was scored 1, based on the assumption that family members might report different life events because of differences in each person's experience.

*Source: Fink, SV: The influence of family resources and family demands on the strains and well-being of caregiving families. Nurs Res 44:139, 1995, with permission.*

Determining interrater reliability is very common in nursing research and is used in many observational studies. Interrater reliability values should be reported in any study in which observational data are collected or when judgments are made by two or more data collectors. In Excerpt 8.5, several researchers judged patient adjustment by using the Global Adjustment to Illness Scale. The interrater reliability coefficient was 0.44, indicating only a moderate amount of agreement. The use of Cohen's kappa to assess interrater reliability is shown in Excerpt 8.6. In this study, interrater reliability was established between a researcher and another individual trained in scoring the Behavior Test of Interpersonal Skills (BTIS). The BTIS measured nurse-expressed empathy and consisted of 13 situations involving nurse-patient interactions. These situations had been role-played and videotaped. Subjects (patients) in the study viewed the recorded situations and responded verbally. High interrater reliabilities were reported between the researcher and the individual who scored the BTIS ($r = 0.90$ to $1.00$).

## VALIDITY

**Validity** is the accuracy with which an instrument or test measures what it is supposed to measure.[1,4] The researcher should not consider whether a test is valid or invalid. Instead, the researcher should ask, "Is it valid for what and for whom?" For example, an anatomy and physiology test is probably not a valid statistics test. An anatomy and physiology test does not measure any aspects of statistics, regardless of how reliable the test might be. With respect to "for whom," a test in anatomy and physiology would be a valid measure for use by college students but not for students in grade school.

An instrument may have excellent reliability even though it may not measure what it claims to measure. However, an instrument's data must be reliable if they are to be valid. Thus, high reliability is a necessary, though insufficient, condition for high validity. Because different instruments and tests are designed for a variety of

**EXCERPT 8.5**

## REPORTING INTERRATER RELIABILITIES

Following completion of the interview, the interviewer judged patient adjustment using the Global Adjustment to Illness Scale (GAIS) (Derogatis, 1975), an observational measure of adjustment designed to identify patients' feelings of distress about their current medical condition. Scale values range from 1 to 100 in 10 deciles, with the top decile representing very good adjustment and the bottom decile representing extremely poor adjustment. In four studies examining interrater reliability and validity of brief interview-rated methods of psychosocial adjustment, Morrow et al (1981) reported that the GAIS most accurately reflected clinical impressions by a majority of professional raters. Interrater reliability coefficients reported for experienced interviewers was 0.44, and evidence of construct validity was provided for the four studies with measures such as The Rating of Psychosocial Functioning ($r = 0.68$–$0.80$). Nurse interviewers collected demographic and illness data from the patient record.

*Source: Houdin, AD, Jocobsen, B, and Lowery, BJ: Self-blame and adjustment to breast cancer. Onc Nurs Forum 23:75, 1996, with permission.*

purposes, different types of validity include content validity, criterion-related validity, and construct validity.

### Content Validity

Content validity is the extent to which an instrument or test measures an intended content area. Usually this type of validity is used in the development of a questionnaire, interview schedule, interview guide, or instrument. The instrument is constructed using concepts from the literature to reflect the range of dimensions of the

**EXCERPT 8.6**

## USE OF COHEN'S KAPPA STATISTIC

Regarding reliability, the non-reactivity of the Empathy categories was demonstrated when no significant differences resulted between subjects' initial scores and scores 6 and 16 weeks later (Gerrard, 1992). There were high positive correlations ($r = .80$) between the Empathy categories. Before the study, interrater reliability was established. Kappa statistic based on a comparison between initial scoring and rescoring 1 week later ranged from 0.93 to $+1.00$ and from 0.90 to $+1.00$ for interrater reliability between the researcher and another individual experienced in scoring the BTIS. Content validity was established with input from health professionals (Gerrard & Buzzell, 1980) and through comparison of the content of actual nurse-patient interactions with BTIS situations (Olson, Iwasiw, & Gerrard, 1991).

*Source: Olson, JK: Relationship between nurse-expressed empathy, patient-perceived empathy and patient distress. Image J Nurs Schol 27:317, 1995, with permission.*

variable being measured. Content validity is then determined by a panel of experts. Experts carefully evaluate all items or questions used by the instrument as well as the instrument's overall appropriateness for use in a proposed study population. Excerpt 8.7 contains the typical sentence in most journal articles, indicating that a panel of experts was chosen to evaluate content validity. In this excerpt, individuals were chosen to establish content validity of the advance directive attitude survey. Excerpt 8.8 provides a more detailed discussion of how (use of literature and members of the Chemical Dependency Issues Task Force) and who (individuals with expertise in substance abuse research, recovering nurses) established content validity.

## Criterion-Related Validity

Criterion-related validity is a measure of how well an instrument measuring a particular concept compares with a criterion, providing more quantitative evidence on the accuracy of the instrument. In some instances, a newer instrument is compared with an older, more reputable, instrument. A correlation coefficient is calculated for each set of scores. The two scores are calculated, with the resulting $r$ being referred to as the validity coefficient. A high validity coefficient indicates high criterion-related validity. In addition, an instrument may be selected for comparison that is expected to measure an attribute or concept that is opposite to the dimension of interest. Criterion-related validity can be divided into two types: concurrent and predictive.

### Concurrent

When a new instrument is administered at about the same time that data are collected on the criterion, concurrent validity is being assessed. A concern with

---

**EXCERPT 8.7**

## CONTENT VALIDITY

**Instrument**

The instrument used to collect data was an adapted version of Nolan and Bruder's (1997) advance directive attitude survey (ADAS). The ADAS was developed in 1996 to measure patients' attitudes toward advance directives on two medical units in a tertiary care teaching hospital. The tool is a 16-item, 4-point Likert scale designed to determine the extent to which advance directives are viewed as positive or negative; respondents answer from 1 (strongly disagree) to 4 (strongly agree). Higher scores indicate more favorable attitudes toward advance directives. The original tool included items about (a) opportunity for treatment choices, (b) effect of advance directives on the family, (c) effect of an advance directive on treatment, and (d) perception of illness. Content validity was established using a panel of experts. Cronbach's alpha for the instrument was 0.74.

*Source: Douglas, R, and Brown, HN: Patient's attitudes toward advance directives. Image J Nurs Schol 34:61, 2002, with permission.*

**EXCERPT 8.8**

## CONTENT VALIDITY

**Measures**

The instruments used in this study were: (a) Demographic and Licensure Information (DLI), administered at Time 1; (b) Lifetime Substance Abuse (LSA), administered at Time 1; (c) Employment History (EH), administered at Time 3; (d) Maintenance of Abstinence (MA), administered monthly; and (e) Current Work Description (CWD), administered at Times 2 and 6. Evidence in support of content validity of all questionnaires was established based on a literature review, review by the National Council of State Boards of Nursing (NCSBN's) Chemical Dependency Issues Task Force, and by experts in substance abuse research. In addition, content validity was established by pilot testing the instruments on 10 recovering nurses.

*Source: Haack, MR, and Yocum, CJ: State policies and nurses with substance use disorders. Image: J Nurs Schol 34:89, 2002, with permission.*

concurrent validity involves comparing the results obtained from one sample with the results of some criterion measured from a different sample. For example, an instrument measuring stress that has been validated in a healthy normal population will not necessarily provide valid results when used to measure stress in hospitalized patients. Excerpt 8.9 illustrates the use of concurrent validity. In this example, concurrent validity was assessed with nine measures of well-being and self-esteem. Validity coefficients were not reported for the nine well-being measures, and a low-to-moderate validity coefficient was associated with self-esteem ($r = 0.54$).

### Predictive

Predictive validity is the ability to predict future events, behaviors, or outcomes. A classic example of predictive validity is the use of Graduate Record Examination (GRE) scores to admit students to graduate school. Many graduate schools require a combined (verbal and quantitative) minimum score of 1000 in the hope that students who achieve that score will have a higher probability of succeeding in graduate school. This topic has been the subject of many research studies in which the questions are asked, "Are GREs a valid measure, and if so, valid for what and for whom?"

## Construct Validity

Construct validity is the extent to which an instrument measures an intended hypothetical concept or construct. The process of validating a construct is by no means easy. Construct validity is the most valuable, yet the most difficult, way to assess an instrument's validity. Researchers take years to provide evidence of construct validity. To establish the amount of construct validity, researchers can perform a number

## USE OF CONCURRENT VALIDITY

Well-being was measured with the Satisfaction with Life Scale (SWLS) (Diener, Emmons, Larsen, & Griffin, 1985) and Purpose in Life Test (PLT) (Crumbaugh & Maholick, 1964). SWLS is a 5-item unidimensional scale that measures subjective global life satisfaction as a cognitive-judgmental process with a 7-point response format ranging from strongly agree to strongly disagree. High scores indicate high satisfaction. Test-retest reliability (0.82), Cronbach's alpha (0.87), concurrent validity with nine measures of well-being, and correlations with self-esteem (0.54) have been reported (Corcoran & Fischer, 1987; Diener et al, 1985). For this sample, the standardized alpha was 0.85 and correlation with self-esteem 0.60.

*Source: Anderson, SE: Personality, appraisal, and adaptational outcomes in HIV seropositive men and women. Res Nurs Health 18:303, 1995, with permission.*

of tasks including hypothesis testing, multitrait-multimethod testing, and factor analysis. Refer to Burns and Grove[4] for a more thorough discussion of construct validity. One of the more popular procedures is to produce correlational evidence showing that the construct has a strong relationship with certain measured variables and a weak relationship with other variables. This type of construct validity is referred to as convergent and discriminant validity.

Excerpt 8.10 provides an example of how construct validity was approached. The researchers want to know if their instrument is measuring sexual health practices (construct validity) or if in fact it is measuring something else. In order to determine this, several measures (i.e., measures of risk-taking, self-expression) are used to evaluate the construct. The researchers then make predictions about the construct in terms of other related constructs.

## CONSTRUCT VALIDITY

### Sexual Health Practices

Sexual health practices included safe sex behaviors and the new construct, SHRB, as well as rates of sexually transmited infections (STI) testing and treatment among the respondents. Safe sex behaviors were measured by responese to the Safe Sex Behavior Questionnaire (SSBQ), a self-report instrument containing 27 items within a 4-point Likert response format. Evidence of construct validity was found through significant correlations between the SSBQ and measures of risk-taking and self-expression (Cole & Slocumb, 1995).

*Source: Rew L, Fouladi, RT, and Yockey, RD: Sexual health practices of homeless youth. Image: J Nurs Schol 34:139, 2002, with permission.*

## UNDERSTANDING THE IMPORTANCE OF PSYCHOMETRIC PROPERTIES ASSOCIATED WITH INSTRUMENTATION

Most research studies use some sort of data collection instrument, often a published, standardized instrument with good reliability and validity. A "good" instrument is essential if research results are to be useful. Assessing the quality of an instrument is done by evaluating the properties of reliability and validity in relation to the instrument being used. This process is called **psychometric evaluation.**

The usefulness of data collection instruments depends on the extent to which researchers can rely on data as accurate and meaningful. Developing instruments or modifying existing instruments requires a certain amount of skill and expertise. Developing psychometrically sound instruments is an important, labor-intensive, and time-consuming task. In the initial search for instruments that might measure a particular concept or construct, one is apt to think about developing one's own instrument. The process of tool development is lengthy and requires considerable research sophistication. Using a newly developed instrument in a study without first evaluating properties of reliability and validity is unacceptable and a waste of time. Identifying whether an instrument used in a study has discussed issues of reliability and validity are important from a researcher's point of view.[4]

At the heart of all measurement is reliability. Reliability is the consistency with which an instrument measures what it is supposed to measure.[1,4] If an instrument is not producing high reliability coefficients ($r = 0.70$ or higher), it is serving no research or evaluation function and jeopardizing the meaningfulness of the data. For example, if a research study reported an alpha coefficient (internal consistency) for the Self-Efficacy Scale (SES) of 0.58, there is concern that the SES measure is not a stable one. Acceptable alpha coefficients vary, depending on the situation and the judgment of the researcher, but normally an alpha coefficient below 0.50 represents poor reliability. A moderate alpha coefficient is considered between 0.50 and 0.70.

Remember, validity is the extent to which an instrument measures what it is supposed to measure.[1,4] Although validity is an important characteristic of an instrument, reliability is necessary before validity can be considered. An instrument that is not reliable cannot be valid. However, an instrument can be reliable without being valid. For example, an instrument may consistently measure anxiety each time the instrument is administered. However, if the concept to be measured is depression, the instrument is not considered valid.

Appropriateness relates to the fit of the instrument to the intended subjects in order to produce valid data. Many times researchers will adapt or modify existing instruments that have been developed for other studies with proven reliability and validity with a specific group of subjects. Examine the similarity between subjects in an original study where the development and construction of the instrument began with those subjects in the current study. For example, would an instrument administered to premenopausal women for measuring depression be valid if administered to homeless youth? Other factors such as culture, socioeconomic level, development level, and language must be considered when attempting to administer the same instrument to two different populations. Question the researcher's decision to adapt and/or modify an instrument that has not been tested for reliability and validity with subjects that are different from those involved in the original development of the instrument.

The process of instrument development begins with previous research, which forms the foundation of the new instrument. If there is no relevant previous research, pilot studies are to be conducted to provide a foundation for the content of the newly developed and/or adapted instrument. Pilot studies help to point out flaws or errors in the construction of the instrument, selection of the sample, and data collection procedures. Pilot testing also gives insight into problems that could be encountered in editing and coding data.

## QUESTIONS TO CONSIDER WHEN CRITIQUING LEVELS OF MEASUREMENT AND ISSUES OF RELIABILITY AND VALIDITY

Identify a research study to critique. Read the study to see if you recognize any key terms discussed in this chapter. Remember that all studies serve as a guide in critiquing levels of measurement and issues of reliability and validity.

1. *Did the study address issues of reliability? If so, what methods of estimating reliability were used?* Look for key terms such as "stability" for test-retest reliability, "Cronbach's alpha" for internal consistency, and "kappa statistic" for interrater reliability. In many studies, information on reliability and validity associated with instrumentation will be reported from earlier studies. Identify if reliability coefficients (Cronbach's alpha) are calculated for both the current study and those reported in previous research. Perhaps both reliability coefficients are compared with one another.
2. *Did the study address issues of validity? Was there sufficient information available to appraise the instrument's validity? If so, what methods of estimating validity were used?* Look for key terms such as "content validity," "criterion-related validity," and "construct validity." The validity of an instrument is critical to the success of any research study. Identify the reason a particular instrument was chosen. If a study is designed to examine parenting skills but the instrument measures coping skills, the results of the study are of little value. Try to understand the usefulness of the instrument given the context in which it is applied.
3. *Can you identify the main study variable(s)? How were study variables measured: were nominal, ordinal, and interval/ratio levels of measurement used?* Look to see how each variable was measured. Levels of measurement guide the kind of statistical analyses that can be performed.

## QUESTIONS TO CONSIDER WHEN CRITIQUING INSTRUMENTS

Identify a research study to critique. Read the study to see if you recognize any key terms discussed in this chapter. Remember that all studies may not contain all key terms. The following questions serve as a guide in critiquing instruments.

1. *Does the instrument measure what it claims to measure?* If possible, look over the items in the instrument to see if they make sense. Unfortunately, many research studies will not publish entire instruments. In some instances, a few examples of the items are reported. Look to see if there is mention of where the reader can obtain a copy of the instrument. If the instrument has been adopted from another source, that source should be documented in the reference list. If the instrument is an author-developed instrument, an address may be available at the beginning or end of the research report to indicate where a complete copy can be obtained. All publications related to instrument testing should likewise be referenced. For those instruments that are author-developed with little, if any, information regarding reliability and/or validity, an assessment of the instrument is imperative with respect to validity.

2. *Are there instructions on how to obtain, administer, and score the instrument?* Locating existing instruments is not an easy task. Journal articles sometimes publish a copy of the instrument or examples of items within the instrument. Check the reference list to identify the author of the instrument and some of the early work done on establishing reliability and validity. Many times the author's place of employment, address, and e-mail are listed. The computer database Health Psychological Instruments Online is available and can search for instruments that measure a particular concept or construct or for information on a particular instrument. Very often, little, if any, information is presented with respect to how and under what conditions instruments are to be administered and scored.

3. *Are scoring procedures explained in sufficient detail?* Refer to the methods section (instrumentation) of the article to find information on scoring procedures.

4. *Does the instrument yield a total score, or are there several subscales associated with the instrument?* Refer to the methods section (instrumentation) of the article, and identify if a total score and/or subscales are calculated. In many instances, the sentence, "A total score as well as subscale scores are derived from the instrument" is typical. Note that if such a sentence exists, you should be able to identify the names of the various subscale measures.

5. *Has the instrument been pilot-tested?* Pilot testing identifies and corrects any problems before the actual study is implemented in its final form. Advantages of a pilot test include an opportunity to evaluate the psychometric properties of instruments, practice collecting data, uncover questions and/or instructions that might be ambiguous, assess reliability of subjects, and estimate time associated with data collection. The number of subjects needed for a pilot study varies. If the purpose of the pilot study is to uncover questions and/or instructions that might be ambiguous, 10 to 20 subjects may be sufficient. When the purpose of the pilot test is to evaluate the psychometric properties of an instrument, a much larger sample is necessary. Pilot studies are well worth the time and effort. Problems

associated with administering an instrument are costly when they occur after data collection has begun.

## SUMMARY OF KEY IDEAS

1. Measurement is the systematic assignment of numerical values to concepts or constructs to reflect properties of those concepts or constructs.
2. The four levels of measurement are nominal, ordinal, interval, and ratio.
3. The lowest level of measurement, nominal, classifies subjects or objects according to different categories.
4. Ordinal levels of measurement specify the order of items being measured, without specifying how far apart they are (interval size).
5. Interval levels of measurement possess all characteristics of nominal and ordinal scales, in addition to having an equal interval size based on an actual unit of measurement.
6. Ratio levels of measurement represent the highest level. In ratio scales, the categories are different, ordered, and separated by a constant unit of measurement, and an absolute zero point exists.
7. Reliability is the consistency with which an instrument measures what it is supposed to measure. Different types of reliability include test-retest, internal consistency, and interrater.
8. Validity is the accuracy with which an instrument measures what it is supposed to measure. Different types of validity include content, criterion-related, and construct.
9. Instruments may have good reliability even if the instrument does not measure what it claims to measure.

## LEARNING ACTIVITIES

1. A study was conducted to investigate the effect of dual-earner families on the development of preschool children. Information was collected on the following variables: satisfaction with income (measured as dissatisfied versus satisfied); satisfaction with child care (measured as low, moderate, high); income level (measured as $30,000 to $39,999; $40,000 to $49,999; $50,000 to $59,999; $60,000+); mother's age (measured as mother's actual age); and family stress level (measured as none, very little, moderate, a great deal). Which variable(s) represent(s) an interval/ratio level of measurement?

2. Define the following variables using an ordinal scale of measurement: health status, amount of pain, patient satisfaction, age.

3. Comment on the strength of Cronbach's alpha in the following example:

   Cronbach's alpha was calculated for the Barriers to Cessation Scale in three samples. In study 1 (n = 91), alpha was 0.87; in study 2 (n = 25), alpha was 0.81; and in study 3 (n = 156), alpha was 0.83.

4. What information is missing when evaluating the coefficient of stability in this example?

   State anxiety, the transitory situation-specific response to events, was measured by Spielberger, Gorsuch, Lushene, Vagg, and Jacobs' (1983) 20-item State Anxiety Scale, with items rated from 1 to 4. Internal consistencies ranged from 0.92 to 0.95, with a test-retest reliability of 0.90.

5. What type of validity is discussed in the following sentences?

   Pregnancy risk, intrapartal risk, and infant's health status at birth were measured by revisions of the instruments reported by Hobel, Hyvarinen, Okada, and Oh (1973) and updated to reflect current diagnostic procedures. A panel of perinatal nurse specialists, a pediatrician, and an obstetrician validated the new scale. The pregnancy risk scale has 80 items, the intrapartal risk scale has 45, and the infant's health status at birth has 69.

## References

1. Nunnaly, J, and Bernstein, IH: Psychometric Theory, ed 3. McGraw-Hill, New York, 1994.

2. Knapp, TR: Treating ordinal scales as ordinal scales. Nurs Res 42:184, 1993.

3. Knapp, TR: Treating ordinal scales as interval scales: An attempt to resolve the controversy. Nurs Res 39:121, 1990.

4. Burns, N, and Grove, SK: The Practices of Nursing Research: Conduct, Critique, and Utilization, ed 4. Philadelphia, WB Saunders, 2001, pp 223–241, 389–406, 441–447.

5. Huck, SW, and Cormier, WH: Reading statistics and research. HarperCollins Publishers, New York, 1996.

6. Knapp, TR, and Brown, JK: Ten measurement commandments that often should be broken. Res Nurs Health 18:465, 1995.

7. Gable, RK, and Wolf, MB: Instrument Development in the Affective Domain, ed 2. Kluwer Academic Publishers, Boston, 1993.

# Data Collection Methods

James A. Fain, PhD, RN, BC-ADM, FAAN

## LEARNING OBJECTIVES

*At the end of this chapter, you will be able to:*

1. Identify common instruments and methods used to collect data in quantitative and qualitative research.
2. Distinguish between closed-ended and open-ended questionnaires.
3. List the advantages and disadvantages of using questionnaires.
4. Compare and contrast the different types of scaling techniques.

## GLOSSARY OF KEY TERMS

**Closed-ended questionnaire.** Type of format in which subjects are asked to select an answer from several choices.

**Instrument.** A device, piece of equipment, or paper-and-pencil test that measures a concept or variable of interest.

**Likert scale.** Sometimes referred to as a summative scale. Respondents are asked to respond to a series of statements that reflect agreement or disagreement. Most Likert scales consist of five scale points, designated by the words, "strongly agree," "agree," "undecided," "disagree," and "strongly disagree."

**Open-ended questionnaire.** Type of format in which subjects are asked to provide specific answers.

**Questionnaire.** A structured survey that is self-administered or interviewer-administered.

**Response set bias.** The tendency for subjects to respond to items on a questionnaire in a way that does not reflect the real situation accurately.

**Scale.** A set of numerical values assigned to responses that represent the degree to which respondents possess a particular attitude, value, or characteristic.

**Survey.** A method of collecting data to describe, compare, or explain knowledge, attitudes, or behaviors.

Data collection is a major part of the research process. Methods and instruments for data collection must be chosen according to the nature of the problem, approach to the solution, and variables being studied. Whether the researcher is testing hypotheses or seeking answers to research questions, valid and reliable instruments are essential. The purpose of this chapter is to describe various methods of collecting data for both quantitative and qualitative approaches to research.

## QUALITATIVE VERSUS QUANTITATIVE DATA

Data are divided into two categories, qualitative and quantitative. Qualitative data can be observed, written, taped, or filmed. Data collection methods include unstructured interviews, direct observation, case studies, field notes, diaries, or historical documents. Qualitative data are useful for preliminary investigation of new areas and for understanding the results of quantitative analyses. The advantages are that collecting the data does not require prior knowledge of the subject and individual variation can be recorded in depth.

Quantitative data are numerical. Numerical data can be used directly (e.g., weight in pounds, height in inches, age in years) or to form categories (e.g., male or female) that can be formulated into counts or tables. The advantages are that data can be analyzed without extreme effort, comparisons can be made, and hypotheses can be tested with well-developed statistical techniques. If data are collected in a standardized, unbiased manner, insights and results may apply to other populations. The distinction between qualitative and quantitative data is not always clear. In qualitative data, each category is assigned a code. These codes are easily entered into a computer and analyzed using statistical techniques based on counts (e.g., chi-square analysis).

## QUANTITATIVE DATA COLLECTION METHODS

Quantitative data collection methods include the use of instruments. An **instrument** is a device used to record or gather data on a particular concept.[1] An instrument may be a piece of equipment, structured interview, or paper-and-pencil test. Data-gathering instruments used in research studies include questionnaires, rating scales, checklists, standardized tests, and biophysical measures. Methods for collecting data may be based on a form of self-report that asks individuals to complete a questionnaire, survey, or standardized test.

### Surveys and Questionnaires

Surveys are a popular method for collecting data to describe, compare, or explain knowledge, attitudes, and behavior.[2] A **survey** is a series of questions posed to a group of subjects. **Questionnaires** are structured self-administered surveys. The most common way of distributing questionnaires is through the mail, although many research situations allow for face-to-face administration. Mailed questionnaires are economical and reach a large population in a relatively brief time. One disadvantage of using mailed questionnaires is a low return rate. Responses from 60 percent to 80 percent of a sample are considered excellent. Realistically, researchers can expect return rates from 30 percent to 60 percent for most studies.[3] Excerpt 9.1 illustrates the use of a mailed questionnaire to mothers of toddlers to explore factors indicative of maternal confidence. Note the excellent return rate of questionnaires (i.e., 81 percent to 88 percent) for mothers in both the full-term and preterm populations.

**Closed-ended questionnaires** ask subjects to select an answer from among several choices. This technique is often used in large surveys when questionnaires

EXCERPT 9.1

## USE OF MAILED QUESTIONNAIRE

**Methods**

Descriptive correlational and comparative methods were used to investigate the patterns of substance abuse–impaired nurses. A modified Dillman total design method (1978) was implemented to conduct this mailed survey.

**Participants**

Two groups were samples: substance-impaired nurses who consider themselves in recovery (n = 100) and nonimpaired nurses (n = 100). Research questionnaires were mailed to a convenience sample of impaired and nonimpaired nurses throughout the United States. Those willing to participate were mailed the questionnaire throughout the US Postal Service.

A total of 190 questionnaires were sent to impaired recovering nurses; 102 question-naires were returned for a response rate of 54%. Two incomplete questionnaires were eliminated. A total of 176 questionnaires were mailed to nonimpaired nurses; 108 ques-tionnaires were returned, for a response rate of 61%. Three incomplete questionnaires were eliminated, and five questionnaires were eliminated because nurses responded yes to two or more of the five CAGE questions. The number of usable questionnaires for each group was 100.

*Source: West, MM: Early risk indicators of substance abuse among nurses. Image: J Nurs Schol 34:187, 2002, with permission.*

are mailed to subjects. In addition, this type of questionnaire is easily coded. **Open-ended questionnaires** ask subjects to provide specific answers to questions. Open-ended questionnaires are less frequently found in research studies, particularly when quantitative methods for data analysis are planned. The researcher has less control over subjects' answers because there are no fixed choices provided for each ques-tion. An example illustrating the difference between open-ended and closed-ended questions is shown in Table 9.1.

### Developing a Questionnaire

Designing good questions that are easy to answer, while focusing on the issues and information to be collected, is essential to developing a questionnaire. An example of a questionnaire is illustrated in Figure 9.1. The following are guidelines to consider when designing questions:

1. Ask questions that are specific rather than general.[2,4] For example, if you want to know the level of patient satisfaction, the question "Are you satisfied or dissatisfied with the care you received?" is too general and might elicit opinions about other aspects of patient satisfaction. The question, "How would you rate your level of satisfaction regarding being able to have input into your treatment preferences—excellent, very good, good, fair, or poor?" reflects an answer about respect for values, expressed needs, and input into treatment preferences.

## TABLE 9.1 EXAMPLE OF OPEN-ENDED AND CLOSED-ENDED QUESTIONS

**Open-Ended Question**

Describe some reasons to wear a seat belt when riding in a car driven by someone else.

**Closed-Ended Question**

1. How often do you wear a seat belt when riding in a car driven by someone else?
   a. Never
   b. Rarely
   c. Sometimes
   d. Most of the time
   e. Always

**Open-Ended Question**

Explain your beliefs about drinking.

**Closed-Ended Question**

1. During the past 30 days, how many times did you drive a car when you had been drinking alcohol?
   a. 0 times
   b. 1 time
   c. 2–3 times
   d. 4–5 times
   e. 6 or more times

---

We are interested in learning more about you. This questionnaire covers a few personal, health, and demographic variables for those in this course. Please answer each question by circling the answer that best describes you. Please return this form to the instructor when requested.

1. What degrees do you currently have?

|      | Yes | No |
|------|-----|-----|
| BS   | 1   | 0   |
| BA   | 1   | 0   |
| MS   | 1   | 0   |
| MSN  | 1   | 0   |
| JD   | 1   | 0   |
| MD   | 1   | 0   |
| PhD  | 1   | 0   |

Other (specify):

2. Have you taken any of the following exams within the last 5 years?

|       | Yes | No |
|-------|-----|-----|
| GRE   | 1   | 0   |
| GMAT  | 1   | 0   |
| MCAT  | 1   | 0   |
| LSAT  | 1   | 0   |
| MAT   | 1   | 0   |

Other (specify):

3. How many semesters of statistics have you taken?
4. Have you ever used a personal computer to analyze data?

   1    Yes
   0    No

FIGURE 9.1 In-class questionnaire.

Now we would like to know something about your personal habits.

5. How often do you drink coffee?

   | | |
   |---|---|
   | 0 | Rarely or never |
   | 1 | Less than 1 cup per month |
   | 2 | 1–3 cups per month |
   | 3 | 1–6 cups per week |
   | 4 | 1–2 cups per day |
   | 5 | 3–4 cups per day |
   | 6 | 5+ cups per day |

6. How many cigarettes do you smoke per day?

   | | |
   |---|---|
   | 0 | None, never smoked |
   | 1 | None now, former smoker |
   | 2 | Half a pack or less (0–10) |
   | 3 | Between $1/2$ and 1 pack (11–20) |
   | 4 | Over 1 pack and up to $1 1/2$ packs (21–30) |
   | 5 | Over $1 1/2$ packs and up to 2 packs (31–40) |
   | 6 | Over 2 packs |

7. If you smoke, at what age did you begin smoking?
   Please answer if you have ever smoked regularly, even if you have quit. Leave it blank if you have never smoked.

8. How often do you participate in some sort of physical exercise or sport?

   | | |
   |---|---|
   | 0 | Rarely or never |
   | 1 | Less than once a month |
   | 2 | 1–3 times per month |
   | 3 | 1–3 times per week |
   | 4 | 4–6 times per week |
   | 5 | Every day |

To help us understand the different groups of people answering these questions, we need to know a little about your background characteristics.

9. How old were you on your last birthday?
10. Which birth order are you? (Give number; e.g., 1 if first, 3 if third, and so on)
11. Gender:
    F Female          M Male
12. How tall are you? _____ feet _____ inches
13. How much do you weigh? _____ lb
14. Are you currently certified in cardiopulmonary resuscitation (CPR) by either the American Heart Association or the American Red Cross?

    | | |
    |---|---|
    | 1 | Yes |
    | 0 | No |

15. Have you ever been told by a doctor that you had any of the following conditions?

    | | Yes | No |
    |---|---|---|
    | Heart disease | 1 | 0 |
    | High blood pressure | 1 | 0 |
    | High cholesterol | 1 | 0 |
    | Emphysema | 1 | 0 |
    | Cancer | 1 | 0 |

16. Compared with other people your age, how would you rate your health?

    | | |
    |---|---|
    | 4 | Excellent |
    | 3 | Good |
    | 2 | Fair |
    | 1 | Poor |

FIGURE 9.1 In-class questionnaire.

2. Use simple language.[2,4] Make sure the style is appropriate to the education and knowledge of respondents. If you want to know how the respondent thinks lung cancer rates are changing, you could ask a layperson, "Do you think lung cancer is increasing, decreasing, or staying the same?" For an epidemiologist, such basic language would make the question hard to answer. In this case, you should specify period of time, morbidity and mortality rates, race, age, and gender. The question, "In the last 5 years, do you think the incidence of respiratory cancer in white males under 65 years of age has increased, decreased, or stayed the same?" assumes a specific respondent.

3. Each question should represent one concept.[2,4] Avoid asking two (or more) questions at the same time. For example, the question "Do you wear seat belts when driving your car?" is really asking several questions: "Can you drive a car?", "Do you own a car?", and "Do you wear seat belts?" If the answer to the original question is "No," it could mean "No, I can't drive or don't have a driver's license" or "Yes, I can drive, but no, I don't wear my seat belt when I drive." The question, "When you are in a car, how often do you fasten the seat belt—always, sometimes, or never?" is appropriate.

4. Delimit any reference to time.[2,4] For example, if you ask "Do you exercise often?" it is not clear what "often" means. A more specific question is, "In the past week, how often did you exercise—once, twice, or three times; more than three times?"

5. Phrase questions in as neutral a way as possible.[2,4] Try not to let content, structure, or wording favor a certain answer. For example, ask "Do you agree or disagree with the following statement" rather than "Don't you think that . . .?" Make sure there are the same number of positive and negative answers, so that respondents will not feel influenced to choose the more heavily weighted point of view.

### Designing Good Answers

Asking good questions also involves specifying good answers. Questions can be designed to elicit three main types of answers: open-ended, categorical, and continuous.

**Open-ended responses.** An open-ended question elicits an answer consisting of a free-form statement or essay in which the respondent chooses what to say. Such answers are useful either in the early stages of drafting questions or at the end of a questionnaire in order to enrich or to help interpret shorter responses. Most open-ended responses are not analyzed by using a computer. If such free-form data are to be analyzed by computers, responses need to be coded after the questionnaires have been returned. Coding responses is a tedious and time-consuming task.

**Categorical responses.** A categorical response is a type of closed answer that respondents are asked to choose from a limited number of alternatives. When writing categorical responses, answer choices should not leave out any of the most important possibilities. To allow for answers that are rare (occurring less than 5 percent of the time) or that the researcher has not considered, a category such as

"Other: Specify:" can be placed at the end of the list. Answers should also be mutually exclusive.

Additionally, categories should not overlap. For example, the question, "How old are you: 18 to 21, 21 to 35, 36 to 65, 65 and over?" has two categories that overlap. In this example, if respondents choose more than one answer, the answers may not be mutually exclusive. It is better for the researcher to think of such a question as a *series* of questions that allow yes/no answers. For example, the question, "Have you had any of the following conditions or illnesses—diabetes, hypertension, high cholesterol, heart attack?" should really be considered as four separate questions.

**Continuous responses.**   Continuous responses can accommodate a large range of values, representing a continuum. Each value can be entered directly and does not need to be coded. Examples include age, weight, height, blood pressure, and so forth. Researchers should specify the unit of measurement used in each value and the level of precision desired (how many decimal places). For example, a study of nutrition in newborns should ask for weight to the nearest half ounce and age to the nearest month. For a similar study among older adults, weight to the nearest pound and age in years at the last birthday are sufficient.

## Ordering the Questions

A questionnaire is a collection of questions in which the whole becomes more than the sum of its parts. In addition to wording each question carefully, it is important to plan the order in which questions are asked. Dillman[3] specifies five principles for ordering questions:

1. Start with the topic that the respondent will consider most useful or important.
2. Group questions that are similar in content. Within content area, group questions of the same type. For example, on a given topic, group questions requiring yes/no answers.
3. Take advantage of relationships among groups of questions to build continuity throughout the questionnaire.
4. Questions about sensitive topics should be placed about two-thirds of the way into the questionnaire. Within a topic area, put the questions that are easier to answer first and those that are likely to be more sensitive or objectionable last.
5. Demographic questions that the respondent might consider boring or personal should be placed at the end of the questionnaire. A respondent might consider demographic questions (e.g., age, sex, marital status, income) intrusive if they are presented at the beginning of a questionnaire. After completing the questionnaire, however, respondents might not consider the demographic questions as offensive.

## Scales

A **scale** is a set of numerical values assigned to responses, representing the degree to which subjects possess a particular attitude, value, or characteristic. The purpose of a scale is to distinguish among people who show different intensities of the entity to be measured. Scales are created so that a score can be obtained from a series of items. Several formats are used in creating scales for rating a set of items. Three common types of scaling techniques include Likert, semantic differential, and visual analogue.

### Likert Scales

**Likert scales,** also called summative scales, require subjects to respond to a series of statements to express a viewpoint. Subjects read each statement and select an appropriately ranked response. Response choices commonly address agreement, evaluation, or frequency. Likert's original scale included five agreement categories: "strongly agree (SA)," "agree (A)," "uncertain (U)," "disagree (D)," and "strongly disagree (SD)." The number of categories in the Likert scale can be modified: it can be extended to seven categories (by adding "somewhat disagree" and "somewhat agree") or reduced to four categories (by eliminating "uncertain").

There is no correct number of response categories. Some researchers believe the "uncertain" option should be omitted to force subjects to make a choice. Other researchers believe subjects who do not have strong feelings should be given an option to express that attitude. When the forced-choice method is used, responses that are left blank are generally interpreted as "uncertain." Frequency categories for Likert scales may include terms such as "rarely," "seldom," "sometimes," "occasionally," and "usually." However, these terms are adaptable and should be selected for their appropriateness to the stem question.[5] Table 9.2 displays several four-, five-, and six-point Likert responses for choices addressing agreement, frequency, and evaluation.

Each choice along the scale is assigned a point value, based on the extent to which the item represents a favorable or unfavorable characteristic. Point values could be SA = 5, A = 4, U = 3, D= 2, SD = 1 or SA = 2, A = 1, U = 0, D = −1, SD = −2. The actual values are unimportant as long as the items are consistently scored and follow scoring guidelines. The use of Likert scales are presented in Excerpt 9.2.

Some items within an instrument may be worded negatively to avoid creating a **response set bias,** the tendency for subjects to respond to items based on irrelevant criteria in a way that inaccurately reflects the situation. Instruments dealing with attitudes about psychological or social issues are particularly vulnerable to response sets. For example, subjects who are asked to agree or disagree with a set of statements may tend to respond in a socially acceptable way (social desirability response set). To avoid the possibility of response set biasing, the researcher may balance the occurrence of positively and negatively worded items on an instrument in order to reduce the tendency for subjects to agree or disagree in a uniform way. A good example is the Personal Resource Questionnaire (PRQ), a two-part measurement of multidimensional characteristics of social support. PRQ-I provides descriptive information about the person's resources and level of satisfaction with these resources. PRQ-II contains 25 items divided into five subscales: intimacy, social integration, nurturance, worth, and assist/guidance. PRQ-II is shown in Table 9.3. The intensity of each item is measured on a seven-point Likert scale, with response

TABLE 9.2 EXAMPLES OF LIKERT RESPONSES

| | | |
|---|---|---|
| Strongly disagree | Strongly disagree | |
| Disagree | Disagree with reservations | |
| Agree | Agree with reservations | |
| Strongly agree | Strongly agree | |
| | | |
| Almost never | Never | Always |
| Occasionally | Rarely | Frequently |
| Usually | Infrequently | Sometimes |
| Almost always | Sometimes | Rarely |
| | Frequently | Never |
| | Often | |
| | | |
| Excellent | Excellent | Excellent |
| Good | Good | Very good |
| Fair | Satisfactory | Good |
| Poor | Unsatisfactory | Fair |
| | Poor | Poor |
| | | |
| Not at all | None | Great deal |
| A little | Very little | Moderate |
| Moderately | Moderately | Somewhat |
| Quite | A great deal | Poor |
| Extremely | | |
| | | |
| Almost none | None | A little |
| Some | A little | Some |
| Most | Some | Moderate amount |
| Almost all | A great deal | Great deal |
| | | |
| Very satisfactory | Very satisfactory | |
| Satisfactory | Somewhat satisfactory | |
| Unsatisfactory | Somewhat unsatisfactory | |
| Very unsatisfactory | Very unsatisfactory | |
| | | |
| Extremely satisfied | | |
| Satisfied | | |
| Dissatisfied | | |
| Extremely dissatisfied | | |

choices ranging from "strongly agree" (7) to "strongly disagree" (1). Items are numbered 1 to 25 and scored in a straightforward manner. Mean scores for each subscale are calculated (sum divided by items in subscale); higher scores indicate greater perceived social support in each of the five dimensions. Items 4, 6, 7, 10, and 24 are worded negatively and must be recoded ($7 = 1$, $6 = 2$, $5 = 3$, $4 = 4$, $3 = 5$, $2 = 6$, $1 = 7$) to reflect the positive direction of the other 20 items. Subscales associated with the PRQ-II are as follows: Intimacy: items 1, 5, 10, 15, 19; Social Integration: items 2, 6, 11, 16, 20; Nurturance: items 7, 12, 17, 21, 23; Worth: items 3, 8, 13, 18, 24; Assistance/Guidance: items 4, 9, 14, 22, 25.

**EXCERPT 9.2**

## USE OF LIKERT SCALES

**Measures**

Everyday stressors were measured with the Everyday Stressors Index, a 20-item tool which assesses common problems experienced on a daily basis by mothers of young children. Areas assessed include financial concerns, role overload, employment problems, parenting worries, and interpersonal conflict. Mothers rather how much each problem worried, upset, or bothered them from day-to-day on a 4-point Likert scale ranging from *not at all bothered* (1) to *bothered a great deal* (4). The ratings are summed for a total score.

Self-esteem was assessed by the Rosenberg Self-Esteem Scale (RS-E), a 10-item measure of global self-esteem. Repondents rated each of the items on a 5-point Likert scale from *strongly disagree* (1) to *strongly agree* (5). A summary score was obtained by reversing the ratings for the five negative items and adding them to the five positive items.

*Source: Lutenbacher, M: Relationship between psychosocial factors and abusive parenting attitudes in low-income single mothers. Nurs Research 51:158, 2002, with permission.*

---

TABLE 9.3 PERSONAL RESOURCE QUESTIONNAIRE (PRQ): PART II

Below are some statements with which some people agree and others disagree. Please read each statement and circle the response most appropriate for you. There is no right or wrong answer.
- 1 = Strongly Disagree
- 2 = Disagree
- 3 = Somewhat Disagree
- 4 = Neutral
- 5 = Somewhat Agree
- 6 = Agree
- 7 = Strongly Agree

**Statements**

1. There is someone I feel close to who makes me feel secure.
   1     2     3     4     5     6     7
2. I belong to a group in which I feel important.
   1     2     3     4     5     6     7
3. People let me know that I do well at my work (job, homemaking).
   1     2     3     4     5     6     7
4. I can't count on my relatives and friends to help me with problems.
   1     2     3     4     5     6     7
5. I have enough contact with the person who makes me feel special.
   1     2     3     4     5     6     7
6. I spend time with others who have the same interests that I have.
   1     2     3     4     5     6     7
7. There is little opportunity in my life to be giving and caring to another person.
   1     2     3     4     5     6     7

## TABLE 9.3 PERSONAL RESOURCE QUESTIONNAIRE (PRQ): PART II

8. Others let me know that they enjoy working with me (job, committees, projects).

   1       2       3       4       5       6       7

9. There are people who are available if I needed help over an extended period.

   1       2       3       4       5       6       7

10. There is no one to talk to about how I am feeling.

   1       2       3       4       5       6       7

11. Among my group of friends we do favors for each other.

   1       2       3       4       5       6       7

12. I have the opportunity to encourage others to develop their interests and skills.

   1       2       3       4       5       6       7

13. My family lets me know that I am important for keeping the family running.

   1       2       3       4       5       6       7

14. I have relatives or friends that will help me out even if I can't pay them back.

   1       2       3       4       5       6       7

15. When I am upset there is someone I can be with who lets me be myself.

   1       2       3       4       5       6       7

16. I feel no one has the same problems as I.

   1       2       3       4       5       6       7

17. I enjoy doing little "extra" things that make another person's life more pleasant.

   1       2       3       4       5       6       7

18. I know others appreciate me as a person.

   1       2       3       4       5       6       7

19. There is someone who loves and cares about me.

   1       2       3       4       5       6       7

20. I have people to share social events and fun activities with.

   1       2       3       4       5       6       7

21. I am responsible for helping provide for another person's needs.

   1       2       3       4       5       6       7

22. If I need advice, there is someone who would assist me to work out a plan for dealing with the situation.

   1       2       3       4       5       6       7

23. I have a sense of being needed by another person.

   1       2       3       4       5       6       7

24. People think that I'm not as good a friend as I should be.

   1       2       3       4       5       6       7

25. If I got sick there is someone to give me advice about caring for myself.

   1       2       3       4       5       6       7

*Source: Brandt, PA, and Weinert, C: The PRQ: A social support measure. Nurs Res 30:277, 1981.*

The Role Questionnaire (RQ) is a 14-item rating scale that has two subscales: role conflict and role ambiguity. Eight items make up the role conflict scale, and six items make up the role ambiguity scale. Excerpt 9.3 discusses how items associated with role ambiguity need to be reverse-scored to reflect the direction of the other eight items. Examples of role ambiguity items include: "I know exactly what is expected of me," "I feel certain about how much authority I have," and "Clear, planned goals exist for my job." By reverse-scoring the six role ambiguity items (e.g., 7 = 1, 6 = 2, 5 = 3, 4 = 4, 3 = 5, 2 = 6, 1 = 7), higher scores would indicate higher levels of role ambiguity. The eight role conflict items are already

**EXCERPT 9.3**

## REVERSE SCORING OF ITEMS IN A QUESTIONNAIRE

### Instrumentation

The Role Questionnaire (RQ) is a 14-item rating scale constructed to assess perceived levels of role conflict and role ambiguity. It was developed by Rizzo, House, and Lirtzman (1970). Each statement is rated on how it applied to you and your present job. Respondents were asked to rate each item on a 7-point Likert scale. A score of 1 indicated that the statement was not true of one's job. As items that measure role ambiguity were worded positively, they had to be scored in a reverse direction. Higher scores were indicative of higher levels of role conflict and role ambiguity. Psychometric testing has been conducted for the RQ.

*Source: Fain, JA: Perceived role conflict, role ambiguity, and job satisfaction among nurse educators. J Nurs Educ 26:233, 1987, with permission.*

worded positively so that higher scores indicate higher levels of role conflict. Examples of role conflict items include: "I have to do things that should be done differently," "I receive an assignment without the proper support," and "I receive incompatible requests from two or more people."

### Semantic Differential Scales

The semantic differential scale is composed of a set of scales, using pairs of adjectives that reflect opposite feelings. The technique was developed by Osgood, Suci, and Tannenbaum[7] to measure attitude, beliefs, or both. Subjects are asked to select one point on the scale that best describes their view of the concept being measured. The scale is different from Likert scales in two ways:

1. Only two extremes are labeled.
2. The continuum is based not on agree/disagree but rather on opposite adjectives that express the respondent's feelings.

The example shown in Figure 9.2 illustrates a seven-point semantic differential scale that explores womens' feelings about the labor and delivery experience in childbirth. The middle section represents a neutral position.

The semantic differential scale is scored by assigning values from 1 to 7 to each of the spaces within each adjective pair, with 1 representing the negative extreme and 7 the positive extreme. To avoid biases or a tendency to check the same column in each scale, the order of negative and positive responses are varied randomly. For example, in Figure 9.2, ratings of painful/not painful, slow/fast, lonely/shared, and unprepared/prepared place the negative value on the left. In the other four scales, the positive values are on the left. A total score can be obtained by summing the scores for each rating. Lower total scores usually reflect negative feelings toward the concept being measured; higher scores usually reflect positive feelings. If the researcher decides that higher numbers represent a positive word value, the negative high score items need to be reverse-scored. A score of 7 for the adjective pair "satisfying/unsatisfying" would be scored as a 1 when it was summed, and the adjective

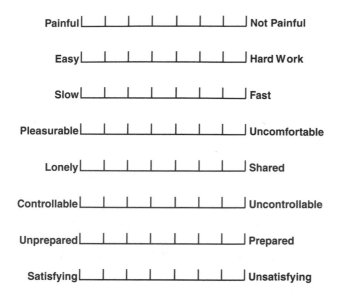

**FIGURE 9.2** Example of a semantic differential scale describing the labor and delivery experience for women.

pair "unprepared/prepared" would remain as a score of 7. Excerpt 9.4 describes the use of a semantic differential scale. Women who participated in the study were asked to look at a pair of words and rate their feelings about the 13 different concepts on a seven-point scale. The semantic differential scale is different from the Likert scale in that only two extremes are labeled. Second, the continuum is not based on agree/disagree but on opposite adjectives that express the respondent's feelings.

## EXCERPT 9.4

### USE OF THE SEMANTIC DIFFERENTIAL SCALE

**Power as Knowing Participation in Change Test (PKPCT)**

The PKPCT is a semantic differential instrument with four subscales—awareness, choices, freedom to act intentionally, and involvement in creating changes—and a total score. Each subscale is composed of a list of 13 bipolar adjectives. One of the adjective pairs in each list duplicates an earlier item pair, consistent with semantic differential theory. Each subscale item is scored from 1 to 7, with total subscale scores ranging from 13 to 91. Higher scores indicate relatively more power. Women participating in 1997 and 2000 qualitative studies of hypothyroid-like symptoms and fatigue noted that powerlessness was significant in their experiences; thus, the PKPCT was chosen to describe powerlessness.

*Source: Dzurec, LC, Hoover, PM, and Fields, J: Acknowledging unexplained fatigue of tired women. Image: J Nurs Schol 34:41, 2002, with permission.*

**Directions:** Please place an X at the point on the line that best reflects how much pain you experienced with the venipuncture.

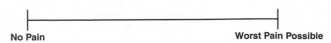

No Pain                                    Worst Pain Possible

FIGURE 9.3   Example of the visual analogue scale (VAS).

## Visual Analogue Scales

The visual analogue scale (VAS) is useful for measuring subjective phenomena (e.g., pain, fatigue, shortness of breath, anxiety). The scale is unidimensional, quantifying intensity only. The VAS is 100 mm long, with anchors at each end to indicate the extremes of the phenomenon being assessed. Subjects are asked to mark a point on the line indicating the amount of the phenomenon experienced at that time. The intensity of the phenomenon is scored by measuring the millimeters from the low end of the scale to the subject's mark.[8] The VAS is a reliable and valid measure for assessing subjective patient experiences. An example of a VAS is shown in Figure 9.3. Use of the VAS is illustrated in Excerpt 9.5.

## Q Methodology

Q Methodology (or Q sort) is an example of a sorting technique used to characterize opinions, attitudes, or judgments of individuals through comparative rank ordering.[9] The technique involves giving an individual a set of cards containing a series

### EXCERPT 9.5

## USE OF VISUAL ANALOGUE SCALE

**Instrument**

I used a horizontal VAS to measure the dependent variable of preoperative anxiety. The VAS previously was reported to be a valid and reliable measure of self-reported preoperative anxiety among a sample of 40 female ambulatory surgery patients.

This VAS consists of a 10-cm horizontal line with defined ends representing extreme limits of preoperative anxiety. The left end of the line represents "no sensation" and the right end represents "as much anxiety as could possibly be." Each subject self-reported the level of preoperative anxiety by making a vertical mark across the line at the point that represented his or her level of anxiety. The research assistant read the following directions to each subject: "This line represents the amount of worry, anxiety, concern, or fear which patients may feel before surgery. The left end of the line represents no worry, anxiety, concern, or fear. The right end of the line represents as much worry, anxiety, concern, or fear as can be. Please make a vertical mark on this line to represent how much worry, anxiety, fear, or concern you feel right now."

*Source: Gaberson, KB: The effect of humorous and musical distraction on preoperative anxiety. AORN J 62:784, 1995. Reprinted with permission. Copyright © AORN, Inc, 2170 S Parker Road, Suite 300, Denver, CO 80231.*

of written items, such as statements or phrases, each item being placed on a separate card. The individual is asked to sort the cards into piles according to some scaled criterion. The number of cards should range from 40 to 100, depending on the research question.[10] The number of piles is usually 5 to 10, ranging from low priority to high priority. The researcher specifies how many cards are to go into each pile so that the subject is faced with forced choices. Subjects may replace any card or move any card to another pile any time during the sorting process until they are satisfied with the results. Subjects are advised to first select those cards that go into the extreme categories. The method is supposed to yield a normal distribution of responses, with fewer statements in the extreme category.

In Zax's[11] study exploring postpartum concerns of teenage mothers, subjects were asked to sort through cards and place them in 5 piles, from least to greatest postpartum concerns among teenagers. Each statement was preceded by, "I am worried about . . ." The Q sort items are shown here. Although considerably fewer than 40 cards were used in this study, it was a beginning attempt to explore self-expressed concerns of first-time teenage mothers during the first 3 postpartum months.

> When my body will look normal again.
> Having my body feel normal again.
> How to take care of my baby.
> How my baby has been acting.
> How I can take care of my baby and do other important things too.
> How things are different with my friends.
> How things are different with my boyfriend.
> Making love.
> School.
> How things are different with my family.
> How I'll be able to do household chores.
> What it was like being in labor and giving birth.
> How my boyfriend feels about my baby.
> How I feel emotionally.

## Instruments

Phenomena measured by psychosocial instruments (e.g., coping, stress, self-concept, self-esteem, motivation) are studied widely in nursing. Many psychosocial instruments have already been developed, tested, and refined to measure a particular variable or concept. Selecting an appropriate instrument is critical for the researcher. The method of measurement must closely fit the conceptual definition of the variable or concept. Instruments consist of a series of items that may be analyzed either as a total score or independently as separate subscales. Despite the type of instrument sought, certain kinds of information should be available about any standardized instrument.

Psychosocial instruments usually include guidelines for scoring and interpreting scores. Guidelines for scoring include information on criteria for acceptable

**EXCERPT 9.6**

## INFORMATION ON HOW TO SCORE AND INTERPRET THE MODIFIED FATIGUE SYMPTOM CHECKLIST (MFSC)

**Measures**

Modified Fatigue Symptom Checklist (MFSC)

Participants described their levels of fatigue using the modified fatigue symptom checklist (MFSC; Pugh, 1993). The MFSC is a norm-referenced, 30-item, Likert scale with a potential range of scores from 30 to 120 (item range = 1–4). Higher scores indicate more fatigue. The instrument includes six subscales:

1. subjective weariness
2. decreased concentration
3. psychoogical
4. physical: lower body
5. physical: head and neck
6. physical: generalized

Pugh modified an earler version of the instrument, the fatigue symptom checklist (FSC; Yoshitake, 1971), to improve clarity of directions and ease of administration. Internal consistency reliability estimates for the total MFSC checklist and the subscales range from 0.73 for the physical subscale to 0.91 for the total checklist. Based on the psychometric analyses of the MFSC completed by Pugh, and on the conceptual fit between Pugh's definition of fatigue and our definition in the study, the MFSC was chosen as an appropriate measure of fatigue. In our study, internal consistency reliabilities for the MFSC ranged from 0.57 (physical: head and neck symptoms) to 0.95 (total checklist).

*Source: Dzurec, LC, Hoover, PM, and Fields, J: Acknowledging unexplained fatigue of tired women. Image: J Nurs Schol 34:41, 2002, with permission.*

responses, the number of points to be assigned to various responses, the procedures for computing total scores, and, usually, normative data on a wide range of population groups. Journal articles usually do not provide a copy of the questionnaire or other instrument used in the study, nor do they give detailed guidelines for scoring and interpreting scores. A typical research report is shown in Excerpt 9.6, with a discussion of the Modified Fatigue Symptom Checklist.

The construction of an instrument is complex and time-consuming. The development of an effective instrument requires an in-depth knowledge of the phenomena under study and considerable skill in measurement. Beginning researchers should use instruments that have already been developed, ones with established reliability and validity. Standardized instruments are developed by experts in a particular area of study.

## Biophysical Measures

Nursing research includes variables measured with physiological instruments. Various monitoring devices have been developed to measure vital signs and other

## USE OF TECHNOLOGY TO MEASURE BIOPHYSICAL VARIABLES

**Instruments**

Maximal inspiratory pressure was defined as the maximal negative pressure that the subject could generate and maintain for 1 second when inspiring against an occluded airway (Black and Hyatt, 1979). It was measured with a direct pressure transducer ($+300$ mm Hg, model P23, Gould Instruments, Ballain Villiers, France), which was amplified (model 7P122, Grass Instruments, Quincy, MA) and recorded on a strip-chart recorder. The mouth pressure signal was calibrated against a column of water before each test. The mouth pressure transducer was connected by stiff polyethylene tubing to a one-way valve attached to a straight disposable mouthpiece (Vitalograph, Lenexa, KS) with a 1.7 mm diameter leak. The leak prevented subjects from closing their glottis or using their buccal muscles to create artificially high pressures.

*Source: Hopp, LJ, et al: Incremental threshold loading in patients with chronic obstructive lung disease. Nurs Res 45:196, 1996, with permission.*

physiological data. These devices yield quantitative data that are easily analyzed. For example, maximal inspiratory pressure is used to indicate inspiratory muscle strength, which provides an index of performance for patients with chronic obstructive lung disease. Excerpt 9.7 shows an example of how maximal inspiratory pressure was measured.

## QUALITATIVE DATA COLLECTION METHODS

### Interviews

An interview schedule, sometimes called an interview guide, is a list of topics or an open-ended questionnaire administered to subjects by a skilled interviewer. The presence of the interviewer allows for probing of subjects' responses and decreases the possibility of vague answers. Interviewing is often used in qualitative studies to elicit meaningful data; however, open-ended questionnaires may be used with other instruments to generate both qualitative and quantitative data, as shown in Excerpt 9.8.

Audio and video recordings may be used to complement interviews. Researchers must consider the possibility that subjects might be sensitive to the presence of audio and video equipment and should ask for the subject's permission to tape. In Excerpt 9.9, the researcher has audiotaped a phenomenological interview (a qualitative research approach) and provided the reader with the list of questions asked.

### Participant Observation

This type of qualitative data collection is used in ethnographic research. The technique (see Chapter 13 for discussion) involves direct observation through involve-

EXCERPT 9.8

## USE OF OPEN- AND CLOSED-ENDED QUESTIONNAIRES TO COLLECT DATA

**Instruments and Procedure**

The self-administered instruments used in the study included the Women's Roles Interview Protocol (WRIP) and a demographic questionnaire requesting information on age, marital status, number of children, educational level, income, ethnic background, and perceived adequacy of income. The WRIP was developed to stimulate participant responses related to central roles (e.g., work, spousal, and maternal roles), the extent of involvement in each role, descriptions of role likes and dislikes, and perceived levels of stress in each role. The WRIP includes 43 closed- and open-ended questions related to the stressful and satisfying aspects of the work environment and to strategies employed in coping with perceived stress in the work environment. The instrument has been used as both an interview guide and a self-administered questionnaire. In different research settings, the decisions about mode of administration have been based on the educational level of participants, recommendations of collaborators, and preference of participant representatives.

*Source: Meleis, AI, Messias, DK, and Arruda, EN: Women's work environment and health: Clerical workers in Brazil. Res Nurs Health 19:53, 1996, with permission.*

ment with subjects in their natural setting, participating in their lifestyle activities. Through participation and observation, data are collected in an unstructured manner as field notes written in a journal. The key element in participant observation is involvement with subjects in their environment and development of a trusting relationship.

## Focus Group Interviews

Focus groups are acceptable subjects for in-depth interview. The technique serves a variety of purposes, with the ultimate goal of observing the interactions among focus group members and detecting their attitudes, opinions, and solutions to specific topics posed by the facilitator.[12] Focus groups are designed to be nonthreatening so participants can express and clarify their views in ways that are less likely to occur one-on-one. There is a sense of "safety in numbers."[13] Focus groups have a value similar to that of an open-ended question; however, with the latter, there is no ability to probe participants for meaning.

Recruiting subjects to participate in a focus group interview is critical. The use of purposive sampling is most often employed when individuals known to have a desired expertise are sought. Recruitment may be sought through the media, posters, or advertisements. Incentives (i.e., money, gifts, certificates, coupons, and so on) may need to be provided to ensure attendance by a sufficient number of participants.[13]

| EXCERPT 9.9 |
| --- |

## USE OF AUDIOTAPING DURING INTERVIEW

In-depth, face-to-face audio-taped interviews were conducted by the researcher with each of the participants, in an interview room on the psychiatric unit. The interviews lasted approximately 1–2 hours, although for some participants, the interview was broken into shorter segments and completed over 2–3 days. The very nature of the phenomenological questioning makes it difficult to design a structured questionnaire because questions emerge and are derived as the understanding of the phenomenon emerges. However, in using vanManen's (1990) method, he points out that the "interview process needs to be disciplined by the fundamental question that prompted the need for the interview in the first place." He suggests that often researchers give in to the temptation to "let the method rule the question rather than the research question determining what kind of (interview) method is most appropriate." To avoid this pitfall, four questions were posed to serve as a general interview guide.

1. I'm interested in what people see as important or meaningful experiences in their lives. As you reflect back over your life, what are some of these for you?
2. What would you say have been some of the successes in your life? The disappointments? What were you doing at these times?
3. If you were to tell your life story, how would you describe the things, the events, or whatever that have given you a sense of meaning and purpose in your life? How do these influence or relate to your feeling that life is not worth living?
4. Has that sense of meaning or purpose changed over the years? In what way? How do you experience meaning in your life now?

*Source: Moore, SL: A phenomenological study of meaning in life in suicidal older adults. Arch Psych Nurs 11:29, 1997, with permission.*

A focus group is typically made up of 6 to 12 individuals who are asked to discuss a particular topic led by a facilitator. Fewer participants may result in an inadequate discussion. Focus group discussions are recorded either manually, by having someone take notes, or by audiotape. If taped, the discussion is transcribed. A transcript of the discussion becomes the data of the focus group interview.

Excerpt 9.10 presents an example of a study using a focus group interview. Anderson and colleagues[14] reported on diabetes care and education issues among Latinos with diabetes. The study involved 42 patients receiving diabetes care from the Community Health and Social Services Clinic in Detroit. The 42 patients were divided into 4 focus groups, with 47 issues identified and prioritized.

## QUESTIONS TO CONSIDER WHEN CRITIQUING DATA COLLECTION METHODS

Identify a research study to critique. Read the study to see if you recognize any key terms discussed in this chapter. Remember that all studies may not contain all key

**EXCERPT 9.10**

## USE OF FOCUS GROUP INTERVIEW

The overall goal of this project was to develop culturally appropriate diabetes education and care programs for Latinos with diabetes. The purpose of using focus groups was to identify issues and themes that could guide the development of diabetes care and education programs and materials.

Forty-two patients receiving diabetes care from the Community Health and Social Services Clinic in Detroit were enrolled in this study. The majority were of Mexican heritage. Participants were compensated for their participation in the focus groups and invited to attend a free series of educational classes about diabetes care. Both of these incentives were considered useful for attracting participants. The focus groups were conducted by two leaders, both of whom were bilingual. Both leaders were familiar with focus group methodology and Latino culture. Focus group questions were generated by the Michigan Diabetes and Research and Training Center (MDRTC) project team based on questions used in an earlier focus group study. The questions were then reviewed and revised by Latino health professionals. Open-ended questions were used to elicit a wide range of responses.

**Example of Focus Group Questions**
1. Please introduce yourself briefly and say a few words about yourself.
2. Please tell us a little bit about your diabetes, how long you have had it, how it is treated, etc.
3. I would like you to tell us about how diabetes affects the following areas of your life. (Discuss each of these areas separately, one at a time: family relationships, community relationships, work situations, recreation activities, spiritual or religious life.)
4. What kinds of changes have you made or tried to make in the way you eat to take care of your diabetes? Have these changes been difficult?
5. Have you changed your level of physical activity to take care of your diabetes? If so, how?

*Source: Anderson, RM, et al: Using focus groups to identify diabetes care and education issues for Latinos with diabetes. Diabetes Educ 24:618, 1998, with permission.*

terms. The following questions[1,12,13] serve as a guide in critiquing data collection methods:

1. *What types of instruments and/or scales were used to measure the main study variables?* Authors should describe and justify instrumentation used in a study. If you do not know how instruments and/or scales are used, information is lacking that is vital to understanding the data they produce. In quantitative studies, data collected usually take the form of statistical operations when being analyzed. See Chapter 10 for a discussion of the most commonly encountered statistics. In qualitative studies, data are elicited through interviews and participant observation. Refer to Chapters 12 to 14

for a more detailed discussion of data collection as it relates to a qualitative approach to research.

2. *Was the data collection process described clearly?* Data collection procedures should be explained in detail. It is not sufficient to read that a questionnaire or survey was used. Readers need to know the details regarding administration of questionnaires, surveys, and scales. It is important to determine if the questionnaires/surveys were administered to individuals or groups, by the researcher or by research assistant(s), with scripted instructions, under conditions that were similar for all subjects, and if all sections or parts of the questionnaire/survey were to be completed and returned.

## SUMMARY OF KEY IDEAS

1. Questionnaires are self-reported forms or interviews designed to collect information.
2. A scale is a set of numerical values assigned to responses, representing the extent to which subjects possess a particular attitude, value, or characteristic.
3. Likert scales consist of a series of statements in which subjects select an appropriately ranked response that reflects their agreement or disagreement.
4. Semantic differential scales measure subjects' feelings about a concept, based on a continuum that extends between two extreme opposites.
5. The visual analogue scale is a 100-mm line used to measure subjective phenomena.
6. Psychosocial instruments for measuring concepts or phenomena in nursing are the most commonly used quantitative method of data collection.
7. Interviews and observation are common methods of data collection in qualitative research.
8. Focus groups present researchers with opportunities to observe the interactions among participants and record their attitudes and opinions.

## LEARNING ACTIVITIES

1. Complete the in-class questionnaire in Table 9.2. As a class, tally the results, and share these with one another. Identify which questions were open-ended, categorical, and continuous responses. Were the questions and answers meaningful and interesting?

2. Design a questionnaire. Write a paragraph that introduces the questionnaire to the respondent and that explains how to answer the questions. This paragraph should be encouraging but general. Provide enough specific information. Include a variety of answers to questions that represent open-ended, categorical, and continuous variables.

## References

1. Polit, DF, Beck, CT, and Hungler, BP: Essentials of Nursing Research: Methods, Appraisal, and Utilization, ed 5. Lippincott Williams & Wilkins, Philadelphia, 2001, pp 263–267, 271, 389.
2. Fink, A: The Survey Handbook. Sage Publications, Thousand Oaks, CA, 1995.
3. Dillman, DA: Mail and Telephone Surveys: The Total Design Method. John Wiley, New York, 1978.
4. Fink, A, and Kosecoff, J: How to Conduct Surveys: A Step by Step Guide. Sage Publications, Beverly Hills, CA, 1985.
5. Spector, PE: Summated Rating Scale Construction: An Introduction. Sage Publications, Newbury Park, CA, 1992.
6. Lutenbacher, M: Relationship between psychosocial factors and abusive parenting attitudes in low-income single mothers. Nurs Research 51:158, 2002.
7. Osgood, CE, Suci, GJ, and Tannenbaum, RH: The Measurement Meaning. University of Illinois Press, Urbana, IL, 1957.
8. Gift, AG: Visual analogue scales: Measurement of subjective phenomena. Nurs Res 38:286, 1989.
9. Stephenson, W: The Study of Behavior. Q Technique and its Methodology. University of Chicago Press, Chicago, 1975.
10. Tetting, DW: Q sort update. West J Nurs Res 10:757, 1988.
11. Zax, S: Postpartum concerns of teenage mothers: An exploratory study. Unpublished master's thesis, Yale University School of Nursing, 1985.
12. Burns, N, and Grove, SK: The Practice of Nursing Research: Conduct, Critique, and Utilization, ed 4. WB Saunders, Philadelphia, 2001, pp 424–426, 671.
13. Gillis A, and Jackson, W: Research for Nurses: Methods and Interpretation. FA Davis, Philadelphia, 2002, pp 234–239, 618.
14. Anderson, RM, et al: Using focus groups to identify diabetes care and education issues for Latinos with diabetes. Diabetes Educ 24:618, 1998.

# 10 Analyzing the Data

James A. Fain, PhD, RN, BC-ADM, FAAN

## LEARNING OBJECTIVES

*At the end of this chapter, you will be able to:*

1. Differentiate between descriptive and inferential statistics.
2. Compare and contrast the three measures of central tendency.
3. Compare and contrast the three measures of dispersion.
4. Distinguish between parametric and nonparametric procedures.
5. Evaluate a researcher's choice of descriptive and inferential statistics in published research.

## GLOSSARY OF KEY TERMS

**Analysis of variance (ANOVA).** A parametric procedure used to test whether there is a difference among three group means.

**Chi-square.** A nonparametric procedure used to assess whether a relationship exists between two nominal level variables; symbolized as $x^2$.

**Confidence interval.** A range of values computed from sample data that estimates a population parameter.

**Correlation.** A measure that defines the relationship between two variables.

**Descriptive statistics.** Statistics that describe and summarize data.

**Homogeneity of variance.** Situation in which the dependent variables do not differ significantly between or among groups.

**Inferential statistics.** Statistics that generalize findings from a sample to a population.

**Level of confidence.** Probability level in which the research hypothesis is

accepted with confidence. A 0.05 level of confidence is the standard among researchers.

**Mean.** A measure of central tendency calculated by summing a set of scores and dividing the sum by the total number of scores; also called the average.

**Measures of central tendency.** Descriptive statistics that describe the location or approximate center of a distribution of data.

**Measures of dispersion.** Descriptive statistics that depict the spread or variability among a set of numerical data.

**Median.** A measure of central tendency that represents the middle score in a distribution.

**Mode.** The score or value that occurs most frequently in a distribution; a measure of central tendency used most often with nominal-level data.

**Negative correlation.** Correlation in which high scores for one variable are paired with low scores for the other variable.

**Negatively skewed.** Referring to distribution of scores in which the tail is to the left and the mean is larger than the median.

**Outlier.** Data point isolated from other data points; extreme score in a data set.

**Parameter.** Numerical characteristic of a population (e.g., population mean, population standard deviation).

**Positive correlation.** Correlation in which high scores for one variable are paired with high scores for the other variable, or low scores for one variable are paired with low scores for the other variable.

**Positively skewed.** Referring to distribution of scores in which the tail is to the right and the mean is smaller than the median.

**Probability.** Likelihood that an event will occur, given all possible outcomes.

**Range.** A measure of variability that is the difference between the lowest and highest values in a distribution.

**Robust.** Referring to results from statistical analyses that are close to being valid even though the researcher does not rigidly adhere to assumptions associated with parametric procedures.

**Skewed distribution.** A distribution of scores with a few outlying observations in either direction.

**Standard deviation (SD).** The most frequently used measure of variability; the distance a score varies from the mean.

**Symmetrical distribution.** A distribution of scores in which the mean, median, and mode are all the same.

**t-test.** A popular parametric procedure for assessing whether two group means are significantly different from one another.

**Variance.** Measure of variability, which is the average squared deviation from the mean.

The purpose of data analysis is to answer research questions, test hypotheses, or both. The research design and type of data collected determine selection of appropriate statistical procedures. Once data have been collected, statistical procedures describe, analyze, and interpret quantitative data. Application of the appropriate statistics helps the researcher decide if the results and conclusions of the study are justified. Despite how well researchers conduct a study, inappropriate analyses can lead to inappropriate conclusions. Many different statistical procedures are used to analyze data. This chapter provides an overview of the most commonly used statistics that describe and examine relationships and that test for differences.[1] A consumer of nursing research needs to interpret and apply statistical data applicable to nursing practice. This can be accomplished by reading and evaluating data analyses.

## USING STATISTICS TO DESCRIBE

Statistical procedures are classified into two categories, descriptive and inferential statistics. **Descriptive statistics** describe, organize, and summarize data. **Inferential statistics** make generalizations about populations, based on data collected from samples. Descriptive statistics include measures of central tendency and measures of dispersion. **Measures of central tendency** describe the location or approximate the center of a distribution of data. A distribution consists of scores and numerical values and their frequency of occurrence. Measures of central tendency include the mean, median, and mode. **Measures of dispersion** are descriptive statistics that depict the spread or variability among a set of numerical data. Measures of dispersion are described by the range, variance, and standard deviation. Two additional measures of dispersion that are not frequently found in the literature are percentile and interquartile range.

## Measures of Central Tendency

### Mean

The **mean** is the most commonly used measure of central tendency and is often associated with the term "average." The mean is calculated by adding all the scores in a distribution and dividing the total by the number of scores. One major characteristic of the mean is that the calculation takes into account each score in the distribution.

In defining the mean with a formula, the following notation is used. The symbol that represents the mean is $\overline{X}$, read as "X bar." $\Sigma$, the Greek letter "sigma," is used to denote the sum of values.

When data represent either an interval or a ratio scale, the mean is the preferred measure of central tendency. The mean is a stable and reliable measure. If equal-sized samples are randomly selected from the same population, the means of those samples will be similar to each other as compared with either the medians or modes.

Excerpt 10.1 includes a table with the results of a study conducted to examine the influence of family resources and demands on the well-being of families providing care to an elderly parent. Descriptive statistics included the mean, standard deviation, potential range, and actual range for six variables. Note that the mean is designated as M and the standard deviation as SD. Within the article, information is provided on how each concept was measured, along with the format used in creating scales for each variable. Scoring methods associated with each scale are not always included in journal articles, because of page limitations. The researcher needs to locate the original publication where major properties and scoring methods associated with the scale are discussed.

The mean is very sensitive to extreme values, or "outliers." An **outlier** is a data point isolated from other data points. In a distribution of scores with outliers, the mean is "pulled" in the direction of those extreme values. For example, in the distribution of ages: 23, 22, 25, 26, 29, 27, and 23, the mean age is 25. Suppose the 29 becomes 50. The age 50 years is considered an outlier. The mean age is now 28, yet the median and mode remain the same.

### Median

The **median** (Mdn) is the middle score or midpoint of a distribution. Researchers sometimes call it the 50th percentile; 50 percent of the distribution falls below or

## EXCERPT 10.1

### USE OF THE MEAN, STANDARD DEVIATION, AND RANGE AS MEASURES OF CENTRAL TENDENCY

**Description of Study Variables**

| Variable | M | SD | Potential Range | Actual Range |
|---|---|---|---|---|
| Family social support | 97.13 | (12.11) | 35–140 | 70–125 |
| Internal family system | 44.70 | (6.90) | 0–60 | 29.5–57.5 |
| Family life changes | 3.99 | (2.31) | 0–10 | 0–9 |
| Amount of help | 14.85 | (12.04) | 0–80 | 1–55 |
| Caregiver's appraisal | 28.11 | (12.83) | 0–88 | 5–59 |
| Family strains | 4.26 | (2.55) | 0–10 | 0–10 |

Source: Fink, SV: The influence of family resources and family demands on the strains and well-being of caregiver's families. Nurs Res 44:139, 1995, with permission.

above the midpoint. The median is calculated by first arranging the scores in rank order. If there is an odd number of scores, the median is the middle score. For example, if a set of scores on a pain scale administered to five patients is 4, 5, 7, 8, and 9, the median is 7. If an even number of scores appears in the distribution, the median is the point halfway between the two middle scores. For example, if the set of scores on the pain scale was 4, 5, 5, 7, 7, and 9, the median is $(7 + 5/2) = 6$. Thus, the median is not necessarily one of the scores in the distribution.

One major characteristic of the median is that it does not take into account each score in the distribution. The median is not sensitive to extreme scores. For example, if a set of scores on a coping scale administered to five patients is 12, 15, 22, 31, and 35, the median score is 22. The mean for this distribution of scores is 23. However, if one value changes and the set of scores is 12, 15, 22, 31, and 125, the median is still 22, whereas the mean is now 41.

The median is an appropriate measure of central tendency when the data represent a skewed distribution. A distribution that has outlying observations in one direction is a **skewed distribution**. A **symmetrical distribution** is one in which the mean, median, and mode are all the same (Fig. 10.1). Skewed distributions have off-centered peaks and longer tails in one direction. The mean, median, and mode do not coincide in skewed distributions; rather, their relative positions remain constant. The mode is closest to the peak of the curve, as this is where the most frequent scores are found. The mean is closest to the tail, where the relatively few extreme scores are located. For this reason, the mean score in **positively skewed** distributions lies toward the high score values; the mean in the **negatively skewed** distribution falls close to the low score values (see Figure 10.1). In a skewed distribution, the median always falls somewhere between the mean and the mode.

The word "median" is abbreviated as "Mdn." Excerpt 10.2 includes a table in which the mean (M) and median (Mdn) are presented for two variables measured on an interval-ratio scale: age and years of education. The mean age of the sample was 56.58 years, with a median of 55. The mean number of years of education was 11.04

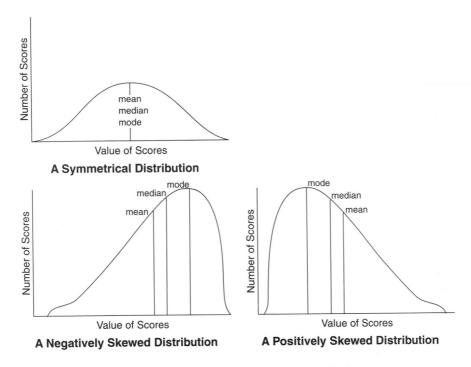

FIGURE 10.1 Measures of central tendency in normal and skewed distributions.

### EXCERPT 10.2

## USE OF MEAN AND MEDIAN AS MEASURES OF CENTRAL TENDENCY

**Demographic and Background Information of Sample**

|  | M | SD | Range | Median | No. | % |
|---|---|---|---|---|---|---|
| N = 65 |  |  |  |  |  |  |
| Age (yr) | 56.58 | 14.02 | 29–90 | 55 | — | — |
| Education (yr) | 11.04 | 3.08 | 3–18 | 12 | — | — |
| Race |  |  |  |  |  |  |
| Black |  |  |  |  | 27 | 49 |
| White |  |  |  |  | 28 | 51 |
| Admission route |  |  |  |  |  |  |
| Emergency department |  |  |  |  | 29 | 53 |
| Doctor's office |  |  |  |  | 4 | 7 |
| Transfer |  |  |  |  | 22 | 40 |
| Annual income (n = 44) |  |  |  |  |  |  |
| <$10,000 |  |  |  |  | 18 | 41 |
| $10,000–$24,999 |  |  |  |  | 14 | 24 |
| $25,000–$40,000 |  |  |  |  | 7 | 12 |
| >$40,000 |  |  |  |  | 5 | 9 |

*Source: Warner, CD: Somatic awareness and coronary artery disease in women with chest pain. Heart Lung 24:436, 1995, with permission.*

years, with a median of 12. In both examples, the mean and median were almost identical, indicating a normal distribution. If the median age was 65, this would represent a negatively skewed distribution.

## Mode

The **mode** is the most frequently occurring score in a distribution. It is an appropriate measure of central tendency for nominal data. A distribution of scores may have more than one mode. Data with a single mode are called unimodal; data with two modes, bimodal. In Excerpt 10.3, the authors display a frequency distribution for the variables age, race, number of sexual partners in the last 12 months, and living situations. In a frequency distribution, the most frequently occurring score (mode) can be identified. Of the 225 subjects who participated in the study, the most frequent number of sexual partners in the last 12 months was 1 (n = 126). Also, the most frequent age category was 20 to 21 years (n = 99). Excerpt 10.4 provides more

---

**EXCERPT 10.3**

## FREQUENCY DISTRIBUTION
### Demographic Characteristics of the Sample

| Characteristic | Response | f | % |
|---|---|---|---|
| Age | 18–19 | 57 | 25.1 |
| | 20–21 | 99 | 43.6 |
| | 22–23 | 53 | 23.3 |
| | 24–25 | 18 | 7.9 |
| Race | White | 21.2 | 93.4 |
| | Black | 2 | .9 |
| | Other | 13 | 5.8 |
| Number of sexual partners in last 12 months | 0 | 6 | 2.6 |
| | 1 | 126 | 55.5 |
| | 2 | 34 | 15.0 |
| | 3 | 23 | 10.1 |
| | 4 | 10 | 4.4 |
| | 5 or more | 26 | 11.3 |
| Do you live | At home/family origin | 110 | 48.5 |
| | In dormitory | 68 | 30.0 |
| | With friends/ roommate(s) | 31 | 13.7 |
| | Other | 18 | 7.9 |

*Source: Cole, FL, and Slocumb, EM: Factor influencing safer sexual behaviors in heterosexual late adolescents and young adult collegiate males. Image J Nurs Schol 27:217, 1995. Copyrighted material of Sigma Theta Tau, used with permission.*

EXCERPT 10.4

## SAMPLE CHARACTERISTICS REPORTED WITHIN TEXT OF ARTICLE

**Sample**

As shown in [the Table], respondents ranged in age from 18 to 25 years; the mean was 21.5 years old. Thirty-eight (16.8%) were freshmen, 52 (23%) were sophomores, 63 (27.9%) were juniors, and 73 (32.3%) were seniors. The majority (148) stated that they were Catholic; however, 15 (7%) were Protestant, 25 (11.8%) were members of other religious affiliations, and 24 (11.4%) indicated no religious affiliation. Nine (4.1%) stated they were very religious, 98 (44.7%) somewhat religious, 72 (32.9%) not very religious, 32 (14.6%) not at all religious, and 8 (3.7%) antireligious. The model respondent was white (212), had only one sexual partner in the preceding 12 months (126), and lived with their family of origin (110).

*Source: Cole, FL, and Slocumb, EM: Factor influencing safer sexual behaviors in heterosexual late adolescents and young adult collegiate males. Image J Nurs Schol 27:217, 1995, with permission.*

detail about the sample within the article and also reports the modal response for race and living situation.

### Comparing the Mean, Median, and Mode

Researchers choose a measure of central tendency depending on the level of measurement, shape, or form of the distribution of data and research objective.

#### Level of Measurement

The use of the mean is appropriate with interval-ratio and sometimes ordinal data (see Chapter 8). The mean is a more precise measure than the median or mode because it takes into account every score in a distribution. The mean is also the most stable of the three measures. If a number of samples are randomly drawn from a target population, the mean varies less, compared with the median and mode. The median is an ordinal statistic based on ranks. Applying the mean to ordinal data must yield meaningful results. Likewise, it makes little sense to compute a median for nominal data (e.g., marital status, religious affiliation). Because the mode requires only a frequency count, it can be applied to any set of data at the nominal, ordinal, or interval-ratio level of measurement.

#### Shape of the Distribution

The shape or form of the distribution is another factor that influences the researcher's choice of a measure of central tendency. In skewed distributions (see Figure 10.1), the mean, median, and mode do not coincide, although their relative positions remain constant in moving away from the peak toward the tail. The order is always from mode, to median, to mean. In a skewed distribution, the median always falls somewhere between the mean and mode. It is this characteristic that makes the median the most appropriate measure of central tendency for describing a skewed distribution.

## Research Objective

Regardless of the purpose of the study, the researcher uses the mode as a preliminary indicator of central tendency. If a more precise measure of central tendency is warranted, the median or mean is used. To describe a skewed distribution, the researcher chooses the median to give a balanced picture of the extreme scores or outliers. In addition, the median is sometimes used as a point in the distribution at which scores can be divided into two categories containing the same number of respondents. The mean is preferred over the median because the mean is easily used in more advanced statistical analyses.

## Measures of Dispersion

### Range

The **range** is the simplest measure of dispersion. It is calculated by subtracting the lowest score in the distribution from the highest score. Excerpt 10.1 illustrates examples of how the range is reported. The researcher reports the potential and actual ranges for each dependent variable. In this case, the variable caregiver appraisal has a potential range of 0 to 88. Based on the results of the study, subjects scored between 5 (lowest score) and 59 (highest score).

The range is considered an unstable measure because it is based on only two values in the distribution. It is extremely sensitive to outliers and does not take into account variations in scores between extremes.

### Variance and Standard Deviation

The variance and **standard deviation** are measures of dispersion. Both measures are based on deviated scores. A deviated score is defined as the difference between a raw score and the mean of that distribution ($x^2 = X - \overline{X}$). Raw scores below the mean have a negative deviation, whereas raw scores above the mean have a positive deviation. The sum of the deviated scores in a distribution always equals 0. Thus, if researchers use deviated scores in calculating measures of variability, they must find ways to get around the fact that the sum of the deviated scores in a distribution always equals 0. Each deviated score is squared, so that all numbers become positive.

The sum of the squared deviations divided by the number of scores is referred to as the **variance.** Mathematically, the variance is the average squared deviation from the mean. By itself, the variance is not very meaningful. Because each of the deviated scores is squared, the variance is expressed in units that are squares of the original units of measure. For example, if heart rate is measured in beats per minute, the variance is in units of beats$^2$ per minute$^2$. To understand what beat$^2$ per minute$^2$ means, researchers need to calculate the square root of the variance. This will convert beats$^2$ per minute$^2$ back to the original unit of measure (beats/minute).

The square root of the variance is referred to as the standard deviation (SD). As an index that summarizes data in the same unit of measurement as the original data, the SD is the most commonly reported measure of dispersion. Like the mean, the standard deviation is the most stable measure of variability and takes into account each score in the distribution. To calculate the SD, two formulas can be used. The first formula involves finding out the deviated scores. Each deviated score is squared, added up, and divided by (N − 1). This is a measure of variability, called variance. In its present form, this measure of variability is not useful.

An example of the calculation follows. Suppose a researcher was interested in calculating the variance and standard deviation for the variable age. Age has a variance of 193.33 square years (year$^2$). Most people would have trouble interpreting a square year. By taking the square root of the variance, the variable is returned to its original scale of measurement (years). The resulting statistic is an SD of 13.90 years. The SD, like the mean, is sensitive to outliers. It is an appropriate measure of dispersion for distributions that are symmetrical, not skewed.

An alternate formula can be used to calculate the standard deviation to eliminate the tedious task of working with negative and positive numbers. This formula gives the same results with fewer calculations.

## Comparing the Range, Variance, and Standard Deviation

The range, although quick and simple to obtain, is not very reliable. Although the range is calculated from two scores in a distribution, both the variance and SD take into account every score in a distribution. Despite its relative stability, the variance is not widely used because it cannot be employed in many statistical analyses. In

CALCULATION OF THE SAMPLE VARIANCE AND STANDARD DEVIATION USING THE DEVIATED SCORES

| X | $x^2 = (X - \overline{X})$ | $(X - \overline{X})^2$ |
|---|---|---|
| 33 | 33−38 | $(-5)^2 = 25$ |
| 68 | 68−38 | $(30)^2 = 900$ |
| 28 | 28−38 | $(-10)^2 = 100$ |
| 33 | 33−38 | $(-5)^2 = 25$ |
| 28 | 28−38 | $(-10)^2 = 100$ |
| 56 | 56−38 | $(18)^2 = 324$ |
| 42 | 42−38 | $(4)^2 = 16$ |
| 29 | 29−38 | $(-9)^2 = 81$ |
| 38 | 38−38 | $(0)^2 = 0$ |
| 25 | 25−38 | $(-13)^2 = 169$ |
| $\Sigma X = 380$ | $\Sigma x^2 = (X - X) = 0$ | $\Sigma x^2 = (X - X)^2 = 1740$ |

$\overline{X} = 38.0$

Variance $(S^2) = \dfrac{1740}{9} = 193.33$ square years

Standard Deviation $(s) = \sqrt{\dfrac{1740}{9}} = 13.9$ years

| X | X² | |
|---|---|---|
| 33 | 1089 | $s = \sqrt{\dfrac{\Sigma X^2 - \dfrac{(\Sigma X)^2}{N}}{N-1}}$ |
| 68 | 4624 | $s = \sqrt{\dfrac{16,180 - \dfrac{(380)^2}{10}}{9}}$ |
| 28 | 784 | $s = \sqrt{\dfrac{16,180 - 14,440}{9}}$ |
| 33 | 1089 | $s = \sqrt{\dfrac{1740}{9}}$ |
| 28 | 784 | $s = 13.9$ years |
| 25 | 625 | |
| $\Sigma X = 380$ | $\Sigma X^2 = 16,180$ | $S = 13.9$ years |

contrast, the SD squares the deviated scores and returns them to their original units of measure. Calculating the SD is the initial step for obtaining other statistical measures, especially in the context of statistical decision making.

## INFERENTIAL STATISTICS

Inferential statistics focus on the process of selecting a sample and using the information to make generalizations to a population. Information contained in a sample is used to make inferences concerning a parameter. A **parameter** is a numerical characteristic of a population (e.g., population mean, population standard deviation). Researchers estimate the parameters of a population from a sample. For example, suppose a researcher randomly samples 125 people with type 1 diabetes and measures changes in blood glucose levels. If the mean blood glucose level is 70 mg/dL, this represents the mean sample statistic. If researchers were able to study every individual with type 1 diabetes, an average blood glucose level could be calculated. This would represent the parameter of the population. Researchers are rarely able to study an entire population. The use of inferential statistics allows researchers to make inferences about the larger population (all individuals with type 1 diabetes) from studying the sample (125 randomly selected people with type 1 diabetes).

Inferential statistical procedures are divided into two types. The first involves the estimation of parameters. A parameter estimation is evaluated by a single number or an interval. For example, a researcher might calculate a sample mean and use its value (age of 18) to estimate the mean age of female drivers. Because the estimate consists of a single value, it is called a point estimate. Alternatively, the mean age could be estimated by saying that it is some age between 16 and 22. This is an interval estimate and is associated with some amount of confidence. Confidence associated with an interval estimate is called the confidence interval. A **confidence interval** is a range of values that has some specified probability (e.g., 0.95 or 0.99) of including a particular population parameter.

The second type of inferential statistical procedure is hypothesis testing, which allows the researcher to formulate a hypothesis concerning the parameter, sample the population of interest, and make objective decisions about the sample results of the study. Central to hypothesis testing is a discussion of probability. Probability helps evaluate the accuracy of a statistic and test a hypothesis. Research findings are often stated and communicated using probability. Two types of hypothesis testing include parametric and nonparametric procedures.

## Probability

**Probability** is an essential concept for understanding inferential statistics. Probability is a means of predicting (e.g., "There is a 50 percent chance of rain the rest of the week." or "This operation has an 80 percent chance of success."). Probability is a system of rules for analyzing a set of outcomes. Probability is the likelihood that an event will occur, given all possible outcomes. The lowercase p signifies probability. For example, the probability of getting heads with the single flip of a coin is 1 out of 2, or 1/2, or 0.5. Therefore, the probability is expressed as 50 percent, or $p = 0.5$. The probability of getting a four when a die is thrown is 1 out of 6, 1/6, or $p = 0.17$. Conversely, the probability of not rolling a four is 5 out of 6, 5/6, or $p = 0.83$.

To establish whether an outcome is statistically significant, the researcher must set up a confidence level. A **level of confidence** is a probability level in which the null hypothesis can be rejected with confidence and the research hypothesis can be accepted with confidence. Researchers use 0.05 as the standard level of confidence; that is, researchers are willing to accept statistical significance occurring by chance 5 times out of 100. The 0.05 level of confidence is graphically depicted in Figure 10.2. As shown, the 0.05 level of confidence is found in the small areas of the "tails." These are the areas under the curve that represent a distance of $\pm1.96$ SD from a mean difference of 0. A 1.96 SD in either direction represents 2.5 percent of the sample mean differences $(50\% - 47.5\% = 2.5\%)$. In other words, 95 percent of the sample differences falls between $-1.96$ SD and $+1.96$ SD from a mean difference of 0.

Confidence levels can be set up for any amount of probability. For example, a more stringent confidence level is 0.01. Using this level of confidence, there is 1 chance out of 100 that the sample difference could occur by chance (1%). The 0.01 level of confidence is represented by the area that lies 2.58 SDs in both directions from a mean difference of zero.

The magnitude of p does not indicate the amount of validity associated with each research hypothesis. Avoid using terms such as "highly significant" or "more significant." Once the level of significance is chosen, it represents a decision rule. The

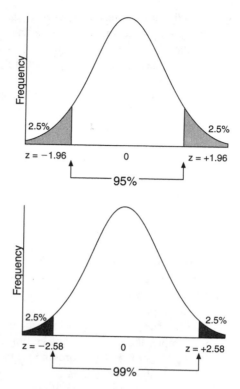

**FIGURE 10.2** Graphic representation of 0.05 and 0.01 levels of confidence.

decision rule is dichotomous: yes or no, significant or not significant. Once the decision is made, the magnitude of p reflects only the relative amount of confidence that can be placed in that decision.

## PARAMETRIC VERSUS NONPARAMETRIC STATISTICAL TESTS

Different statistical tests are appropriate for different sets of data. A decision in choosing an appropriate statistical test depends on whether a researcher selects a parametric or nonparametric procedure. Parametric procedures require assumptions to be met for statistical findings to be valid. General assumptions associated with parametric procedures include the dependent variable being measured on an interval-ratio scale that is normally distributed in the population and groups being mutually exclusive (independent of each other). Random sampling allows every member of the population to have an equal and independent chance of being selected for a sample. If randomization is used, the assumption of independence is met. Specific statistical techniques may have specific assumptions.

Nonparametric tests make no assumptions about the shape of the distribution and are referred to as "distribution-free" tests. Nonparametric tests are usually used when data represent an ordinal or nominal scale. Moreover, nonparametric tests involve simpler and fewer calculations. The major drawback to nonparametric tests is that they are less powerful than parametric tests. Figure 10.3 distinguishes between descriptive and inferential statistics and their various subtypes.

## USING STATISTICS TO EXAMINE RELATIONSHIPS

### Correlations

A **correlation** is a measure that defines the relationship between two variables. For example, a researcher might be interested in knowing the relationship between smoking and lung capacity. Using correlational techniques, a researcher can determine the nature and size of relationships between variables. The correlation coefficient (r) is an index that describes the relationship between two variables.

The correlation coefficient is a decimal between +1.0 and −1.0. The sign (+ or −) preceding the coefficient shows whether the correlation is positive or negative. A **positive correlation** shows that high scores on one variable are paired with high scores on the other variable. Conversely, low scores on one variable are paired with low scores on the other variable. For **negative correlation,** low scores on one variable are paired with high scores on the other variable, and high scores on one variable are paired with low scores on the other variable. A negative correlation reflects an inverse relationship between two variables.

To judge the strength or size of the correlation, consider the actual number of the correlation coefficient (0.63) and the p value (<.05). The closer the coefficient is to either +1.0 or −1.0, the higher or stronger the correlation. The closer the coefficient is to zero, the lower or weaker the correlation. The direction of the relationship does not affect the strength of the relationship. A correlation of −0.85 is just as high or strong as +0.85. The following categories show the strength of the correlation coefficients:

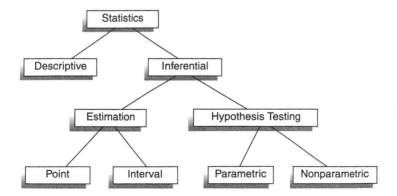

FIGURE 10.3 Descriptive and inferential statistics.

0.90–1.0: Very high
0.89–0.70: High
0.69–0.50: Moderate
0.49–0.26: Low
0.25–0.00: Little, if any

### Pearson Product-Moment Correlation

The Pearson Product-Moment correlation, or simply the Pearson r, is a common correlational technique researchers use to examine the relationship between two variables. The Pearson r is a parametric procedure using interval-ratio data. Refer to Munro[2] for calculation of the correlation coefficient (r).

### Correlation Matrix

Researchers can present correlations in a table format or within the text of an article. A specialized form of a correlation table is the correlation matrix. The correlation matrix presents all possible combinations of the study variables. Excerpt 10.5 is an example of a correlation matrix in which the numbers across the top correspond to the study variables listed on the left-hand margin of the table. The number 4 across the top represents the variable-perceived susceptibility. Each number in the table represents the correlation coefficient between the variables corresponding to the row and column in which the variable is located. The correlation of 0.38 represents a correlation between attitudes toward condoms and safe sex behaviors. Note that the author has a 1.00 in the diagonal to show that correlating a variable with itself is always 1.00.

A researcher often displays correlation coefficients within the text of an article, as shown in Excerpt 10.6. The Pearson r between family well-being and length of time was negatively correlated (r = −0.23). It was reported that the more years a family provided care to an elderly parent, the lower the amount of family well-

---

### EXCERPT 10.5

### CORRELATION MATRIX WITH 1.00 IN THE DIAGONAL

**Zero–Order Correlations Among Predisposing Factors and Safe Sex Behaviors**

|                            | 1      | 2      | 3      | 4     | 5     | 6     |
|----------------------------|--------|--------|--------|-------|-------|-------|
| 1. Self-Esteem             | 1.00   |        |        |       |       |       |
| 2. Internal Health LOC     | .21*   | 1.00   |        |       |       |       |
| 3. Chance Health LOC       | −.14*  | .21*   | 1.00   |       |       |       |
| 4. Perceived Susceptibility| −.17** | −.08   | .04    | 1.00  |       |       |
| 5. Attitudes toward Condoms| .08    | .02−   | .15**  | .05   | 1.00  |       |
| 6. Safe Sex Behavior       | −.08   | .16**  | .01    | −.05  | .38*  | 1.00  |

Note: LOC – Locus of control
* p<.01
** p<.05

Source: Cole, FL, and Slocumb, EM: Factor influencing safer sexual behaviors in heterosexual late adolescents and young adult collegiate males. Image J Nurs Schol 27:217, 1995. Copyrighted material of Sigma Theta Tau, used with permission.

## EXCERPT 10.6

### PEARSON CORRELATIONS PRESENTED WITHOUT A TABLE

Pearson product moment correlations were used to examine the relationships between the study variables and the length of time the family had provided assistance and family SES. Length of time was significantly and negatively related to family well-being, $r = -.23$, $p<.05$, but was not related to any of the independent variables. Socioeconomic status was significantly related to internal system resources, $r = .25$, $p<.05$, and the family well-being, $r = .40$, $p<.01$.

*Source: Fink, SV: The influences of family resources and family demands on the strains and well-being of caregiving families. Nurs Res 440:139, 1995, with permission.*

being. Length of time was defined as the number of years families provided care to an elderly parent. Family well-being was measured by forming a composite score that combined several scores on different measures. The score reflected outcomes of family process in terms of the individuals' perceptions of family health, their satisfaction with the family's functioning, and perceived health and well-being. In addition, a positive correlation ($r = 0.25$) was found between internal family resources and family well-being. The stronger the sense of internal strengths and ability to work together in solving problems, the higher the increase in family well-being.

## USING STATISTICS TO TEST FOR DIFFERENCES

### t-Test

The **t-test** is an inferential statistical procedure used to determine whether the means of two groups are significantly different. If the sample means are far enough apart, the t-test will yield a significant difference, allowing the researcher to conclude that the two groups do not have the same mean. For example, suppose a researcher wanted to know if patients who had open heart surgery using the internal mammary artery as a graft had more chest pain postoperatively than those using the saphenous vein as a graft. The variable chest pain is measured on a ratio scale using the visual analogue scale (VAS) (see Chapter 9). An example of data from five subjects might look like the following.

Based on the group means, it appears that the five patients who had a saphenous

| Group 1<br>Internal Mammary Artery Graft | Group 2<br>Saphenous Vein Graft |
|:---:|:---:|
| 4 | 6 |
| 3 | 5 |
| 5 | 8 |
| 6 | 7 |
| 8 | 10 |
| $\Sigma X = 26$ | $\Sigma X = 36$ |
| $\overline{X}_1 = 5.2$ | $\overline{X}_2 = 7.2$ |

vein graft had more intense chest pain postoperatively ($\overline{X}$ = 7.2 versus $\overline{X}$ = 5.2). Both sample means provide the best estimate of the two population means. Some amount of error is inevitable because the means of 7.2 and 5.2 correspond to samples. The statistical question becomes: Is the difference between the two sample means large enough for the researcher to conclude that the population means are different from one another? The t-test will answer this question.

### Assumptions

Assumptions associated with the t-test include those associated with parametric procedures. In addition, both groups must have similar variances with respect to the dependent variable. This is related to the assumption implied by the null hypothesis that the groups are from a single population. This assumption is referred to as **homogeneity of variance.**

### Forms of the t-Test

Several forms of the t-test exist. Researchers use the independent t-test when scores in one group have no logical relationship with scores in the other group. Researchers refer to an independent t-test as the pooled t-test, when comparing two independent groups and the four assumptions have been met. If the variances of the groups are significantly different (violation of the assumption of homogeneity of variance), the t-test is calculated using the separate t-test, which takes into account the fact that the variances are not equal; it is a more conservative measure.

Excerpt 10.7 reports the results of seven t-tests. Each t-test compared group means on seven variables. The mean prepregnancy weight of group 1 (135.69) was compared with the mean prepregnancy weight of group 2 (129.81). Group 1 comprised those primigravidas who increased their prepregnant weight by 25 percent or less. Group 2 comprised those primigravidas who increased their prepregnant weight by more than 25 percent. The asterisk and footnote at the bottom of the table indicate that a statistically significant difference was found between the prepregancy weights of group 1 and group 2. There was also a statistically significant difference in percent of weight gain between groups 1 and 2 (20.60 percent and 33.21 percent, respectively). Those in group 2 had a higher percent of weight gain than those in group 1. No significant differences were found between groups 1 and 2 on the variables age, gestation, height, delivery weight, and birth weight (p:0.05).

The second form of the t-test is the dependent t-test, also called the correlated t-test, matched t-test, or t-test for paired comparisons. This is an appropriate test for situations in which scores in the first group can be paired with a score in the second group. The classic example is a pretest-posttest design, in which a single group of subjects is measured twice. An example of a correlated t-test is the two-group study that matches subjects. Excerpt 10.8 displays another situation in which a logical relationship occurs between scores in both groups: husband and wife responses. The purpose of this study was to determine if there were differences in the levels of adjustment, support, symptom distress, hopelessness, and uncertainty reported by women and their spouses during the recurrent phase of breast cancer. A significant

**EXCERPT 10.7**

## USE OF SEVERAL t-TESTS IN ONE TABLE

**Means, Standard Deviations, and t-Tests of Demographic Characteristics by Group**

| Variables | Group 1 | Group 2 | t value | p |
|---|---|---|---|---|
| | Mean [SD] | Mean [SD] | | |
| Age (years) | 25.75  (4.83) | 25.83  (4.81) | −0.08 | 0.94 |
| Gestation (weeks) | 38.85  (1.20) | 39.27  (1.16) | −1.83 | 0.07 |
| Height (inches) | 64.61  (2.22) | 64.73  (2.42) | −0.25 | 0.80 |
| Prepregnancy weight (lbs) | 135.69 (15.43) | 129.81 (14.83) | 1.98 | 0.05* |
| Delivery weight (lbs) | 163.69  (18.3) | 172.71 (21.25) | −2.33 | 0.09 |
| Percent of weight gain | 20.60  (3.52) | 33.21  (5.45) | −14.02 | 0.001* |
| Birth weight (grams) | 3,266 [351.54] | 3,384 [327.47] | −1.77 | 0.08 |

*Denotes statistically significant variables between groups.

Source: Purfield, P, and Morin, K: Excessive weight gain in primigravidas with low-risk pregnancy: Selected obstetric consequences. J Obstet Gynecol Neonat Nurs 24:434, 1995, with permission.

difference was found between levels of uncertainty about the illness, with husbands reporting significantly more uncertainty (M = 84.2 versus 80.0) than their wives. Women also, in contrast to their husbands, reported higher levels of social support (M = 98.6 versus 91.9). On the adjustment measure, significant differences were found between women's and husband's levels of emotional distress, with women reporting more distress (M = 0.50 versus 0.38) than their husbands.

When reading journal articles, the researcher never has to know how to calculate the various forms of the t-test or use a t table to determine whether a significant difference exists. In Excerpts 10.8 and 10.9, there is a column labeled p. The actual probability of each test can be evaluated. If the probability level is 0.5 or less (p<0.05), there is a statistically significant difference between the two means. In some instances, the researcher will not report the actual probability level, only that the p<0.05. Munro[2] reviews the calculation of the t-test.

## Analysis of Variance

**Analysis of variance (ANOVA)** is an inferential procedure used to determine whether there is a significant difference among three or more group means. The difference between the t-test and ANOVA is the number of groups being compared. A simple, or one-way, ANOVA refers to one independent variable with several levels. For example, the variable nursing specialty can be defined as having three levels (i.e., pediatric nursing, community-health nursing, medical-surgical nursing). A two-way ANOVA represents two independent variables with several levels.

### Assumptions

Assumptions associated with ANOVA include those associated with parametric procedures, including homogeneity of variance. In ANOVA, the independent

**EXCERPT 10.8**

## DISPLAY OF SIX PAIRED t-TESTS

**Comparison of Women's and Husband's Scores on the Major Study Variables (n = 74 couples)**

| Variable | Women | Husband | Paired t | p |
|---|---|---|---|---|
| Uncertainty (MUIS)[a] | | | | |
| M, SD | 80.0 (16.9) | 84.2 (15.7) | 2.08 | <.05 |
| Range | 43–148 | 41–121 | | |
| Hopelessness (HS) | | | | |
| M, SD | 3.5 (3.4) | 3.8 (3.7) | .59 | .56 |
| Range | 0–16 | 0–17 | | |
| Social Support (SSQ)[b] | | | | |
| M, SD | 98.6 (11.3) | 91.9 (10.6) | 4.01 | <.001 |
| Range | 73–120 | 69–114 | | |
| Symptom Distress (SDS) | | | | |
| M, SD | 25.0 (8.2) | 26.0 (7.9) | 1.45 | .15 |
| Range | 13–48 | 13–46 | | |
| Emotional Distress (BSI) | | | | |
| M, SD | .50 (.33) | .38 (.36) | 2.50 | <.02 |
| Range | .02–2.3 | 0–1.5 | | |
| Role Adjustment (PAIS) | | | | |
| M, SD | 30.0 (15.8) | 27.2 (160) | 1.31 | .19 |
| Range | 4–73 | 5–68 | | |

[a] Scores obtained on a modified version of the MUIS.
[b] Scores obtained on a modified version of the SSQ.
*Source: Northouse, LL, Laten, D, and Reddy, P: Adjustment of women and their husbands to recurrent breast cancer. Res Nurs Health 18:515, 1995, with permission.*

variable must be measured on a nominal scale. In some instances, the researcher will recode a continuous variable like age into several categories (i.e., 13 to 19, 20 to 26, and 27 to 33).

Most standard parametric statistical procedures (i.e., t-test and ANOVA) list fairly restrictive assumptions that are required to be met if the chosen statistical test is to be valid. A statistical procedure that is appropriate even when its assumptions have

**EXCERPT 10.9**

## ANOVA SUMMARY TABLE WITHOUT SS

**Analysis of Variance Summary for Anxiety**

| Source | df | MS | F | p |
|---|---|---|---|---|
| Between groups | 2 | 3.85 | 0.56 | .58 |
| Within groups | 43 | 6.91 | | |
| Total | 45 | | | |

*Source: Gaberson, KB: The effect of humorous and musical distraction on preoperative anxiety. AORN J 62:784, 1995, with permission.*

been violated is said to be **robust,** or thought of as a robust statistic. It is not uncommon for researchers to use parametric procedures for data that are measured on an ordinal scale or data that violate the assumption of normality. The degree of risk depends on how severely the assumptions are broken. It is probably safe to use parametric procedures to analyze ordinal data with roughly equal unit sizes, but these procedures are not reasonable to use for nominal data.

### Concept of Variance

In ANOVA, variation is examined to determine whether between-group variance is greater than within-group variance. In conducting ANOVA, both types of variation (between-group and within-group) add up to total variation. Scores within each group vary among one another from the group means and are termed within-group variance. The distance among group means is called between-group variance. If the between-group variance is larger than the within-group variance, scores in the different groups are far enough apart for a researcher to conclude that the group means are significantly different. If the between-group variance is smaller than, or about the same as, the within-group variance, the group means are not significantly different. The F-statistic is a three- or four-digit number that indicates the size of the difference between the groups, relative to the size of the variation within each group. The larger the F-statistic (greater between-group variance), the greater the probability of finding a statistically significant difference among the group means.

Results of an ANOVA are presented in an ANOVA summary (Table 10.1). Table 10.1 has five columns: Source (source of variation), SS (sums of squares), df (degrees of freedom), MS (mean square), and F (F-statistic).[1,3] Refer to Munro[2] for calculation of the ANOVA.

The most important number in the entire ANOVA summary is the single value in the F column. The F value is calculated by dividing the MS associated with between-group variance by the MS associated with within-group variance (27.8 divided by 1.2 = 23.16). As displayed in the table, if a significant difference among the sample means is found, an asterisk next to the calculated F value indicates significance. As in the t-test, the researcher never has to know how to calculate an ANOVA summary. The actual probability of the ANOVA can be evaluated by examining the probability level. If the probability is 0.05 or less ($p < 0.05$), there is a statistically significant difference among the means. In some instances, the researcher reports not the actual probability level but rather that $p < 0.05$.

TABLE 10–1  ANOVA SUMMARY TABLE

| Source | SS | df | MS | F |
|--------|------|----|------|--------|
| Between | 55.6 | 2 | 27.8 | 23.16* |
| Within | 14.4 | 12 | 1.2 | |
| Total | 70.0 | 14 | | |

*$p < 0.05$.*

The summary table in Excerpt 10.9 is similar to the table in Excerpt 10.2, except that there is no SS column. In this study, the author investigated the effect of humorous distraction on preoperative anxiety. The dependent variable was preoperative anxiety measured by a VAS. Subjects were assigned to one of three groups. The first group was exposed to a 20-minute audiotaped comedy routine. The second group was exposed to a 20-minute audiotape of slow, quiet instrumental music. The third group was a control group. A one-way ANOVA revealed no significant differences among the three group means (F = 0.56, df = 2/43, p = 0.58).

## NONPARAMETRIC STATISTICAL TESTS

### Chi-Square

**Chi-square** analysis is the most commonly reported nonparametric statistic that compares the frequency of an observed occurrence (actual number in each category) with the frequency of an expected occurrence (based on theory or past experience). The chi-square statistic is the appropriate test when variables are measured on a nominal scale and the researcher counts the number of items in each category.

### Assumptions

Assumptions associated with chi-square analyses include the use of frequency data, categories that are mutually exclusive, and a theoretical basis for categorization of variables. Chi-square analyses use nominal (categorical) data. Frequency data represent the actual number of subjects or elements in each category. The chi-square test compares counts, not means. Data that are not normally distributed and that violate the assumptions underlying parametric statistics can be categorized to use the chi-square statistic. Each category is mutually exclusive when subjects are assigned to one category. Theoretical reasons for categorizing variables ensure that the analysis will be meaningful and prevent the researcher from having to recategorize subjects to find relationships between variables. Research questions and methods for analysis are established prior to data collection.

### TYPES OF CHI-SQUARE TESTS

The two types of chi-square tests are the one-sample and the independent samples tests. The one-sample test is used when a researcher is interested in the number of responses, objects, or subjects that fall into two or more categories. This type of chi-square test compares the set of observed frequencies with the corresponding set of theoretical frequencies that define a specific distribution. This type of test is called a "goodness-of-fit" test. If the two sets of frequencies differ by an amount that can be attributable to sampling error, then there is said to be a "good fit" between the observed data and what would be expected. If sampling error cannot adequately explain the discrepancies between the observed and expected frequencies, then a "bad fit" is said to exist, with a significant difference between the two.[3] For example, a researcher might compare the number of cesarean sections in a local community hospital (observed frequencies) with reported national rates for all community hospitals (theoretical norms). In this example, use of the one-sample chi-square is appropriate.

The independent samples chi-square test is used to determine if two categorical variables are independent of one another. Tests of independence examine the extent of association or relationship between two categorical variables. Researchers frequently compare two or more samples on a categorical response variable. Because the response variable can be composed of two or more categories, there are several options to which the independent samples chi-square test can be applied.

The independent samples chi-square test is calculated with frequency data tabulated in a series of rows and columns called a contingency table. Figure 10.4 illustrates a $2 \times 2$ contingency table (two rows and two columns). Each frequency tabulated in the table must be independent and must represent a different individual or unit of observation classified according to two variables. For example, a researcher might want to know if there is a relationship between type of dietary instruction and fasting blood glucose levels. Data from two groups of individuals with diabetes (experimental and control groups) are cross-tabulated with average fasting blood glucose levels. Blood glucose levels can be measured on an interval-ratio scale. Use of chi-square analyses require that data be tabulated as frequencies. In this example, blood glucose levels are recoded into two categories: less than and greater than the upper limit of normal blood glucose values (Figure 10.4). The independent samples chi-square test can also be used for a larger number of rows or

|  | Average Blood Glucose Levels less than 120 mg/dL | Average Blood Glucose Levels greater than 120 mg/dL |
|---|---|---|
| **Experimental Group:** 6 sessions with the RD to review meal planning |  |  |
| **Control Group:** Customary patient education |  |  |

FIGURE 10.4 $2\times2$ contingency table.

EXCERPT 10.10

## REPORTING RESULTS OF CHI-SQUARE TESTS IN TABLE

**Sociodemographic Differences Between Men and Women**

| | Men (n = 77) | | Women (n = 50) | | | |
|---|---|---|---|---|---|---|
| | *M* | *SD* | *M* | *SD* | *Statistic* | *p* |
| Age | 34.5 | 7.8 | 30.5 | 7.6 | $t = -2.89$ | <.01 |
| Socioeconomic status | 38.33 | 15.25 | 23.86 | 12.74 | $t = -5.56$ | <.01 |
| | *No. (%)* | | *No. (%)* | | | |
| Race | | | | | $X^2 = 8.30$ | .01 |
|   Caucasian | 59 (76.6) | | 26 (52.0) | | | |
|   Afro-American,Hispanic | 18 (23.4) | | 24 (48.0) | | | |
| Education | | | | | $X^2 = 26.01$ | <.01 |
|   Graduate degree | 8 (10.4) | | 2 (4.0) | | | |
|   College graduate | 14 (18.2) | | 3 (6.0) | | | |
|   1–3 yrs college | 31 (40.3) | | 10 (20.0) | | | |
|   High school graduate | 18 (23.4) | | 14 (28.0) | | | |
|   7th–11th grade | 6 (7.7) | | 21 (42.0) | | | |
| Source of HIV infection | | | | | $X^2 = 76.15$ | <.001 |
|   Gay/bisexual contacts | 54 (70.1) | | 0 | | | |
|   Heterosexual contacts | 3 (3.9) | | 31 (62.0) | | | |
|   Blood transfusions | 4 (5.2) | | 7 (14.0) | | | |
|   Intravenous drug use | 16 (20.8) | | 12 (24.0) | | | |

*Source: Anderson, SE: Personality, appraisal, and adaptational outcomes in HIV seropositive men and women. Res Nurs Health 18:303, 1995, with permission.*

columns (e.g., $2 \times 3$, $3 \times 4$, $5 \times 6$, $7 \times 7$). Refer to Munro[2] for calculation of the chi-square statistic.

As with other statistical procedures, the actual probability associated with the chi-square is evaluated to determine if there is a statistically significant difference. It is often difficult for the reader to know what the actual computed expected cell frequencies are, as these data are not usually reported in tables. Excerpt 10.10 illustrates one format for presenting the independent samples chi-square test. Researchers actually displayed the observed frequencies for three variables (e.g., race, education, and source of HIV infection). Results of the chi-square analyses indicated that a greater proportion of men had gay/bisexual contacts as their source of infection. In addition, women were younger (note results of t-test analysis) and less educated (note results of chi-square analysis).

## QUESTIONS TO CONSIDER WHEN CRITIQUING DESCRIPTIVE AND/OR INFERENTIAL STATISTICS

Identify a research study to critique. Read the study to see if you recognize any key terms discussed in this chapter. Remember that all studies may not contain all key

terms. The following questions[4] serve as a guide in critiquing descriptive and/or inferential statistics:

1. *Were appropriate descriptive statistics used?* Statistics used in descriptive research include measures of central tendency and measures of dispersion. Descriptive statistics summarize important features of numerical data and do not infer anything beyond the data.

2. *Are the reported descriptive statistics appropriate to the level of measurement for each variable?* Remember that nominal and ordinal data can be described by frequency counts; interval/ratio data can be added or subtracted. Tests of statistical inference that require mathematical manipulation should be applied only to variables on the interval/ratio scale. Because ordinal data occur frequently in the behavioral and social sciences, many researchers believe that psychological scales approximate equal intervals fairly well, with results providing satisfactory and useful information.[5,6]

3. *Were appropriate statistics used to answer the research questions or test study hypotheses?* Statistics can be categorized by the purposes for which they are used. As described in this chapter, the function of some statistics is to describe a set of data (using statistics to describe); others are used to examine relationships between or among sets of data (using statistics to examine relationships), and still others are used to detect whether differences exist between groups of data (using statistics to test for differences). Do not get stuck on various statistics reported in research studies. If a particular statistical technique is unfamiliar, look it up a text, or ask a friend or colleague. If tables are used in the research report, look over the data (i.e., raw scores sometimes reported as totals, averages, ranges, frequencies, or standard deviations), and identify if the author has described the findings within the text.

4. *Is the sample size adequate?* Power analyses are used to identify appropriate sample sizes based on the type of statistical analyses performed. Other nursing research textbooks describe power analysis in more detail, but several pieces of information need to be available to readers of research reports. First, a clear explanation of how the sample size was derived needs to be provided. If the number of subjects imposes limitations on the study, these need to be stated.

5. *If tables were used in the research report, were results clearly and completely stated?* Look over the entire table before trying to absorb specific information contained in the table. All tables should be adequately referenced within the research report, with author(s) directing the reader's attention to particular sections of the table. Is the title of the table adequate in describing the content of the table? Have any of the numerical pieces of data within the table been subjected to statistical tests of significance? If so, are the results adequately marked and is appropriate information provided concerning how to interpret the results?

## SUMMARY OF KEY IDEAS

1. Descriptive statistics are used to summarize measures of central tendency (mean, median, mode) and dispersion (range, variance, standard deviation).
2. Inferential statistics focus on determining how likely it is that results based on a sample are the same that would be obtained for the population.
3. Researchers need to establish the level of measurement for data collected in order to select appropriate statistical procedures.
4. Parametric and nonparametric procedures are two types of statistical tests. Parametric procedures require assumptions to be met in order for statistical findings to be valid. Nonparametric procedures make no assumptions about the shape of the distribution and are often described as "distribution free."
5. Parametric statistical tests include Pearson correlations, the t-test, and ANOVA.
6. The Pearson r (Pearson Product-Moment Correlation) is a measure that defines the relationship or association between two variables.
7. The t-test is a parametric procedure that determines if there is a significant difference between two group means.
8. ANOVA is a parametric procedure that determines if there is a significant difference among three or more means.
9. Chi-square analysis is a nonparametric procedure used to assess whether a relationship exists between two categorical variables.
10. A statistical procedure that is appropriate even when the assumptions are violated is said to be robust.

## LEARNING ACTIVITIES

1. Using the data in Excerpt 10.2, write three or four sentences describing the sample characteristics using measures of central tendency (mean, median, mode) and measures of dispersion (range, variance, standard deviation).

2. As a researcher, collect data on marital status (measured as married or not married); family stress level (measured as low, moderate, and high); height (measured as inches); and satisfaction with care (measured as very satisfied, somewhat satisfied, somewhat dissatisfied, and very dissatisfied). Identify the appropriate measures of central tendency and dispersion for each of these variables.

T-TEST FOR LENGTH OF SECOND STAGE OF LABOR IN MINUTES BY WEIGHT GROUP

| Groups | n | M (in minutes) | SD | t value | p |
|--------|-----|----------------|-------|---------|-------|
| ≤25% | 50 | 72.42 | 46.69 | | |
| | | | | −2.05 | 0.02* |
| ≥25% | 46 | 93.28 | 52.87 | | |

*p<.05

3. Interpret the results of the following t-test. "Groups" refer to primigravidas who increased their prepregnant weight by 25 percent or less and those who increased their weight by 25 percent or greater.

4. Use the results in the table and write two or three sentences describing the findings.

## References

1. Burns, N, and Grove, SK: The Practice of Nursing Research: Conduct, Critique, and Utilization, ed 4. WB Saunders, Philadelphia, 2001, pp 499–567.
2. Munro, BH: Statistical Methods for Health Care Research, ed 4. Lippincott Williams & Wilkins, Philadelphia, 2000.
3. Huck, SW, and Cormier, WH: Reading Statistics and Research, ed 2. HarperCollins Publishers, New York, 1996.
4. LoBiondo-Wood, G, and Haber, J: Nursing Research: Methods, Critical Appraisal, and Utilization, ed 4. Mosby-Year Book, St. Louis, 1998, pp 365, 383.
5. Knapp, TR: Treating ordinal scales as interval scales: An attempt to resolve the controversy. Nurs Res 39:121, 1990.
6. Knapp, TR: Treating ordinal scales as ordinal scales. Nurs Res 42:184, 1993.

# Selecting a Research Design: Quantitative Versus Qualitative

Paula T. Lusardi, PhD, RN, CCRN, CCNS

## LEARNING OBJECTIVES

*At the end of this chapter, you will be able to:*

1. Understand the links among philosophy, theory, and research questions, with regard to selection of design.
2. Define and explain the purpose of research design.
3. Describe characteristics of a good research design.
4. Compare and contrast significant quantitative/qualitative aspects of research designs.
5. Understand a selected group of designs from both quantitative and qualitative perspectives.
6. Appreciate the process that underlies research design selection.

## GLOSSARY OF KEY TERMS

**Analytic epidemiological studies.** Studies concerned with testing hypotheses to determine if specific exposures are related to the presence or absence of specific diseases or disorders.

**Assumptions.** Statements that are believed to be true; usually based on a person's values and beliefs.

**Control.** Elements built into a design to reduce or eliminate interpretations of the cause of the results. These elements include the use of randomization, manipulation of experimental conditions, and use of comparison or control groups.

**Control group.** The group that does not receive the experimental treatment in an experiment.

**Descriptive epidemiological studies.** Studies concerned with the distribution and patterns of disease or disability in a population.

**Double-blinded study.** Treatment assignment (to either experimental or control group) is unknown to patients and health-care providers.

**Experimental group.** The group that receives the "new" treatment in an experiment.

**Extraneous variable.** Any variable that is not directly related to the purpose of the study but that may affect the dependent variable; sometimes termed intervening or confounding variables.

**Internal validity.** Refers to whether the independent variable made a difference.

**Paradigm.** Organizing framework that contains a set of assumptions or values that underlie how scientists view reality, truth, and research.

**Qualitative research.** Research directed at the discovery of meaning rather than cause and effect.

**Quantitative research.** Research directed at the discovery of relationships and cause and effect. Methods used are based on the scientific method of inquiry.

**Randomized clinical trial (RCT).** A prospective study evaluating the effectiveness of an intervention/treatment in a large sample of patients. Essential features of a clinical trial include use of an experimental and control group, randomization, blinding of patients and health-care providers, and sufficient sample sizes.

**Research design.** Set of guidelines by which a researcher obtains answers to questions.

**Single-blinded study.** Treatment assignment (to either experimental or control group) is unknown to patients.

A research design is a guide chosen by the researcher to answer questions or test hypotheses. Selection of an appropriate design compels the researcher to address critical issues to ensure that the data produced are credible and interpretable within a chosen perspective. The design is the crucial link connecting the researcher's framework and questions with resultant data. Core assumptions and level of inquiry guide the choice of design.[1,2] **Assumptions** are statements or principles that are taken as truth, based on a person's values and beliefs. In other words, how a researcher views reality guides the researcher's choice of questions and the resultant methodology.

Research designs are also a function of the level of knowledge development in the area of inquiry.[3,4] The level of inquiry at which research questions are stated corresponds with the level of sophistication of nursing knowledge concerning variables in a study. If little is known about a particular topic, an exploratory design is used. The focus is on describing and understanding a phenomenon. If the particular phenomenon is well defined and measured, a more structured design may be appropriate to answer research questions or test hypotheses.

Based on these assumptions, this chapter addresses the structure and selection of a research design, presenting contrasting quantitative and qualitative perspectives. Despite the simplicity of this quantitative-qualitative dialectic,[5,6] information presented assists the researcher in wading through the morass of issues tied to design selection.

## QUANTITATIVE VERSUS QUALITATIVE RESEARCH

The terms "quantitative" and "qualitative" are defined in a variety of ways. Researchers often define quantitative research as that which uses numbers to represent reality. **Quantitative research** is directed at the discovery of relationships and cause and effect. Methods used are based on the scientific method of inquiry (see Chapter 1). Quantitative refers to measurement and analysis of causal relationships between variables at a particular point in time. Inquiry is within a value-free context.[7,8]

**Qualitative research** is directed at the discovery of meaning rather than cause and effect. Qualitative research involves the use of language, concepts, and words rather than numbers to represent evidence from research. The word "qualitative" also implies an emphasis on process and meanings in context.[9] The focus is on the creation of social experience and emergent meanings, the relationship between participant and researcher, and the environmental issues that may shape inquiry. Process and meaning are not measured but may be described in terms of intensity, patterning, and frequency.[10]

Quantitative and qualitative research also refer to a researcher's world view, or paradigm. Although defined in several ways, a **paradigm** is an organizing framework that contains a set of assumptions or values that underlie how scientists view reality, truth, and research.[11,12] Within the quantitative-qualitative perspectives, these views are profoundly different.

## QUANTITATIVE AND QUALITATIVE APPROACHES TO DESIGN SELECTION

Assumptions underlying quantitative and qualitative paradigms reveal divergent views of reality. Derived from material by Denzin and Lincoln,[10] Guba and Lincoln,[13] Leininger,[14] and Munhall and Boyd,[15] Table 11.1 presents major quantitative and qualitative contrasts emerging from the nature of reality, view of humans, root source of knowledge, and subsequent research orientation. Review this table and classify your own beliefs.

Researchers often believe in the predominance of one paradigm over another. Depending on whether they emerge from a quantitative or a qualitative perspective, researchers may ask questions in significantly different ways. Belief in the elements of a quantitative perspective would direct the researcher to ask questions focused on relationships among variables, with an outcome orientation. In this case, a resulting design would be more structured. Belief in the characteristics that compose a qualitative paradigm would guide the researcher toward process-oriented exploratory questions. A more flexible design is more appropriate here.

For example, nurses might ask significantly different questions to research postoperative pain management, depending on their perspective. From a quantitative perspective, pain is viewed as a single reality, one that can be captured objectively. The nurse might ask questions focused on the pain as well as its relationship to other variables such as preoperative teaching and amount of pain medication used by the patient. Measurement of pain and related variables at specified times might be the focus of these questions. The nurse might ask, "What is the relationship among timing of pain medication, amount of medication, and pain relief (as measured by a visual analogue scale) in a postoperative population?"

TABLE 11.1 NATURE OF REALITY AND THE CONDUCT OF RESEARCH: QUANTITATIVE VERSUS QUALITATIVE

| Quantitative | Qualitative |
|---|---|
| *Nature of Reality* ||
| Reality obtainable in objective terms | Social construction of reality |
| Single reality | Multiple realities |
| Parts separate and manipulable | Parts interrelated |
| Variables independent of each other | Variables dependent on each other |
| Context free and objective | Context interrelated and subjective |
| Narrow in scope | Broad, inclusive in scope |
| *View of Humans* ||
| Human data collected is objective | Subjective data |
| Human is made of parts | Holistic view |
| *Root Source of Knowledge* ||
| Logical positivism and empiricism | Research traditions: Anthropology Social psychology Philosophy |
| Use of observation | Intuition, Gestalt |
| Psychological and biophysical facts | Social interactions, values, culture |
| *Orientation of Research* ||
| Outcome, product-oriented | Process, phenomena, person-oriented |

Quantitative design is structured so that measurement and testing are prominent characteristics. Research emerging from this perspective centers on explanation, verification of facts, testing of theoretical relationships, and prediction of events.

From a qualitative perspective, the nurse would consider the patient an active participant in a socially constructed context. Many realities might exist for this patient regarding the pain experience. The nurse would be interested in discovering how the patient is encountering the pain experience. Research is process-oriented, with a focus on the patient's perspective of the pain experience in a social context. The nurse might ask, "What is the lived experience of the pain experience for the postoperative patient?" The design is flexible, to capture social and thinking processes. Research emerging from this perspective could center on understanding from the patient's viewpoint, discovery of social processes, and description of happenings.

## What is a Research Design?

A **research design** is a flexible set of guidelines by which a researcher obtains answers to inquiries. The research design answers the question: "What is the best approach to answer my research question in order to provide the most accurate and interpretable data?"

Research designs may be defined from a broad or narrow perspective. From a broad perspective, the design suggests approaches for observation and analysis but does not specifically tell the researcher what to do. Researchers regard design as the total strategy for the investigation, connecting theoretical perspective and problem identification with data collection and analysis. From a limited perspective, researchers consider design as a precisely conceived blueprint that brings empirical evidence to bear on the research problem. It provides methodological direction, such as sampling and random assignment.

In addition, research designs are also characterized from a quantitative and qualitative perspective. Historically, research designs were addressed from a quantitative perspective and were often associated with the term "experimental."[16,17] Quantitative and qualitative research designs have specific purposes. The purpose of quantitative research designs is to provide guidance to test theory and validate information.[18] The purpose of qualitative research designs es is to establish a thorough description of social life.[15,19] Additionally, these approaches sensitize others to social experiences, develop concepts and theory, and strengthen instrument development.[20]

A research design is a general, nonspecific approach to a particular study or precise question. Specifics constitute the specific plan. Just as a soccer player must link general rules of the game to a specific strategy of play, the research design guides the researcher's specific plan. The researcher's plan includes specification of procedures or strategies, such as site selection, selection of essential instruments, timing and types of observations, sampling techniques, and data analysis.

## Characteristics of a Research Design

Specification of a research design allows the researcher to make judgments about the adequacy of a design for answering questions or testing hypotheses. The ability to judge the adequacy of a research design is grounded in specific characteristics. Specified properties lay the basis of design structure and are evident in the design (Table 11.2).

Elements of a research design are a function of two assumptions. First, evidence of the fit between a researcher's paradigm and the data produced is essential. Additionally, characteristics of design should reflect the level of knowledge in the area of inquiry. Although there is general agreement on the essential characteristics of design, the significance of particular attributes are often weighted differently, depending on the researcher's philosophical perspective and purpose of research. Researchers from diverse paradigms often define characteristics differently or emphasize the importance of one characteristic over another. Consequently, the following discussion views design characteristics on a continuum, with quantitative emphasis on one end and qualitative on the other.

### Design as a Function of Philosophy, Theory, and Question Fit

A design is a function of the interrelationship among a researcher's philosophical perspective, theory, and question (Table 11.3). Early in the research process,

---

TABLE 11.2 CHARACTERISTICS OF A RESEARCH DESIGN

Philosophy, theory, question, design fit
Level of concept and knowledge development
Study purpose/focus
Structure and control of phenomena being investigated
Trustworthiness of findings
Researcher involvement with the subjects or participants

---

philosophical assumptions and theoretical approaches are addressed and questions are developed. This process guides the choice of design. The linkage among theory, question, and design should be evident in a research study.[2,12] For instance, a design from a quantitative perspective may be oriented to measurement and explanation of relationships among variables,[8,19,21] whereas a qualitative approach may reveal exploration, description, and understanding.[13-15] Consequently, the assumptions that underlie the researcher's perspective will guide both the questions asked and the guiding theoretical perspective (if one is stated).[1]

### Design as a Function of Knowledge Advancement, Concept Development, and Research Question

Design is also a function of the level of concept development and knowledge development in the area of inquiry (Table 11.4). Questions emerge from this foundation.[3,4,22,23] Linkages among level of knowledge, concept development, and questions asked should be evident. For instance, if theoretical and empirical work may have accumulated in an area of inquiry, then concepts may be more fully developed or measured, and questions might be those of testing and verification.[7,24] The researcher is concerned with the measurement of phenomena and the relationships among variables in the area of inquiry. If theory testing is a priority, a correlational or experimental design may be possible and appropriate. If little is known about the phenomena,[25] the appropriate question is one of discovery.[7,15,24] The researcher is then concerned with the meaning and understanding of phenomena in the area of inquiry.[23] Theory may be used as a guide. If theory development is a priority, then the design will be descriptive or exploratory.

### Design as a Function of Study, Purpose, or Focus

The purpose, or focus, of the research study is reflected in the design. The purpose, closely linked to philosophical perspectives, is manifested in study focus, questions

---

TABLE 11.3 CHARACTERISTICS OF DESIGN: PHILOSOPHY, THEORY, QUESTION, DESIGN FIT

| Quantitative | Qualitative |
| --- | --- |
| **Often little emphasis on philosophy** | **Emphasis on philosophical bases** |
| Theory developed a priori | Theory developed initially or during study |
| Emphasis on theory-question link | Emphasis on philosophy-theory-question link |
| Theory testing | Theory as a guide |

TABLE 11.4 LEVEL OF CONCEPT AND KNOWLEDGE DEVELOPMENT

| Quantitative | Qualitative |
|---|---|
| Comprehensive level of knowledge of phenomenon | Less knowledge of phenomenon |
| Measurement of concepts evident | No measurement of concepts |
| Often precise in measurement; usually not much rich description | Rich description |

asked, and type of data sought (Table 11.5). If the purpose of the study is to explain relationships among variables or predict happening from the objective facts, the design should be quantitatively oriented. If the study proposes to understand and describe subjective meaning from the participant's perspective, the design should be more loosely structured and qualitatively oriented.

## Design as a Function of Control of Phenomena Investigated

Designs are created with varying amounts of control. **Control** refers to those elements built into a research design to reduce or eliminate interpretations of the cause of results. These elements include use of randomization and of comparison or control groups and manipulation of experimental conditions. The more control demanded by the inquiry, the more highly structured the design (e.g., experimental designs). The less control desired, the less structured the design (e.g., field studies) (Table 11.6).

Control in quantitative work is important. Quantitative researchers focus on determining the true relationship between independent and dependent variables. Making solid linkages among variables and ruling out alternative explanations to a causal interpretation is crucial.[26] The design is structured to keep variation at a minimum through such techniques as homogeneity of sample and controlled environment. The research design guides strategies that ensure results that reflect the relationship among studied variables rather than the impact of unwanted influences.

TABLE 11.5 RESEARCH PURPOSE/GOAL

| Quantitative | Qualitative |
|---|---|
| *Study Purpose* | |
| Develop explanation and prediction from "facts" | Develop understanding and meaning from participants |
| *Study Focus* | |
| Objects, subjects, cases | Participants, informants, other people |
| *Types of Data Sought* | |
| Objective; exclusive | Subjective/some objective; inclusive |

TABLE 11.6 STRUCTURE AND CONTROL OF THE SITUATION

| Quantitative | Qualitative |
| --- | --- |
| Control important | Control unimportant |
| Measured variables | Description of phenomena |
| Ruling out alternative explanations and controlling error | Inclusive understanding |
| Experimental designs | Exploratory designs |

The concept of control in a qualitative work has little significance. Researchers are intrigued by participants' understanding of their life experiences in a social context. Research design is flexible in order to attain an inclusive understanding of particular phenomena in a naturalistic setting over time.

### Design as a Function of Trustworthiness of Findings

Trustworthiness is the internal validity or credibility of findings. Trustworthiness of findings answers the questions: "Can persons believe the results of this study?" and "Are the data valid and reasonable?" Many factors related to research can be biased, including the researcher, participants, measurement tools, sampling techniques, data collection procedures, and/or data analysis. Quantitative and qualitative research have strategies that control threats to credibility (bias) in order to produce trustworthy data (Table 11.7).

Quantitative designs focus on internal validity. **Internal validity** refers to solid linkages among variables that rule out alternative explanations.[1] Quantitative designs guide sampling and issues of control to ensure that all groups are equal at the onset of the study to minimize influence of other variables. A discussion of internal validity is presented later in this chapter. Qualitative designs focus on the trustworthiness of participants' responses. Although several factors are important in establishing the trustworthiness of findings (e.g., credibility, fittingness, adaptability, confirmability), credibility of participants' responses lays the foundation for validity.[13,20,27] Guided by design selection, three dominant activities increase the probability that credible findings are produced: prolonged engagement with participants, persistent observation, and triangulation of data sources.[20]

TABLE 11.7 TRUSTWORTHINESS OF FINDINGS

| Quantitative | Qualitative |
| --- | --- |
| Internal validity | Credibility |
| Link among variables; "hard" objective substantiation; internal validity indicators | Function of participants' confirmation completeness of information; researcher's self-reflection |
| Statistical significance, which enables generalizability | Generalizability not an aim of research |

*Design as a Function of Researcher Involvement with Subjects or Participants*

The type of design assumes a specific relationship between the researcher and study subjects or participants. The role of the researcher is often on a continuum, ranging from observer of subjects to participant with informants.[28] In a quantitative approach, researcher involvement is usually as an objective observer, maintaining distance from the research subjects. Objective data are collected with one or more instruments. In a qualitative approach, the researcher is involved as a participant observer. As an insider, the researcher becomes involved with participants in order to understand a problem or situation from the participant's perspective. Often, the researcher is considered the research instrument (Table 11.8).

## CLASSIFICATION OF RESEARCH DESIGNS

Research designs are classified from various perspectives: experimental versus nonexperimental,[18] extent to which variance is controlled,[8] extent to which knowledge is known in the area of inquiry,[3,29] field versus laboratory designs,[18,26] discovery (process) versus verification (outcome),[15,24,30] and deductive versus inductive.[7,31] However, a supposition of this discussion is that research designs may also be classified as quantitative or qualitative. Despite the simplicity of approach, the structure of a research design can be thought of as a continuum. Research designs include elements that reflect quantitative or qualitative viewpoints (Table 11.9). This classification is neither mutually exclusive nor exhaustive.

For example, quantitative designs develop from a strong theoretical base, emerge from questions regarding explanation and relationships between and among variables, and generally derive from evolving knowledge in the area of inquiry. Qualitative approaches emerge from a strong research tradition and perhaps theoretical base, evolve from questions about understanding and description of phenomena, and generally emerge from evolving knowledge.

Consequently, quantitative designs focus on approaches that emphasize explanations of variables, verification of data, measuring variables, use of instruments for data collection, statistical significance, and internal validity.[7] Qualitative designs emphasize understanding social action, discovery of information, meaning of concepts, participatory involvement of researcher as a means of data

---

TABLE 11.8  RESEARCHER/PARTICIPANT RELATIONSHIP

| **Quantitative** | **Qualitative** |
|---|---|
| Little involvement; observer; detachment from subject; outsider perspective | Participant; participant-observer; involved; insider perspective |
| *Tools (Instruments) for Investigation* | |
| Questionnaires; structured interviews; psychometrically sound instruments | "Tool" is usually the researcher; uses variety of sources to collect data |

collection, and trustworthiness of findings as corroborated by the participants in the research.

## Quantitative Designs

Quantitative designs are approaches used to verify data through prescriptive testing, hypothesis testing, correlation, and sometimes description. These designs manifest varying amounts of control over phenomena and error, beginning with the most highly controlled designs and moving to more flexible designs.[3,4]

The more highly controlled designs emphasize causal relationships, whereas the more flexible designs emphasize relationships among variables or variable description. Brink and Woods[3] put experimental or quasiexperimental designs at the highest level and sometimes refer to these designs as level III. "Why" questions guide design selection at this level. Correlational designs are sometimes called level II designs, and they focus on questions of relationships among variables to guide design selection. Finally, exploratory or descriptive designs (level I) ask the question "What is . . .?" or "What are . . .?"

### Experimental and Quasiexperimental Designs

Experimental designs are classified as either true experimental or quasiexperimental.[18] Experimental and quasiexperimental designs have several common characteristics. Both approaches require a robust scientific and theoretical base, a significant level of control, and measurement of concepts using valid and reliable instruments. Most important, both research designs require manipulation of the independent variable, with this manipulation effect being measured on the dependent variable. Although random assignment and a control group are essential for the true experimental design, these characteristics are not required for quasiexperimental designs.

#### TRUE EXPERIMENTAL DESIGN

A true experimental design is an experiment in which the researcher tries to assess whether an intervention or treatment (independent variable) makes a difference in a measured outcome (dependent variable). Designed to answer questions that "test" theory and assess causal relationships, three essential elements must be present:

---

TABLE 11.9 DESIGN STRUCTURE AS A FUNCTION OF QUANTITATIVE-QUALITATIVE DIMENSIONS

| Quantitative Dimension | Qualitative Dimension |
|---|---|
| Strong theoretical base | Strong philosophical perspective |
| Explanation among variables | Understanding of human action |
| Objective approach to phenomena | Subjective approach |
| Measurement of variables | Meaning of concepts |
| Precision in measurement | Description of phenomena |
| Control of error: internal validity | Trustworthiness of findings |

---

control, random assignment, and manipulation of the independent variable. Consequently, subjects are randomly assigned to either an experimental or a control group. Comparisons are made between the **experimental group** (those who receive the experimental intervention) and the **control group** (those who do not receive this intervention). The outcome is measured by the effect on the dependent variable.

The essence of an experiment is the abiity of the researcher to manipulate and control variables so that rival hypotheses are ruled out as possible explanations for the observed reponse. An **extraneous variable** (sometimes called intervening or confounding variable) is any variable that is not directly related to the purpose of the study but that may affect the dependent variable. Extraneous variables can be external factors emerging from the environment and the experiment or internal factors that represent personal characteristics of the subjects of the study. When extraneous variables are not controlled, they exert a confounding influence on the independent variable in such a way that their separate effects are obscured.

For example, a researcher is concerned about patients' pain relief after surgery and wonders if there is a better way to treat postoperative pain. Theory-based research suggests that patients have better pain control if they receive 2 to 4 mg of morphine sulfate intravenously (IV) every 1 to 2 hours. Patients in a particular unit have traditionally been given 5 to 8 mg of morphine sulfate intramuscularly (IM) every 3 to 4 hours, as needed. The question is raised, "Will there be a difference in patients' pain relief if some patients receive the traditional method (5 to 8 mg morphine IM every 3 to 4 hours) and others receive the research-based approach of 2 to 4 mg of morphine IV every 1 to 2 hours. Pain is measured on a visual analogue scale of 0 to 10. Theory, level of research knowledge, and mode of inquiry dictate an experimental design. Patients are randomly assigned to a control group (the group receiving the traditional medication regimen) or an experimental group (the group receiving the new or experimental intervention). The only difference between these two groups is the difference in the administration of pain medication.

In this example, control over extraneous influences has been achieved by creating control and experimental groups and randomly assigning patients to each group. The independent variable was manipulated through use of an experimental intervention. The hypothesis in this research predicts (based on theory and research) which of the two types of pain interventions will give "better" pain relief.

Campbell and Stanley[18] identify three basic true experimental designs. The classic pretest-posttest control group design is one of the most commonly observed in the literature. The design is shown diagrammatically in Figure 11.1. Pretesting provides the researcher with information about the similarity of experimental and control groups on measures of the dependent variable before the independent variable is introduced.

The pretest-posttest control group design is sometimes referred to as a "before-and-after" design. Schaffner[32] used this type of design to determine the effects of maternal voice audiotape on the behavior and parasympathetic tone of 3- to 5-year-old children experiencing short-stay surgery. Children were randomly assigned to a maternal audiotape group, a children's story tape group, or no-story (control) group. Children's behaviors and responses were measured before and after tapes.

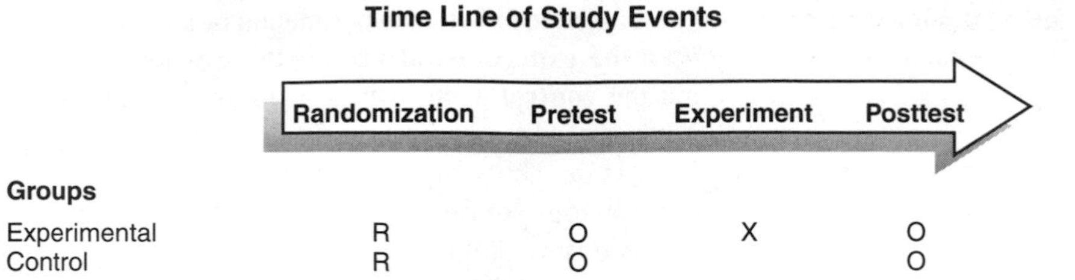

**Time Line of Study Events**

| | Randomization | Pretest | Experiment | Posttest |
|---|---|---|---|---|
| **Groups** | | | | |
| Experimental | R | O | X | O |
| Control | R | O | | O |

O = dependent variable measurement
X = application of the independent variable
R = random assignment to experimental or control group

FIGURE 11.1 Pretest-posttest control group design.

The second true experimental design is the posttest-only control group. Some researchers argue that pretesting is not always necessary, especially when randomization is used. In many nursing studies, it may be inappropriate or impossible to pretest before the independent variable is manipulated. The posttest-only control group is shown in Figure 11.2. Excerpt 11.1 illustrates the use of a posttest-only control group to determine which of two educational approaches has a greater effect on knowledge of AIDS and HIV and on attitudes of women participating in the Women's, Infants, and Children program. The design is slightly different from that of Figure 11.2 in that subjects were assigned to three groups instead of two groups. No pretest was administered.

Wikblad and Anderson[33] compared the effects of dressings on wound healing in 250 patients undergoing heart surgery. Patients were randomly assigned to a control group receiving conventional absorbent dressings or to one of two experimental groups receiving either a semiocclusive hydroactive wound dressing or an occlusive hydrocolloid dressing. The conventional dressing was more effective than the

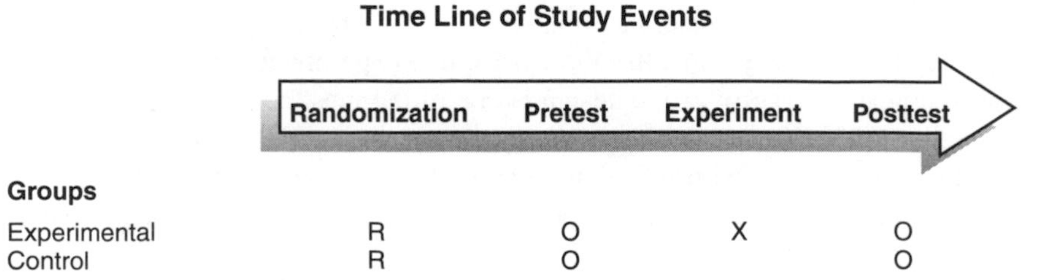

**Time Line of Study Events**

| | Randomization | Pretest | Experiment | Posttest |
|---|---|---|---|---|
| **Groups** | | | | |
| Experimental | R | O | X | O |
| Control | R | O | | O |

O = dependent variable measurement
X = application of the independent variable
R = random assignment to experimental or control group

FIGURE 11.2 Posttest-only control group design.

EXCERPT 11.1

## USE OF POSTTEST-ONLY CONTROL GROUP

**Study Design**

All subjects who agreed to participate completed a modified version of the 1989 CDC Health Risk Survey. The subjects were then randomly assigned using a random numbers table to one of three groups: (1) Control—no specific educational program except an opportunity to read current health department pamphlets about AIDS for 15 minutes and ask questions (n = 73); (2) Video-tape instruction—*The Subject is AIDS* by ODN Productions (n = 71); (3) Nurse educator encounter—a standardized presentation on AIDS/HIV transmission and prevention by a black community health nurse (n = 73). Each program lasted 15–18 minutes. After the educational program was completed, the subjects then completed a posttest questionnaire to ascertain short-term knowledge gain and attitude changes.

*Source: Ashworth, CS, et al: An experimental evaluation of an AIDS educational intervention for WIC mothers. AIDS Educ Prev 6:154, 1994, with permission.*

hydroactive dressing in wound healing. There was no significant difference between the conventional dressing and the hydrocolloid dressing. This experimental design measured a dependent variable after intervention only. There was no pretesting. Sometimes the posttest-only control group designs are referred to as "after-only designs."

A third true experimental design is the Solomon Four-Group design. This design combines the aforementioned approaches into one design and allows the researcher to control for the effect of the pretest. This is done by conducting the experiment twice, once with pretests and once without pretests. The main disadvantage of this design is the difficulty involved in actually conducting two studies. More time and effort are required to conduct two experiments simultaneously. There is also the problem of recruiting increased number of subjects of the same kind that would be tested twice. The Solomon Four-Group design is shown in Figure 11.3. For other variations of true experimental designs, refer to Campbell and Stanley.[18]

QUASIEXPERIMENTAL DESIGNS

Like the experimental design, a quasiexperimental design dictates manipulation of the independent variable. The outcome is "predicted" by theory and research. However, random assignment and/or control groups are absent.

Often, nurse researchers are obliged to use a quasiexperimental design because of the nature of the study or clinical setting. Additionally, the nurse may find it impossible to develop a control group or to randomly assign patients to groups owing to the nature of the clinical setting. Although the researcher may use control and experimental groups in quasiexperimental designs, these designs may use convenience (no random assignment) sampling or matched groups.

Several different quasiexperimental designs are outlined in the research literature. Campbell and Stanley[18] illustrate more than 10 different quasiexperimental designs.

**Time Line of Study Events**

| | Randomization | Pretest | Experiment | Posttest |
|---|---|---|---|---|
| **Groups** | | | | |
| **1.** Experimental | R | O | X | O |
| **2.** Control | R | O | | O |
| **3.** Experimental | R | | X | O |
| **4.** Control | R | | | O |

O = dependent variable measurement
X = application of the independent variable
R = random assignment to experimental or control group

FIGURE 11.3  Solomon Four-Group design.

The most common and basic type seen in nursing research is the nonequivalent control group design, also called a comparison group. When reading a research report, do not get confused with the true experimental pretest-posttest control group design (see Figure 11.1). With nonequivalent groups, there is no randomization of subjects into groups. The researcher selects two samples from two similar available groups. The nonequivalent control group is shown in Figure 11.4.

Refer to the previous example of the researcher interested in patients' pain relief after surgery. Suppose that two surgical floors (6-East and 7-West) decide to change their approach to pain medication intervention. Nurses on 6-East decide to use 2 to 4 mg of morphine IV every 1 to 2 hours for the postoperative population; 7-West still wants to continue using 5 to 8 mg of morphine IM every 3 to 4 hours. Both floors have similar numbers of surgical patients. Unfortunately, the researcher cannot create control and experimental groups because of the nature of the clinical setting. It is decided to group all the patients and compare the pain relief received

**Time Line of Study Events**

| | Pretest | Experiment | Posttest |
|---|---|---|---|
| **Groups** | | | |
| Experimental | O | X | O |
| Comparison | O | | O |

O = dependent variable measurement
X = application of the independent variable

FIGURE 11.4  Nonequivalent control group design.

from the different interventions. In this example, the researcher must assign patients to groups randomly. Patients are assigned as a function of the floor location (or by convenience); consequently, the groups are nonequivalent. The research question focuses on which of the two medication interventions might be "best" for pain relief.

A more elaborate quasiexperimental design might test each group before and after the intervention. Similar to the before-and-after experimental design, this approach allows the researcher to compare the before-and-after scores within each group (within-group comparison). Additionally, the researcher may compare scores of one group against those of another (across-group comparison). This design is called "quasiexperimental before-and-after." For other variations of quasiexperimental designs, refer to Campbell and Stanley[18] and Cook and Campbell.[26]

## Randomized Clinical Trials

**Randomized clinical trials (RCTs)** is the most widely accepted approach to evaluating the effectiveness of an intervention/treatment in a large sample of patients. RCTs require the researcher to adhere strictly to principles of experimental design. Clinical trials typically use a pretest-posttest control group design, follow subjects in time (prospective), collect outcome data after an extended period, and frequently sample from multiple sites.[6] Essential features of clinical trials include use of an experimental and control group, randomization, blinding of patients and health-care providers, and sufficient sample sizes.[6]

Experimental designs typically involve two groups, experimental and control. Sometimes there may be three groups, where more than one intervention/treatment is presented. The experimental group receives the intervention/treatment, and the control group usually receives the standard, customary care. Use of a control group enables the researcher to compare the performance of the treatment group(s) to that of a group that did not receive the intervention/treatment but was exposed to the same passage of time.

A major feature of the clinical trial is that patients are assigned to the treatment group(s) by a method that maximizes the probability that the two groups will be similar in demographic characteristics that may influence either the response to the intervention/treatment or various outcome measures. With randomization, treatment group assignment is based on probability alone and not on the health-care provider's preference.

Blinding of patients and health-care providers is important because it reduces biasing of perceptions or ways of acting on everyone's part. Blinding means that the treatment assignment is not known to certain individuals. In a **single-blinded study,** the treatment assignment is unknown to patients; in a **double-blinded study,** the treatment assignment is unknown to the patients and to the health-care providers. In double-blinded studies, the treatment assignment is revealed only if there are serious or unexpected side effects from the intervention/treatment.

Sufficient sample sizes are required in clinical trials to ensure that the effectiveness of the intervention/treatment can be detected by statistics used to compare the groups' outcomes. With small samples, the study is said to lack statistical power, meaning the study has a low chance of confirming a difference between groups that really does exist. If the study has adequate statistical power, it is important to conduct a power analysis to determine the appropriate number of subjects needed to have a certain chance (usually 80 percent) of detecting a significant difference if one actually does exist. Refer to other research textbooks for a detailed discussion of power analysis.

Excerpt 11.2 displays part of the methods section of a randomized clinical trial. The purpose of the study was to test the effectiveness of the Safety Intervention Protocol among abused women. Seventy-five women were randomly assigned to the experimental group (intervention group), and 75 women were assigned to the control group receiving standard care. Women randomized to the experimental group were offered the standard services plus six safety intervention telephone calls. Strategies for adopting safety behaviors were discussed on each telephone call. The first telephone call occurred within 48 to 72 hours of the initial visit. Remaining calls occurred at 1, 2, 3, 5, and 8 weeks following intake. The intervention ended with the sixth telephone call. Both groups were monitored at 3 months and 6 months. At the 3- and 6-month follow-up, no information on safety was provided to the experimental group.

Evaluating the effectiveness of an intervention/treatment utilizing an RCT is considered the "best" form of evidence, or "gold standard," for clinical research. However, it is important to realize that not all clinical researchable questions can be answered with RCTs. Other research designs can also generate very useful and valid scientific information.

## VALIDITY IN RELATION TO RESEARCH DESIGN

Two kinds of validity related to research design are internal validity and external validity. External validity refers to the extent to which the results of a study can be generalized from the study sample to the larger population (see Chapter 7). Internal validity refers to whether the independent variable actually made a difference. Did

---

### EXCERPT 11.2

### EXAMPLE OF METHODS SECTION FROM A RANDOMIZED CLINICAL TRIAL

**Design**

A two-group randomized control design was followed. Prior to data collection, a power analysis determined the sample size. Using a previous study by McFarland and associates (1998) that found the safety intervention highly effective with a group of pregnant women, a medium treatment effect was predicted. To detect a medium treatment effect size of 0.45 with 80% power, 60 women were needed in each group (Lipsey, 1990). To allow for 25% attrition, 75 women were recruited for each group.

*Source: McFarlane, J, et al: An intervention to increase safety behaviors of abused women: Results of a randomized clinical trial. Nurs Res 51:347, 2002, with permission.*

the intervention or treatment lead to the results, or were the results a response to extraneous variables? Extraneous variables present threats to internal validity because they offer competing explanations for the relationship between independent and dependent variables. True experiments have a great amount of internal validity because of the use of control groups and randomization. Campbell and Stanley[18] have identified several types of threats to internal validity that can be experienced in clinical studies.

## History

History refers to the confounding effects of specific events, other than the experimental treatment that occurs after the introduction of the independent variable or between the pretest and posttest.[18] For example, if a researcher studies the effect of an educational intervention to increase compliance with the American Diabetes Association (ADA) diet regimen, history may be more influential to compliance than is the educational intervention. History can also refer to more global events. For example, a researcher interested in health promotion among adolescents studies the effect of an educational program for increasing the use of seat belts. If, during the course of the study, the state passes a law mandating seat belt use, that also represents a history effect.

## Maturation

A second threat to internal validity is maturation, biological or psychological processes that occur with the passage of time and that are independent of any external events.[18] Maturation is a concern in many areas of clinical research, especially in studies involving long periods between measurements. For example, a researcher studying children might encounter physical and developmental changes, unrelated to an intervention, that may influence performance.

## Testing

The third threat to internal validity is the potential effect of pretesting or repeated testing on the dependent variable. Individuals usually score higher when they retake an achievement or intelligence test. Testing effects refer to improved performance or increased skill occurring because of familiarity with measurements.[18] For example, subjects may actually learn information by taking a pretest, thereby changing their responses on a posttest, independent of any instructional intervention.

## Instrumentation

Instrumentation effects involve the reliability of measurement (see Chapter 8). The effect of any change in the observational technique or measurement instrument might account for observational differences. In particular, the problem of instrumentation becomes crucial when human beings are used as judges, observers, raters, coders, or interviewers. Observers can become more experienced at measurement between the pretest and the posttest. This threat to internal validity can be addressed by documenting test-retest and interrater reliabilities.

## Statistical Regression

Statistical regression is also associated with reliability of a test. When measures are not reliable, there is a tendency for extreme scores (see Chapter 10) on the pretest to regress toward the mean on the posttest.[18] This effect occurs in the absence of intervention. Extremely low scores tend to increase; extremely high scores, to decrease. Statistical regression is of concern when groups are selected on the basis of extreme scores. For example, a researcher wanting to examine the effect of self-efficacy on subjects who comply and on those who do not comply with their diet regimen might assign subjects to two groups based on their pretest scores (e.g., extent of compliance). The effect of the regression will be to move both groups toward their combined average in posttests. The amount of statistical regression is directly related to the extent of measurement error in the dependent variable.

## Mortality

Researchers are often faced with the fact that subjects drop out of a study before it is completed. Mortality, or attrition, refers to the loss of subjects from both experimental and control groups for various reasons.[18] Researchers should determine whether attrition occurs for random or biased reasons and if one particular group is affected more than others.

## Nonexperimental Designs

Nonexperimental research is clearly distinguishable from experimental and quasi-experimental research in that it does not manipulate the independent variable. In nonexperimental designs, the researcher observes the actions of variables as they occur in the natural state. The major purpose of nonexperimental research is to uncover new knowledge and describe relationships among variables. This type of research is also a rich source of data that help the researcher to formulate questions to use in an experimental or quasiexperimental design. These designs are used to answer level I and II questions of Brink and Woods.[3] Several different types of nonexperimental designs are described in the literature. Two basic categories of nonexperimental designs are descriptive and correlational.

### Descriptive Designs

Descriptive designs gather information about conditions, attitudes, or characteristics of individuals or groups of individuals. The purpose of descriptive research is to describe the meaning of existing phenomena at a specific time and to explore relationships among phenomena. Enumeration and brief description of characteristics are the key elements in this design. For example, a researcher decides to survey the religious affiliations of patients because there has been little pastoral care at a particular institution. A brief description and enumeration of affiliations will help support the need for further religious support within the institution.

Walcott-McQuigg and coworkers[34] present an example of a descriptive study. The purpose of the study was to seek from college-educated African-American women factors that they perceived influenced their individual weight control behavior and to identify factors that influenced African-American women collectively. Factors were described briefly, and response frequencies were recorded.

Excerpt 11.3 illustrates the use of a descriptive design whose purpose was to describe the sexual health practices of homeless adolescents. A survey was administered to a convenience sample of 414 homeless young men (244) and young women (170) aged 16 to 20 years, the majority of whom were Anglo-American. Excerpt 11.3 displays descriptive statistics associated with various demographic characteristics.

## Correlational Designs

A correlational design arises from a level of knowledge needing further refinement of variable measurement or clarification of relationships among variables. Unlike the experimental and quasiexperimental designs, the independent variable is not manipulated. However, this design gives support to later work, using more sophisticated designs that explicate causal relationships. Correlational research investigates the relationship among two or more variables. The researcher can use this approach to describe relationships, predict relationships, or test relationships supported by clinical theory. In correlational studies, no attempt is made to control or manipulate the variables under study.

Correlational research can be conducted retrospectively or prospectively. Retrospective research involves examination of data collected in the past, often obtained from medical records or survey. Many epidemiological studies use retrospective data. Prospective research involves the examination of variables through

---

**EXCERPT 11.3**

## EXAMPLE OF A DESCRIPTIVE DESIGN

### Design and Sample

A descriptive design was used. A convenience sample of 425 homeless youth aged 16-20 years responded to a survey administered at a street outreach program in central Texas. Data were analyzed from a final sample of 414 youth (mean age = 18.5, SD = 1.2 years) who provided complete data sets. The mean number of months the respondents reported being homeless was 33.1 (SD = 16.8, Min = 0.25, Max = 96). The majority were young men (58.9%), Anglo-American (75.4%), and heterosexual (65%). Sexual orientation was reported as reason from leaving home by 18% of the respondents. Other reasons for leaving home included parental disapproval of drug use (28%), emotional abuse (18.6%), physical abuse (16.2%), and sexual abuse (12.1%). Half of the respondents (50.8%) reported a history of sexual abuse.

*Source: Rew, L, Fouladi, F, and Yockey, RD: Sexual practices of homeless youth. Image J Nurs Schol 34:139, 2001, with permission.*

direct recording in the present. Prospective studies are more reliable than retrospective ones because of the potential for greater control of data collection methods.

### Descriptive Correlational Design

The purpose of a descriptive correlational study is to describe and explain the nature of existing relationships, without necessarily clarifying the underlying causal factors in the relationship. This type of study is essentially exploratory and often targets the generation of hypotheses. Cassellein and Kerr[35] used a descriptive correlational design to examine the relationship between success with a recommended cardiac lifestyle and satisfaction with a cardiac rehabilitation program 1 year after completion. Using a variety of tools to evaluate success of lifestyle and satisfaction in the program did not yield a statistically significant separation of groups relative to lifestyle on the basis of program satisfaction.

Excerpt 11.4 reports the results of a descriptive correlational design whose purpose was to describe reasons adolescents give for being homeless and to explore the relationship of resilience and selected risk and protective factors in homeless adolescents. In addition to describing the history of homelessness for adolescents who participated in the study, the authors examined relationships between and among several variables (i.e., resilience, loneliness, hopelessness, and social connectedness).

## QUALITATIVE DESIGNS

Qualitative designs are approaches that are used to discover knowledge and to understand the rich descriptions of meanings from social experiences from the participant's perspective. Methods associated with qualitative designs are conducted within a holistic framework and are guided by a philosophical approach. Theory

---

**E x c e r p t   11.4**

### REPORTING RESULTS OF A DESCRIPTIVE CORRELATIONAL STUDY

**Discussion**

The mean resilience score (total/item) for this sample was relatively high (range of 1–7 with 1 being not resilient and 7 being very resilient) at 4.48. This score is slightly lower than the mean score of 5.3 reported by Hunter and Chandler (1999) in their study of students in an inner-city vocational school. Resilience was significantly and negatively correlated with loneliness, hopelessness, and life-threatening behaviors, indicating that homeless youth who feel resilient also tend to feel less lonely, less hopeless, and to engage in fewer life-threatening behaviors than do those with less resilience. Unexpectedly, resilience was also found to be significantly and negatively correlated with connectedness. This finding is in contrast with findings from a study of in-school adolescents in which resilience was positively associated with social connectedness (Resnick et al, 1997).

Source: Rew, L, et al: Correlated of resilience in homeless adolescents. Image J Nurs Schol 33:33, 2001, with permission.

may also guide a study. However, more frequently, theoretical development or refinement results.

Qualitative designs are appropriate when little is known about a subject area, or when something is known but seems inconsistent or does not "ring true."[15] Various approaches exist to understand phenomena. Just as theory and questions dictate the use of specific designs in quantitative approaches, so too they dictate the design of qualitative strategies. Although the study may not be theory-directed, questions do arise that determine specific qualitative strategies. Table 11.10 displays several qualitative designs based on philosophy, theory-research tradition, and questions asked. For a more detailed discussion of phenomenological research, ethnographic research, and grounded theory research, see Chapters 12 through 14.

## OTHER DESIGNS

Numerous other designs exist that do not fit into the aforementioned classification system. Usually these designs originate from specific questions arising from unique purposes.

## HISTORICAL RESEARCH

Historians believe that if we are not familiar with the past, then we will repeat our mistakes in the future. Historical research systematically investigates and critically evaluates information related to past events. Its purpose is not to review literature about past events but to shed light on present events through analysis of cause, effects, and trends of historical events. The goal is to create new insights, not to rehash historical information. Qualitative and quantitative approaches and data collection techniques are used. Daisy[36] presents interesting insights into both the experience and the process of the historical method and its parameters.

TABLE 11.10  COMPARISONS OF SELECTED TYPES OF QUALITATIVE STRATEGIES

| Philosophy | Theory/Research Tradition | Type of Research Questions | Design Methodology |
|---|---|---|---|
| Phenomenology | Philosophy | Meaning questions eliciting the essence of experiences | Phenomenological method (variety of types) |
| Historical/cultural; symbolic interaction | Anthropology; sociology | Descriptive questions of values, beliefs, practices of cultural groups; meaning from social encounters | Ethnography; participant observation |
| Symbolic interaction | Sociology | Process and core concept questions; experiences over time or change with stages and phases | Grounded theory |

## Secondary Analysis

Secondary analysis uses previously gathered data to test new hypotheses, explore new relationships among variables, or create new insights. Because the process of data collection is time-consuming and expensive, use of these data is an efficient way to create new insights and new knowledge. However, the data may be deficient or problematic in areas of variables or populations studied. Despite this caveat, a number of groups are attempting to organize and make available databases for secondary analysis. Brown and Semradek[37] offer a comprehensive article discussing major sources, uses, and limitations of secondary data on health-related subjects. The bibliography offers references to secondary resource studies.

Excerpt 11.5 illustrates a write-up from the methods section of a secondary analysis conducted to assess the Living with Heart Failure Questionnaire for sensitivity to different clinical states and responsiveness to varying intensities of clinical intervention. Note that data were collected from nine previous studies, representing eight sites in the United States.

## Meta-Analysis

Meta-analysis is a technique that uses the findings from several studies to create a data set that may be analyzed as a single piece of datum. By applying statistical procedures to these findings, this technique can be a unique approach to integrate knowledge. Meta-analyses are common in nursing literature. Smith, Holcombe, and Stullenbarger[38] generated an integrated literature and meta-analysis to describe intervention effectiveness for symptom management in oncology nursing research. Twenty-eight randomized experimental and control group studies of symptom management were identified from 428 research reports from 1981 to 1990. Using

---

### EXCERPT 11.5

### ILLUSTRATION OF METHODS SECTION FROM A SECONDARY ANALYSIS

**Methods**

A convenience sample of nine experimental or quasiexperimental studies from eight sites in the United States was used in this secondary analysis. Investigators were identified using a "call to Contributors" published in the January 2000 issue of The Journal of Cardiovascular Nursing inviting investigators with existing LHFQ data to contribute data to this analysis. Each investigator was asked to contribute two or more data points (i.e., baseline and a subsequent measure) on 75 or more individuals with heart failure. Data on patient age, sex, marital status, income, education, EF, NYHA functional class, and the setting where the data were collected (i.e., home, hospital) were requested as well.

*Source: Riegel, B, et al: The Minnesota living with heart failure questionnaire: Sensitivity to differences and responsiveness to intervention intensity in a clinical population. Nurs Res 51:209, 2002, with permission.*

outcome measurements, data suggested that interventions were effective in relieving symptoms for managing nausea and vomiting, pain, anxiety, alopecia, infection, and side effects of chemotherapy.

## Epidemiological Research

Epidemiology studies the distribution and determinants of disease and injury frequency in human populations.[39] Epidemiological questions often arise out of clincial experience and public health concerns about the relationship between social practices and disease outcomes.

Epidemiology began as the study of "epidemics," concerned primarily with mortality and morbidity from acute infectious disease. As medical cures and treatments developed to control many of these problems, and as patterns of disease have changed, chronic diseases and disabilities have gained increased prominence in epidemiology. Today, epidemiology encompasses a broader context of "epidemic" and "disease," including studies of AIDS, outbreaks of controlled diseases such as measles, and more chronic conditions like cardiac disease, arthritis, diabetes, traumatic injuries, and birth defects.

Epidemiology includes the basics of experimental, descriptive, and correlational research designs. It is distinguished as a research approach because of its unique concern with the identification of risk factors associated with disease and disability.[39] Risk factors are exposures that increase or decrease the likelihood of developing certain diseases or disorders. Examples of risk factors include lifestyle practices such as smoking, substance abuse, drinking alcohol, and eating foods high in cholesterol or salt; occupational hazards, such as repetitive tasks of heaving, lifting, and operating computers; and environmental influences, such as second-hand smoke, toxic waste, and sunlight.

Epidemiological studies are generally classified as descriptive or analytic.[39] **Descriptive epidemiological studies** are concerned with the distribution and patterns of disease or disability in a population. These studies provide valuable information that can be used to generate hypotheses and set priorities for health-care planning. Descriptive epidemiological studies usually take the form of case reports, correlational studies, or cross-sectional surveys.

**Analytic epidemiological studies** involve testing hypotheses to determine if specific exposures are related to the presence or absence of specific diseases or disabilities. Analytic epidemiological studies allow the researcher to determine if the disease rate is different among those exposed or unexposed to the factor of interest and, thus, establish that certain exposures either increase or decrease one's risk of developing that disease. Analytic studies are broadly categorized as observational or interventional. Observational studies use surveys, interviews, or review of medical records, whereas the researcher documents the natural course of events, noting who is and who is not exposed and who does and does not develop the disease. There is no direct intervention and no control over who receives the exposure. These observational studies take the form of case-control and cohort studies.

## RESEARCH DESIGN SELECTION

How does one select a research design? There are several questions you may want to ask yourself as you move toward understanding design selection. Each question lays a foundation for the next question, so that choice of design emerges from your philosophical approach, theory, and research questions:

1. How do you approach reality? What are your beliefs about the world, nursing, and patient care? Are your thoughts aligned with a quantitative or qualitative paradigm?
2. With what research tradition are you allied? Do you think holistically, or do you think in terms of a medical, sociological, or psychological viewpoint?
3. Is there an existing theoretical framework to guide inquiry of your chosen phenomena of interest? How much research exists in your area of inquiry? Are the concepts labeled, defined, and/or measured?
4. What question are you asking? Is it a "Why" question (level III), a "What is or what are the relationships among variables" question (level II), or a "What is or what are" question (level I)? Is your question more outcome-oriented or process-oriented? Does your question lend itself to a quantitative or qualitative design?
5. What type of research design emerges from this sequence of questions? Does your design fit with your world view, theory, and research question?

## QUESTIONS TO CONSIDER WHEN CRITIQUING RESEARCH DESIGNS

Identify a research study to critique. Read the study to see if you recognize any key terms discussed in this chapter. Remember that all studies may not contain all key terms. The following questions serve as a guide in critiquing research designs:

1. *Was the research design of the study described along with a rationale for the selection?* In the methods section of a research report, the word "design" should appear as a subheading followed by the particular type: experimental, quasiexperimental, or nonexperimental. The author(s) should have clearly described their choice of design. In some research reports, there is no mention of what type of research design was employed. Based on the specific stated purpose of the study, you should be able to judge the type of design.
2. *Is the research design appropriate for answering the research questions and/or testing the hypotheses of the study?* Although research studies have a number of common components (i.e., problem statement, research questions and/or hypotheses, findings/results, conclusions/discussion), procedures specific to a study are to a great extent determined by the particular research design involved. Read over the research study, and evaluate if the type of research question and/or hypothesis posed is suitable to the research design employed in the study.

3. *If the study utilizes an experimental design, was randomization used to assign subjects to the experimental and control groups?* The validity of an experimental design depends on how subjects are assigned to groups and whether a control group was included in the design. Look to see if random assignment has occurred and if the process is described. Random assignment to groups is important because it distributes known and unknown extraneous (confounding) variables equally across groups, ensuring that the composition of groups is unbiased.

## SUMMARY OF KEY IDEAS

1. A research design is a set of guidelines by which researchers obtain answers to inquiries.
2. Quantitative and qualitative approaches to research constitute an organizing framework that contains a set of assumptions or values that underlie how scientists view reality, truth, and research.
3. Quantitative research, which is directed at the verification of relationships, involves measurement and analysis of relationships. Qualitative research is concerned with the discovery of meaning and the use of language, concepts, and words rather than numbers to represent evidence from research.
4. All research designs are classified as experimental or nonexperimental.
5. Experimental designs are classified as true experimental or quasiexperimental. A true experimental design is actually an experiment in which the researcher tries to assess whether an intervention or treatment (independent variable) makes a difference in a measured outcome. Subjects are randomly assigned to an experimental or control group.
6. Three basic types of true experimental designs include pretest-posttest control group design, posttest-only control group, and the Solomon Four-Group design.
7. A quasiexperimental design dictates manipulation of the independent variable. In this type of design, random assignment, control groups, or both, are absent.
8. The basic type of quasiexperimental design is the nonequivalent control group design.
9. In nonexperimental designs the researcher observes the actions of variables as they occur. The major purpose of nonexperimental designs is to uncover new knowledge and describe relationships. Two basic categories of nonexperimental research are descriptive and correlational research.
10. Randomized clinical trials (RCTs) are prospective studies that evaluate the effectiveness of an intervention/treatment in a large sample of patients. Some researchers consider RCTs to be the "best" form of evidence, or the "gold standard" for clinical research.

11. Quantitative designs focus on internal validity. Internal validity refers to whether the independent variable made a difference or whether the results were a response to some extraneous variable(s).
12. Threats to internal validity include history, maturation, testing, instrumentation, statistical regression, and mortality.

## LEARNING ACTIVITIES

1. Identify several articles from research-oriented journals published within the last 5 years that describe experimental and quasiexperimental designs.
   a. Describe the type of research design used in each article. Did it follow the definition of an experimental design, quasiexperimental design, or both, as defined by this chapter? Describe the characteristics that make each study an experiment or quasiexperiment.

   b. In studies describing an experimental design, what two or three groups were being compared? Was there equivalence between or among the groups?

   c. In studies describing an experimental design, were the extraneous variables controlled to the greatest possible extent? Describe how each variable was controlled.

   d. In studies describing a quasiexperimental design, what characteristics of the study make it quasiexperimental rather than experimental? What factors might have influenced the design so that a quasiexperimental approach rather than a true experimental approach would be used?

## References

1. Burrell, G, and Morgan, G: Sociological Paradigms and Organizational Analysis. Heinemann Educational Books, London, 1979.
2. Morgan, G: Beyond Method Strategies For Social Research. Sage, Newbury Park, CA, 1983.
3. Brink, P, and Woods, M: Basic Steps in Planning Nursing Research: From Question to Proposal. Jones & Bartlett, Boston, 1994.
4. Brink, P, and Woods, M: Advanced Design in Nursing Research. Sage, Newbury Park, CA, 1989.
5. Dreher, M: Qualitative research methods from the reviewer's perspective. In Morse, J: Critical Issues in Qualitative Research Methods. Sage, Thousand Oaks, CA, 1994, p 281.
6. Burns, N, and Grove, S: The Practice of Nursing Research: Conduct, Critique and Utilization, ed 4. WB Saunders, Philadelphia, 2001.
7. Kaplan, A: The Conduct of Inquiry. Chandler, Scranton, PA, 1964.
8. Kerlinger, F: Foundations of Behavioral Research. Holt, Rinehart, & Winston, New York, 1986.
9. Berger, P, and Luckman, T: The Social Construction of Reality. Doubleday, Garden City, NY, 1966.
10. Denzin, N, and Lincoln, Y: Handbook of Qualitative Research. Sage, Thousand Oaks, CA, 1994.
11. Kuhn, T: The Structure of Scientific Revolutions, ed 2. University of Chicago Press, Chicago, 1970.
12. Guba, E: The Paradigm Dialogue. Sage, Newbury Park, CA, 1990.
13. Guba, E, and Lincoln, Y: Epistemological and methodological bases of naturalistic inquiry. Ed Com Tech J 30:2, 1982.
14. Leininger, M: Qualitative Research Methods in Nursing. Grune and Stratton, Orlando, 1985.
15. Munhall, P, and Boyd, C: Nursing Research: A Qualitative Perspective. National League for Nursing Press, New York, 1993.
16. Hayes, W: Statistics, ed 3. Holt, Rinehart, & Winston, New York, 1981.
17. Fischer, Sir RA: The Designs of Experiments. Hafner Publishing, New York, 1935.
18. Campbell, D, and Stanley, J: Experimental and Quasiexperimental Designs for Research. Rand McNally College Publishing, Chicago, 1963.
19. Lincoln, Y, and Guba, E: Naturalistic Inquiry. Sage, Beverly Hills, CA, 1985.
20. Knafl, K, and Howard, M: Interpreting, reporting and evaluating qualitative research. In Munhall, P, and Oiler, C (eds): Nursing Research: A Qualitative Perspective. Appleton-Century-Crofts, Norwalk, CT, 1986.
21. Keppel, G: Design and Analysis: A Researcher's Handbook. Prentice-Hall, Englewood Cliffs, NJ, 1982.
22. Kim, HS: The Nature of Theoretical Thinking in Nursing. Appleton-Century-Crofts, Norwalk, CT, 1986.
23. Schwartz-Barcott, D, and Kim, HS: An expansion and elaboration of the hybrid model of concept development. In Rodgers, B, and Knafl, K: Concept Development in Nursing: Foundations, Techniques and Applications. WB Saunders, Philadelphia, 1993.
24. Reichenbach, H: The Rise of Scientific Philosophy. University of California Press, Berkeley and Los Angeles, 1951.
25. Keith, J: Participant observation. In Fry, C, and Keith, J (eds): New Methods for Old Age Research. Center for Urban

Policy, Loyola University Press, Chicago, 1980, p 8.

26. Cook, T, and Campbell, D: Quasi-experimentation: Design and Analysis Issues for Field Settings. Rand McNally College Publishing, Chicago, 1979.

27. Sandelowski, M: The problem of rigor in qualitative research. ANS 8:27, 1986.

28. Gold, R: Roles in sociological field observations. In McCall, G, and Simmons, J (eds): Issues in Participant Observation: A Text and Reader. Random House, NY, 1969, p 132.

29. Diers, D: Research in Nursing Practice. JB Lippincott, Philadelphia, 1979.

30. Diesing, P: Patterns of Discovery in the Social Sciences. Aldine Atherton, Chicago, 1971.

31. Hempel, C: Aspects of Scientific Explanation and Other Essays in the Philosophy of Science. Free Press, NY, 1965.

32. Schaffner, BH: The effect of a maternal voice audiotape on parasympathetic tone and behavior of hospitalized preschool children. Unpublished dissertation, University of Pennsylvania, 1992.

33. Wikblad, K, and Anderson, B: A comparison of three wound dressings in patients undergoing heart surgery. Nurs Res 44:312, 1995.

34. Walcott-McQuigg, JA, et al: Psychosocial factors influencing weight control behavior of African American women. West J Nurs Res 17:502, 1995.

35. Cassellein, P, and Kerr, J: Satisfaction and cardiac lifestyle. J Adv Nurs 21:498, 1995.

36. Daisy, C: Historiography: Searching for Annie Goodrich. West J Nurs Res 13:408, 1991.

37. Brown, JS, and Semradek, J: Secondary data on health-related subjects: Major sources, uses, and limitations. Public Health Nurs 9:162, 1992.

38. Smith, M, Holcombe, J, and Stullenbarger, E: A meta-analysis of intervention effectiveness for symptom management in oncology nursing research. Oncol Nurs Forum 21:1201, 1994.

39. Greenberg RS, et al: Medical Epidemiology, ed 2. Appleton & Lange, Connecticut, 1996, pp 1–15.

# 12

# Phenomenological Research

Gail E. Russell, EdD, RN, CNAA

## LEARNING OBJECTIVES

*At the end of this chapter, you will be able to:*

1. Define phenomenology.
2. Discuss phenomenology as a philosophy and as a research method.
3. Describe phenomenological research methods.
4. Differentiate phenomenological research methods from other qualitative research methods.
5. Describe the relevance of phenomenology to nursing research and practice.
6. Review and critique phenomenological research in nursing.

## GLOSSARY OF KEY TERMS

**Bracketing.** Identification of any previous knowledge, ideas, or beliefs about the phenomenon under investigation.

**Confirmability.** Method used to establish the scientific rigor of phenomenological research. It has three elements: auditability, credibility, and fittingness. Auditability requires the reader to be able to follow the researcher's decision path and reach a similar conclusion. Credibility requires that the phenomenological description of the lived experience be recognized by people in the situation as an accurate description of their own experience. Fittingness requires that the phenomenological description is grounded in the lived experience and reflects typical and atypical elements of the experience.

**Epistemology.** Branch of philosophy that studies the nature and grounds of knowledge.

**Essences.** The true meaning of something; structural units of common understanding of the lived experience under investigation.

**Hermeneutics.** Research strategy used by researchers who believe that language captures the historical, cultural, and immediate essence of lived experience as understood by the individual. Originally developed to study scripture.

**Intentionality.** Ability of the consciousness to create a mental object, to apply that mental object to reality, and to direct activity toward results.

**Intersubjectivity.** Sharing of awareness and understanding among persons in a common lived experience.

**Intuiting.** Refers to the researcher being immersed in the descriptions of the lived experience so that a comprehensive and accurate interpretation is acquired.

219

**Life world.** The inner world of the human being.

**Lived experience.** The focus of phenomenology. It consists of everyday experiences of an individual in the context of normal pursuits. It is what is real and true to the individual.

**Ontology.** Branch of philosophy that studies the nature and relations of being.

**Phenomenological reduction.** Method of conducting phenomenological analysis and synthesis that includes bracketing and intuiting.

**Phenomenology.** A philosophy and research method that explores and describes everyday experience as it appears to human consciousness in order to generate and enhance the understanding of what it means to be human. Phenomenology limits philosophical inquiry to acts of consciousness.

**Saturation.** Point when data collection is terminated because no new description and interpretations of the lived experience are coming from the study participants.

**Phenomenology** is a qualitative research approach applicable to the study of phenomena that influence nursing practice. Researchers use a phenomenological approach to describe experiences as they are lived. In phenomenological terms, these experiences are called the **lived experience**. Nursing practice is guided by a holistic model that reflects the interrelationship of body, mind, spirit, and environment. Because quantitative methods seek only to find answers to parts of the whole, nurse researchers have looked to other philosophies of science and sought additional research methods that are compatible with investigating humanistic and holistic phenomena. Holistic health care is an example of a phenomenological perspective. This chapter provides the nurse researcher with a basic overview of phenomenology as a philosophical movement and applied research method. The researcher interested in conducting a phenomenological study should pursue additional readings to acquire an in-depth understanding of the approach.

## DEFINITION AND PURPOSE

Phenomenology is both a philosophy and a research method that explore and describe everyday experiences in order to generate and enhance the understanding of what it means to be human. Phenomenology is a way of viewing ourselves, others, and everything else that comes in contact with our lives. In this sense, phenomenology is a system of interpreting and studying the world of everyday life.[1] It is the instant when experience, reflection, and ideas come together and make sense to the individual.

## Phenomenology as a Philosophy and Research Method

Philosophy assesses and systematically relates human knowledge and experience from an integrating perspective.[2] Phenomenology is a reflective philosophy; its character lies not in its content but in the way content is attained.[3] Phenomenology is rooted in confrontation with "the things themselves." Phenomenology deals with something self-evident that one wants to approach more closely. Phenomenologists believe that human experience has meaning. To uncover the meaning in human experience, phenomenologists use an analytic-explicating method that is unlike most philosophy methods, which start with abstract and formal definitions. Phenomenologists believe that the true focus of philosophy is the exploration of the inner world of human beings. Phenomenological interpretations derive their entire content immediately and continuously from the human experience.

Phenomenology, as a research method, is a rigorous, systematic investigation of phenomena. The approach is a descriptive, retrospective, in-depth analysis of a conscious lived experience, which is everyday experiences that are real and true to the individual. The purpose of phenomenology is to describe the intrinsic traits or essences of the lived experience. **Essences** are the elements related to the true meaning of something that give common understanding to the phenomenon under investigation.

## DEVELOPMENT OF PHENOMENOLOGY

Phenomenology can be traced back to the 18th century. In 1786, Kant introduced the distinction between *phenomenon,* the appearance of reality in the consciousness, and *noumenon,* the being of reality itself.[4,5] Whatever is known is phenomenon because to be known means to appear to consciousness; whatever does not appear to consciousness cannot be known. Thus, Kant restricted scientific knowledge to appearances.[6] In 1807, Hegel suggested that phenomena provide a basis for a universal science of being. Hegel further asserted that to be fully conscious of self is to be fully conscious of all reality.[6]

The work of Franz Brentano (1838–1917) and Carl Stumpf (1848–1936) constitutes the preparatory phase of the phenomenological movement. Their goal was to reform philosophy in the service of humanity. Description became the basis of their scientific psychology. Brentano developed the concepts of inner perception and intentionality. Inner perception is the awareness of how our own lived experience appears to our consciousness and is different from unreliable introspection. **Intentionality** is the notion that everything that appears to one's consciousness refers to an object—that we do not "hear" without hearing something. Stumpf, a student of Brentano, founded experimental phenomenology and discovered structural connections in the elements of experience.[4,5]

Edmund Husserl (1857–1938), called the "father of phenomenology," was a prominent leader during the second phase of the phenomenological movement. Husserl asserted that in describing the elements of phenomena, the essence of the lived experience was revealed. Husserl introduced the ideas of intersubjectivity and life world, which are central to phenomenology. **Intersubjectivity** describes how subjective awareness and understanding can be shared in a common world. **Life world** is the world of lived experience.

Husserl's phenomenology was a critique of positivists, focusing on the lived experience but excluding its origins and status outside the act of consciousness itself. His aim was to discover the essential structures and relationships of the lived experience and consciousness, uncluttered by scientific or cultural presuppositions. In his early work, Husserl rejected all existing theories of knowledge, those formally developed as philosophical systems and those that pervaded ordinary thinking. In his later works, Husserl expanded the method of phenomenological reduction and excluded not only extraneous knowledge but also beliefs about the objects of consciousness. By suspending previous knowledge, ideas, and beliefs, or by bracketing, Husserl reached to "the things themselves." This left nothing to study but the experience. Concerned with the experiential underpinnings of knowledge, Husserl insisted that the relationship between human consciousness and its objects was not passive. Human consciousness actively constitutes the objects of experience. In so doing, Husserl rebelled against the positivist approach to the study of human experience, which is based on the belief that all human experience can be reduced to objective reality.[4-6] In philosophy, the study of knowledge and how one comes to know and understand is called **epistemology.**

Neo-Husserlian phenomenology evolved along two paths, hermeneutic and existential. Martin Heidegger (1889–1976) advanced the concept of being-in-the-world from the conception of consciousness as intentionality. The nature of being human is awareness or concern about one's own being-in-the-world. This idea enables human beings to care about and take care of others. In Heidegger's view, there is no separation of mind and matter; no world is separate from the consciousness. This was a radical reassessment of what it means to exist as a human being.[3,7] The study of being is a branch of philosophy called **ontology.**

The concept of phenomenological reduction was developed during the time of Heidegger. **Phenomenological reduction** is a method of phenomenological analysis. It is an inductive method and includes bracketing and intuiting. **Bracketing** requires the researcher to identify any previous knowledge, ideas, or beliefs about the phenomenon under investigation. Once the researcher identifies what he or she knows, it must be bracketed or separated out. This part of the reductive process allows the researcher to remain impartial to beliefs or disbeliefs in the existence of the phenomenon. **Intuiting** refers to the researcher being immersed in the descriptions of the lived experience to acquire a comprehensive and accurate interpretation. Intuiting requires the researcher to wonder about the phenomenon under investigation in relation to various descriptions generated. To illustrate the use of these terms, Excerpt 12.1 describes the methodology of a study whose purpose was to examine the lived experience of parents at the death of a newborn weighing less than 500 g at birth. "Eidetic," a term commonly used in phenomenological research, refers to an extraordinarily accurate and vivid recall of events.

Heidegger placed particular emphasis on language as the vehicle with which human beings encounter "being." Language is a way of being; one *is* one's language. The focus on language and written texts is accomplished through hermeneutic analysis.[8] **Hermeneutics,** or text interpretation, is used by researchers who believe language captures the essence of the lived experience as understood by the individual. Hermeneutic analysis was originally developed to study scripture.

Maurice Merleau-Ponty (1908–1961) and Jean-Paul Sartre (1905–1980) are exis-

EXCERPT 12.1

## USE OF THE TERMS BRACKETING AND INTUITING WITHIN A METHODS SECTION OF A JOURNAL ARTICLE

**Method**

An eidetic phenomenological approach was used for this study. In contrast to hermeneutic phenomenology, which is interpretive, eidetic phenomenology is descriptive (Cohen & Omery, 1994). The goal of phenomenology is to describe the meaning of the human experience from the individual's perspective (Cohen & Omery, 1994; Giorgi, 1986). Two essential features of the phenomenological method are bracketing and intuiting. Bracketing is the ongoing attempt to set aside previous knowledge and assumptions about the phenomenon, and intuiting is the ability to understand the phenomena and depends on the investigator's ability to engage with the subject (Swanson-Kauffmann & Schonwald, 1988).

*Source: Kavanaugh, K: Parents' experience surrounding the death of a newborn whose birth is at the margin of viability. J Obstet Gynecol Neonatal Nurs 26:43, 1997.*

tential phenomenologists who greatly influenced philosophical thought. Merleau-Ponty's[9] assertion that perception is the primary reality differs from Heidegger's conception of being-in-the-world. Perceptual consciousness is access to being and knowledge. The world given to perception is the concrete, intersubjectively constituted life-world of immediate experience. Perception is the sensory motor behavior that constitutes the world prior to reflective thought. We are always immersed in the world and perceptually present to it. Even rationality is ultimately founded in perception.[5,8]

Sartre[10] used phenomenology to reconcile the object and the subject. Sartre's goal was to understand because to understand was to change, to go beyond oneself. Like Husserl, Sartre conceives of consciousness as independent of being. By separating reality into being-in-itself and being-for-itself, Sartre formulated dialectic interrelations between consciousness and the world and between consciousness and body.[5]

Other Husserl followers have used phenomenological reduction to explore and understand religion, ethics, sociology, psychology, education, and nursing. These diverse uses constitute a broad phenomenological tradition.

## PHILOSOPHICAL UNDERPINNINGS OF HUMAN SCIENCE AND INTERPRETIVE RESEARCH METHODS

Often a lack of clarity in distinguishing among the phenomenological assumptions underlying human sciences and the phenomenological method exists. Phenomenology is the philosophical foundation of human sciences and interpretive research methods. The aim of human science is understanding and interpreting. The most important concern in human science is meaning that exists rather than material nature. Human sciences differ fundamentally from natural sciences. The aim of the natural sciences is causal explanation, prediction, and control. Natural sciences assume that the world is structured by laws and generalities.[11]

The phenomenological perspective is also the philosophical underpinning of other qualitative research approaches, including ethnography (see Chapter 13) and grounded theory. Table 12.1[12,13] displays differences among the three qualitative research approaches. Although these research approaches differ, they all recognize the importance of the interpretive processes of the study participant and the researcher. The study participant is viewed as a partner in discovery. Theory development and research in the social sciences and in practice disciplines like nursing increasingly emphasize everyday life experience; the importance of multiple, relativistic constructions of reality; and the ambiguity and complexity inherent in both everyday life and the research enterprise. The researcher is also a participant in the research process and not merely an observer. The reflections of the researcher on the data, the process of data generation, and analysis are themselves important sources of data. Researchers are encouraged to maintain a log of these reflections and to examine the "taken-for-granted" assumptions of both participants and researchers.

More disciplines are embracing interpretive approaches, within a collaborative, interdisciplinary research framework. Phenomenology is a continuing intellectual movement that has profoundly influenced nursing and the social sciences.

## CHARACTERISTICS OF PHENOMENOLOGICAL RESEARCH

Phenomenology has appeal as a research approach because it views human beings as subjects rather than objects, as free agents in situations who make choices based on meaning and values and who have responsibility for their own becoming. Van Manen[11] summarized the characteristics of phenomenological research. Phenomenology as a research method is a rigorous, critical, systematic investigation of a human experience in context. The aim of a phenomenological study is to gain a deep understanding of the nature or meaning of everyday experiences. The research question in phenomenology is always, "What is this experience like?" The goal of phenomenological research is to develop rich, full, insightful descriptions of the lived experience. Any experience that presents itself to one's consciousness is a potential topic for phenomenological research. Consciousness is access to the world; whatever falls outside one's consciousness is outside the bounds of possible experience for that person. To be conscious is to be aware of some aspect of a lived experience. Because the focus of phenomenological research is consciousness, phenomenology is always a retrospective reflection on experience.

Phenomenology systematically uncovers and describes the internal meaning structures or essences of an experience. These essences are grasped through the study of the particulars or the instances of experience as they were encountered. In phenomenology, there is less interest in the facts of an experience and more interest in the meaning these facts hold for the person experiencing them. Phenomenology uncovers the meaning in everyday human experience and brings the meaning of being human to the reader through language.

TABLE 12.1 COMPARISON OF QUALITATIVE METHODS USED IN NURSING RESEARCH

|  | Phenomenology | Grounded Theory | Ethnography |
|---|---|---|---|
| Purpose | To come to understand the meaning of a specific human experience | To generate theory about social structures and processes | To describe a culture |
| Intellectual Roots | Philosophy | Sociology | Anthropology |
| Subjects | Persons who have lived the experience | All persons involved in a social process | All persons past and present in a culture |
| Data sources | Interviews; diaries; review of art, music, and literature | Interviews; participant observation; document review | Participant observation; document review |
| Data analysis | Reflection on the data, explication of themes, constitutive patterns, essences of the experience | Constant comparative analysis | Constant comparative analysis |
| Focus of interview and analysis | Common practices, exemplars, paradigm cases | Phases, dimensions, properties of the social structure | Domains, taxonomies, components, cultural terms |
| Research outcome | Full, rich description of a human experience | Integrated, parsimonious theory with concepts that have analytic imagery | Well-described cultural scene |

## Conducting Phenomenological Research

The first step is to identify a lived experience appropriate for phenomenological study. Phenomenology is the appropriate research method in the following circumstances:

1. The goal is to understand the meaning of a lived experience.
2. The lived experience of interest is not well described or understood; there is little, if any, published research; and/or what is published about the lived experience demonstrates the need for greater depth of description.
3. People who are living or have lived the experience are accessible and are a source of rich and descriptive data; literary or artistic portrayals of the lived experience are available/accessible.
4. There is an audience for the research.

**EXCERPT 12.2**

RATIONALE FOR USE OF PHENOMENOLOGICAL APPROACH TO RESEARCH

The aim of this unique study was to explore the meaning of raising a child with HIV infection from the parent/guardian's perspective. The objective was to identify potential long-term pediatric HIV survivors in the preschool and early school age group who were likely to continue to thrive over the 5-year period of study. The researcher chose a qualitative, longitudinal approach in order to maximize the understanding of this unexplored concept from a phenomenological perspective over time. This method also avoids some of the methodological problems associated with data limitations, cultural barriers, and language impediments found in quantitative survey measures.

*Source: Mawn, B: Raising a child with HIV: An emerging phenomenon. Families Syst Health 17:197, 1999.*

5. The available resources and time and the researcher's style and strengths are compatible with this mode of inquiry. The phenomenological researcher must be comfortable with ambiguity, flexible enough to respond to the emergent nature of the process, and willing to accept multiple realities.[14]

Nursing practice offers a rich source of human experience suitable for investigation using the phenomenological method. Nurses can increase their understanding of the patients' experience of illness and of the therapeutic use of self. Excerpt 12.2 is an example of how the author made it explicit to readers why a phenomenological approach was chosen to study the experience of raising a child with HIV infection from the parent/guardian's perspective.

## Sample

It is common to use a small, purposive sample, selected from persons who have lived the experience under study and who are able and willing to describe it. Participants are solicited until there is redundancy in the data, or saturation. **Saturation** refers to the participants' descriptions becoming repetitive, with no new or different ideas or interpretations emerging. Excerpt 12.3 displays the methods section of a phenomenological study with discussion of how women were selected to participate in a study examining and interpreting the menopause experience.

## Ethical Considerations

Munhall[15] describes several ethical considerations unique to interpretive research that are related to the researcher as the research instrument and the participant as an experiencing human being rather than an object for study. There is concern for the nurse as researcher and the potential conflict of professional practice ethics and the ethics of research.

Informed consent is the knowledgeable and expressed choice of an individual to participate in a research project without coercion, deceit, or duress. In the consent document is an explanation of the research and procedures to be used; a description

**EXCERPT 12.3**

## EXAMPLE OF METHODS SECTION WITH DISCUSSION OF SAMPLE

**Design and Method**

Phenomenology was the study method used for examining the reality and perception of the American woman's experience of the menopausal transition. This method was selected with the goal of developing rich, full, and insightful descriptions of the menopausal experience among American women.

## Sample

A multiethnic sample of 15 menopausal American women in Massachusetts was selected from a pool of voluntary participants from Boston and the suburbs. Participants were solicited through professional contacts. Other participants were employees recruited through colleagues at local hospitals. These women offered names of other women they thought also might be interested in participating. The final number of participants was determined when the investigator achieved informational redundancy, also known as data saturation (Lincoln & Guba, 1985), which means that the last participants provided almost no new information.

*Source: George, S: The menopause experience: A woman's perspective. J Obstet Gynecol Neonatal Nurs 31:77, 2002.*

of risks and benefits to the participant; specific permission to tape and record interviews, if appropriate; and an explanation of how the researcher will ensure the confidentiality and the privacy of the participant. The participant's freedom to withdraw from the project without penalty and to ask questions is also stated. Munhall[15] advocates that the consent be renegotiated as the research project proceeds and circumstances change.

Confidentiality can present the nurse researcher with problems of role conflict. The participant may reveal a problem that warrants clinical intervention or administrative corrective action. The study participant should be advised to seek appropriate treatment or to see a person who is in a position to correct the administrative problem.

The institutional review board (IRB) is used by most academic and health service institutions to oversee research activities. Most IRBs deal regularly with quantitative research proposals. However, the phenomenologist may have to educate the IRB about the philosophical underpinnings and design of phenomenological research. Some IRBs have an expedited review process for qualitative research proposals because restricting access to treatment and manipulation of the interventions are not part of these study designs.

### Data Collection

The phenomenological method embraces a unique approach to data collection because the researcher is the primary study instrument. Phenomenology directs the researcher toward an understanding of the self as person as well as toward the study participant as person. Before data are collected, the researcher conducts a reflective self-assessment and articulates the assumptions, knowledge, and ideas that are brought to the research project. Some phenomenological methods require that these be bracketed, or suspended, during the study so that the lived experience can be approached naively, from a fresh perspective. Followers of Heidegger identify assumptions, knowledge, and ideas and bracket them until data interpretation, when data are compared and contrasted with the descriptions of the lived experience obtained from study participants.

Primary data collection techniques in phenomenological research elicit descriptions of lived experience from study participants by means of interviews or written descriptions. Participants are asked, "What is the experience like?" Interviews are usually unstructured. Interaction between the researcher and the participant is focused on achieving a full description of the lived experience. The researcher must be an empathetic and skilled listener and must encourage fuller description by rephrasing the participant's statements. The interview continues until the experience is fully described. Sometimes a second or third interview is needed to elicit full description. The researcher is encouraged to log his or her reflections on the process of the interviews, as a source of valuable data for analysis. Some phenomenologists use literary and artistic expressions of the lived experience under study as another source of data. Interviews are recorded and transcribed verbatim. Excerpt 12.4 shows how data collection (interviewing) occurred in a study exploring the phenomenon of raising a child with HIV from the perspective of parents of long-term pediatric HIV survivors.

---

### EXCERPT 12.4

### DATA COLLECTION—USE OF OPEN-ENDED INTERVIEW QUESTIONS

The investigator conducted 11 of the 12 interviews in English. A Latino social worker, experienced in working with families affected by HIV and trained in qualitative research methods, conducted one interview in Spanish. In the first annual interview of this 5-year project, the researcher utilized a loosely structured, open-ended interview guide. Questions posed elicited demographic information and were followed by the introductory question, "Can you tell me about the first time in your life when you first realized that you or your child had HIV?" If the participant did not elaborate in great detail to this first question, the researcher followed up with a second question, "Since that time, how have you and your family learned to adjust to living with HIV?" Toward the end of the interview, when the participant had exhausted his/her responses to the first two questions, two additional direct questions were asked, "What suggestions would you have for doctors, nurses, social workers, or other providers to better help families like yours?" and "Do you have any suggestions for families who might face the same situation you have gone through?"

*Source: Mawn, B: Raising a child with HIV: An emerging phenomenon. Families Syst Health 17:197, 1999.*

Written descriptions of lived experience are also an important source of material for phenomenological analysis. Study participants are asked to describe in writing the specific experience or daily routine being studied.

## Data Analysis

Several methods for data analysis exist in phenomenological research. All methods require the researcher to engage in a dialogue with the data and use inductive reasoning and synthesis. Tables 12.2 through 12.7 present the most commonly used methods. Regardless of the method selected, the researcher must read and/or listen to the data many times. This phase of analysis has been called "dwelling with the data." The researcher becomes immersed in the participant's descriptions to identify the themes, essences, or meaning structures of the lived experience. Excerpt 12.5 discusses data analysis utilizing Van Manen's method.

A common problem occurs when the researcher rushes the project and describes the lived experience prematurely. One way to avoid this is to analyze early interviews while collecting data. This sometimes necessitates returning to the participants for clarification or elaboration. Mentorship and guidance of the novice researcher by more experienced personnel is essential.

---

### EXCERPT 12.5

## DISCUSSION OF VAN MANEN'S METHOD TO ANALYIS OF QUALITATIVE DATA

**Data Analysis**

Data analysis was ongoing, with data collection until no new information was achieved. The interviews were analyzed to identify themes pertinent to the personal experience of menopause. Themes were extracted from the similarities and differences described to represent broader aspects of these women's experiences. Thematic analysis of data was conducted using hermeneutic application as described by Van Manen (1990). Hermeneutics is an interpretative method because it purports that there is no such thing as uninterpreted phenomena. For example, some women experienced hot flashes, but they may have had different perceptions about this symptom. In other words, the interpretation or the meaning of hot flashes had varying degrees of significance beyond its description. Some women found hot flashes to be embarrassing, whereas others had little reaction to them or took them in stride.

Overarching themes were developed from the identified categories of repeated findings or data that recurred frequently throughout the interviews. Examples of categories included expectations, physical changes, or goals. Expressions, words, or phrases that described some aspect of the experience were listed separately. Similar expressions were grouped together. Further analysis revealed that the participants were addressing these issues as part of a phase of the menopause experience and that some issues were identified in more than one phase.

*Source: George, S: The menopause experience: A woman's perspective. J Obstet Gynecol Neonatal Nurs 31:77, 2002.*

### TABLE 12.2  VAN KAAM'S METHOD

Participants: Large number of persons who have lived the experience under study
Data generation: Written description of the lived experience by participants

**Data Analysis**

1. List each word or phrase (expression) that describes some aspect of the lived experience.
2. Group similar expressions.
3. Test each expression against two criteria.
   a. Does the expression contain an aspect of the experience that may structure the meaning of the experience?
   b. If yes, abstract this expression, and label it.
4. Eliminate any irrelevant expressions.
5. Reduce concrete, vague, and overlapping expressions to more exactly worded descriptive constituents.
6. Cluster common descriptive constituents, and label the cluster with a more abstract expression of the common theme.
7. Check descriptive constituents against a random sample. Each constituent must:
   a. Be expressed explicitly or implicitly in the majority of the sample of the participants' descriptions.
   b. Be compatible with any description in which it is not expressed.
   c. Be proved to be an expression of some external experience that intrudes on the study, if a description is incompatible with a constituent.

*Source: Van Kaam, A: Existential Foundation of Psychology. Doubleday, New York, 1984.*[16]

### TABLE 12.3  GIORGI'S METHOD

Participants: 2 to 10 persons who have lived the experience under study
Data generation: Interview or written description

**Data Analysis**

1. Read the entire disclosure of the lived experience straight through to obtain a sense of the whole.
2. Reread the disclosure to discover the essences of the lived experience under study. Look for each time a transition in meaning occurs. Abstract these meaning units or themes.
3. Examine meaning units for redundancies, clarification, or elaboration. Relate meaning units to each other and to a sense of the whole.
4. Reflect on the meaning units, and extrapolate the essence of the experience for each participant. Transform each meaning unit into the language of science when relevant.
5. Formulate a consistent description of the meaning structures of the lived experience for all participants.

*Source: Giorgi, A: Psychology as a Human Science: A Phenomenologically Based Approach. Harper and Row, New York, 1970.*[18]

## TABLE 12.4 PATTERSON AND ZDERAD'S METHOD

Participant: Individual nurse
Data generation: Reflection on nurse-patient interactions

**Data Analysis**

1. Be open to lived experience (intuitive grasp).
   a. Be aware of own view.
   b. Identify theories, constructs, and assumptions, and set aside.
   c. List different ways of looking at the lived experience.
   d. Be aware of the lived experience wherever it is found, including the arts.
   e. Observe from within the lived experience.
2. Consider many instances of the lived experience (analytic examination).
   a. Compare and contrast.
   b. Identify common elements or themes.
   c. Determine how the elements of the lived experience are interrelated.
   d. Distinguish from and relate to similar experiences.
3. Construct a description and synthesis.
   a. Define.
   b. Use metaphor.
   c. Use analogy.
   d. Isolate central characteristics.
   e. Synthesize in inclusive description.

*Source: Patterson, J, and Zderad, L: Humanistic Nursing. Wiley and Sons, New York, 1976.*[19]

## TABLE 12.5 COLAIZZI'S METHOD

Participants: 2 to 10 persons who have lived the experience under study
Data generation: Lengthy and repeated interviews to facilitate full description

**Data Analysis**

1. Describe the lived experience under study.
2. Collect participant descriptions of the lived experience.
3. Read all participants' descriptions of the lived experience.
4. Extract significant statements.
5. Articulate the meaning of each significant statement.
6. Aggregate the meanings into clusters of themes.
7. Write an exhaustive description.
8. Return to participants for validation of the exhaustive description.
9. Incorporate any new data revealed during validations into a final exhaustive description.

*Source: Colaizzi, P: Psychological research as a phenomenologist views it. In Vaille, R, and King, M (eds): Existential Phenomenological Alternatives for Psychology. Oxford University Press, New York, 1978.*[20]

---

TABLE 12.6 VAN MANEN'S METHOD

---

Participants: Persons who have lived the experience under study
Data generation: See following

**Data Collection and Analysis**

**Turn to the Nature of Lived Experience**

1. Orient to the lived experience.
2. Formulate the phenomenological research question.
3. Explicate assumptions and preunderstandings.

**Experiential Investigation**

4. Generate data.
   a. Use personal experience.
   b. Trace etymological sources.
   c. Search idiomatic phrases.
   d. Obtain experiential descriptions from participants.
   e. Locate experiential descriptions in the arts.
5. Consult phenomenological literature.

**Phenomenological Reflection**

6. Conduct thematic analysis.
   a. Uncover themes.
   b. Isolate thematic statements.
   c. Compose linguistic transformations.
   d. Glean thematic descriptions from artistic sources.
7. Determine essential themes.

**Phenomenological Writing**

8. Attend to spoken language.
9. Vary examples.
10. Write.
11. Rewrite often.

---

*Source: Van Manen, M: Researching the Lived Experience. State University of New York Press, Buffalo, NY, 1990.*[11]

A real difficulty is managing large amounts of narrative data. A system for filing, coding, and retrieving data is a necessary first step in the analysis of data. Early transcription and analysis of recorded interviews help the researcher maintain the essence of the interview. Some computer programs are now available to assist in data management (e.g., Ethnograph, Martin).

QUESTION OF SCIENTIFIC RIGOR

In quantitative research, the researcher is expected to address the validity and reliability of the measurement instruments as a sign of scientific rigor. Although the phenomenologist is also concerned with reliability, validity is not relevant. Because phenomenology is the study of lived experience, it is contextual; no generalizations can be made. It is the nature of the research rather than a limitation of the

**TABLE 12.7 PARSE'S METHOD**

Participants: Selected to achieve saturation of the data
Data generation: Researcher and participant engage in unstructured discussion or dialogue

**Data Analysis**

1. Attentive study of transcribed discussion.
2. Extract an essence of the experience.
3. Move language to a level of abstraction (synthesis).
4. Using creative conceptualization, identify core concepts and their relations with one another.
5. Interpret findings of the study in relation to Parse's man-living-health theory.

*Source: Parse, R: Parse's research methodology with an illustration of the lived experience of hope.*
  *Nurs Sci Q 3:9, 1990.*

method. Guba and Lincoln[17] suggest confirmability as a measure of scientific rigor.
**Confirmability** has three elements: auditability, credibility, and fittingness.

**Auditability.** Auditability requires readers to be able to follow the decision path of the researcher and arrive at the same or comparable (but not contradictory) findings, given the researcher's data, perspective, and situation. Bracketing, the identification of knowledge, presuppositions, and ideas, help to fulfill this element.

**Credibility.** Credibility requires that findings are faithful descriptions or interpretations of the lived experience. The findings are recognized by people in the situation as an accurate description of their own experience. Through multiple interviews with participants and by giving the participants the opportunity to review and amend the descriptions and themes that emerge from the data analysis, this requirement may be met. To enhance credibility, the researcher's experiences in collecting and analyzing data, often recorded as a diary or log, are included in the discussion of the findings. An example of a research article reporting on credibility is presented in Excerpt 12.6.

**EXCERPT 12.6**

## EVALUATING RIGOR OF QUALITATIVE RESEARCH: CREDIBILITY

Credibility required that the description of the experience be recognizable to the participants as an accurate portrayal of their own experience. Credibility was accomplished through an additional contact with participants to verify and validate the data transcribed from the interviews. Member checks were conducted with each participant after the results of the study were written. To avoid misinterpretation or overinterpretation of the data, portions of the respondent's interviews were presented intact, using exact quotes. The participants were asked to respond regarding the accuracy of their account and to contact the research via the telephone, e-mail, or in writing.

*Source: George, S: The menopause experience: A woman's perspective. J Obstet Gynecol Neonatal*
*Nurs 31:77, 2002.*

**Fittingness.** Fittingness is the extent to which study findings fit the data; that is, the findings should be truly grounded in the lived experience under study and reflect the typical and atypical elements of that experience. Using direct quotes from the study, participants help the researcher to meet this element of confirmability. The ultimate test of fittingness is the affirmation of the existence and meaning of the lived experience by the reader.

WRITING PHENOMENOLOGICAL FINDINGS

The final step in any research is the dissemination of the findings. In phenomenology, this means to let the essential structures of the lived experience "be seen" through language.[11] There are several conventions for the write-up of phenomenological research. Bracketing requires the researcher to identify and suspend foreknowledge and preconceived ideas and assumptions, to approach the lived experience under study from a fresh perspective. Therefore, extensive literature review and synthesis does not precede the study. Literature and experience that are part of the researcher's knowledge base and natural attitude are discussed early in the report under the topic of bracketing. A more comprehensive literature review on the themes, essences, and meaning structures of the lived experience uncovered during data analysis is integrated into the discussion of the study findings.

The phenomenologist is not concerned with the frequency or prevalence of a theme but rather that all the possible descriptions and understandings of the experience be uncovered. Numbers, percentages, and statistical measures are not usually used in the analysis and discussion of the findings. Instead, the phenomenologist develops an accurate, integrated, literary description of an experience and its meaning. The use of direct quotes from the participants illustrates the researcher's analysis and affirms the accuracy of the analysis by providing the reader access to the original data.

Finally, writing, editing, rewriting, and returning to the original data is a repeated cycle. It is helpful to have faculty, informed colleagues, or co-researchers to help in this process. It requires concentration, attention to detail, and time to do it well. A rich description of the essence or meaning of a lived experience is the product of a well-done phenomenological study. This description is powerful in itself. It enables the reader of phenomenology to gain greater insight into what it means to be human and to engage in the experience under study. This insight can guide future nursing activities and personal actions.

## CLINICAL RESEARCH EXAMPLE

Pallikkathayil, L, and Morgan, S: Emergency department nurses' encounters with patients who attempt suicide. In Pallikkathayil, L, and Morgan, S (eds): Phenomenology: A Method for Conducting Clinical Research. WB Saunders, Philadelphia, 1991.

**Participants.** Twenty ED nurses.

**Data generation.** Before initiating interviews, the nurse researcher "bracketed" thoughts and feelings. Study participants were asked, "What is your experience in caring for suicide attempters?" All participants were interviewed individually and the interviews were transcribed. All participants were interviewed within a 2-month period of time. The duration of the interviews ranged from 1 hour to 1 hour and 45 minutes. Encounters described by the participants occurred anywhere from 1 week to 15 years before the interview. The transcribed interviews yielded 686 double-spaced pages of text with 20 to 52 pages per participant.

**Analysis of data.** Giorgi's method was used for data analysis. The unit of analysis was the sentence or thought. Decision rules for identifying and coding meaning units were established after many readings of transcripts. As an example of a decision rule, "feelings" was the code for any emotional experience or expression reflecting an affective component regardless of how it was worded. The research team, consisting of a principle investigator and a research assistant, met weekly to review the coding and to reach consensus where questions or discrepancies arose.

To establish intrarater reliability, each investigator recoded unmarked segments from transcripts coded earlier. The intrarater reliability was 100 percent for each investigator. To establish interrater reliability, four unmarked transcripts were coded by a third individual. The interrater agreement was 90 percent.

After coding each participant's interview, the meaning units were summarized into a narrative capturing the essence of the experience of the nurse's encounter with a suicide attempter. Increasing levels of abstraction were reached. Finally, insights achieved from the disclosures were integrated into a description of the consistent meaning structures across all encounters between an ED nurse and a suicide attempter. This became a beginning theory and model depicting the lived experience.

Validity was established by returning to the participants with a follow-up questionnaire constructed from the findings of the study. A sample item from that questionnaire is: "ED nurses often feel angry when they encounter a suicide attempter." Participants indicated their response on a five-point scale ranging from "strongly agree" to "strongly disagree."

**Findings.** The following model of ED nurse–suicide attempter encounter arose from the data. The suicide attempter brings a set of characteristics to the situation: age, gender, initial or repeat attempt, mental illness, individual needs/expectations, health status, personality, coping abilities, and rights. The nurse brings a set of characteristics to the situation also: length of ED experience, personal experience of suicide, age, gender, past experience of suicide intervention, comfort level with the notion of suicide, personal values, professional values, responsibility, task/holistic orientation, education, values/beliefs, coping abilities, and mind set. The nurse and the suicide attempter come together in a system having its own unique characteristics: staffing, time of day/night, institutional procedures, legal mandates, insurance/reimbursement status, ED philosophy, placement/referral processes, follow-up issues, and intensive care unit capacity. Other individuals in the system also influence the nurse-attempter encounter: family, physician, clergy, other team members, police, paramedics, friends, and other patients. The outcome of the encounter depends largely on the fit of the nurse and the attempter. The better the fit, the more positive the outcome for both nurse and attempter.

## QUESTIONS TO CONSIDER WHEN CRITIQUING PHENOMENOLOGICAL RESEARCH

Identify a phenomenological research study to critique. Read the study to see if you recognize any key terms discussed in this chapter. Remember that all studies may not contain all key terms. Table 12.8 outlines the components of phenomenological research. The following questions serve as a guide in critiquing phenomenological research:

---

TABLE 12.8 CONTENT OUTLINE FOR A REPORT OF PHENOMENOLOGICAL RESEARCH

---

### Introduction
Lived experience under study
• What is the lived experience?
• What is the aim/purpose of the study?
• Why is it important to study this lived experience?
Bracketing
• What is the researcher's interest in the lived experience?
• What is the specific context of the lived experience?
Historical/experiential
• What are the researcher's assumptions and preexisting knowledge?
• Define concepts and terms.

### Methods
Research Design Sample
• Criteria for inclusion
• How access to the sample was obtained
Human Subjects' Considerations
• IRB review and approval
• Process of obtaining and maintaining informed consent described
Data Collection
• How were data collected?
• Researcher's log as source of data
Data Analysis
• Description of procedures used to analyze and interpret data
Confirmability
• How was scientific rigor ensured?

### Findings
• Description of themes or essences uncovered
• Themes and essences substantiated with direct quotes from study participants

### Discussion
• Discussion of meanings and understandings explicated
• Related meanings and understandings to scientific literature and researcher's bracketed preknowledge and assumptions

### References

---

*Source: Boyd, C, and Munhall, P: Qualitative research proposals and reports. In Munhall, P, and Boyd, C (eds): Nursing Research: A Qualitative Perspective, ed 2. National League for Nursing, New York, 1993, pp 424–453.*[22]

1. *Is the research phenomenon of interest clearly stated?* A description of the phenomenon along with a statement why the phenomenon requires a qualitative approach should be provided within the opening paragraphs of the research report.
2. *Does the description help you understand the lived experience of study participants?* It is the lived experience that gives meaning to an individual's perception of a particular phenomenon. Look to see if the authors have captured a perception of the lived experience while emphasizing the richness, breadth, and depth of those experiences.
3. *Is the method used to collect data compatible with the purpose of the research?* Phenomenology is a type of qualitative research approach whose purpose is to describe particular phenomena as lived experience. There should be congruency between the methodology and purpose statement.
4. *Is purposive sampling used?* Purposive sampling is used most commonly in phenomenological research. Identify if the method of sampling selects individuals for participation based on their particular knowledge of a phenomenon.
5. *Have the researchers described the procedures for collecting data?* Look to see if the researchers conducted interviews. Data collection involves open-ended, clarifying questions to facilitate the process of participants describing the lived experience.
6. *Have strategies for analyzing the data been described?* Data analysis requires the researcher becoming immersed in the data. A variety of methods, each reflecting a different way to analyze data, are presented in Tables 12.2 through 12.7. Look to see if the researchers have identified one of these methods and followed the procedures for analyzing data.
7. *Do the themes maintain the integrity of the original data? Have the reseachers used examples to support the interpretation?* In preserving the uniqueness of each person's description of the lived experience, verbatim responses from the interviews are used to identify themes and categories.
8. *What evidence is provided that the conduct of the research meets the criteria of rigor?* Participants acknowledge that the findings of the study are understood and viewed as credible and true. The reseacher sends a copy of the transcribed interview to the participants, asking them if the description reflects their experiences. Content may then be added or deleted as appropriate.

## SUMMARY OF KEY IDEAS

1. Phenomenology is both a philosophy and a research method.
2. The purpose of phenomenological research is to describe the meaning of life through the interpretation of the "lived experience."
3. Understanding behavior or experiences requires that the individual interpret the experience for the researcher.

4. Data are collected through interviews, videotapes, or written descriptions by individuals.
5. Data are analyzed through interpretive analysis or hermeneutics.

## LEARNING ACTIVITIES

### Bracketing Exercise

Bracketing helps the researcher become self-aware. This exercise demonstrates to student-researchers why bracketing is a necessary first step in a phenomenological study.

1. Identify a lived experience for phenomenological study, such as: What is it like to be wheelchair-bound? What is it like to be a pregnant teenager?

2. List anonymously your assumptions and beliefs about the experience and give them to your instructor.

3. The instructor collates the assumptions and beliefs into a master list and distributes it to the class.

4. The instructor leads the class discussion of how varying preconceptions would influence:
   a. The research question

   b. The openness of the researcher to different experiences

   c. What data to collect

   d. How to collect data

   e. How to interpret data

## Interview Role-Play Exercise

Role-playing in-depth interview techniques helps student-researchers develop interviewing skills. Special attention is given to the potential of researcher bias in student questions and interactions with study participants and to listening to problems, such as inattention to detail.

1. Students pair off and interview each other on a common experience, such as: What is it like to be a student? What was it like on your first day of clinical nursing?

2. Students record and transcribe their interviews.

3. After listening to the recording and reading the transcript, students identify:
   a. Content areas tha't could have been more fully explored

   b. How the interviewer may actually lead the participant away from sharing valuable data

    c. How to better elicit data

4. Students share portions of the transcript and their analysis with the class.

5. The instructor leads the discussion and further critiques the students' interview technique.

## References

1. Wagner, H: Phenomenology of Consciousness and Sociology of the Life World: An Introductory Study. University of Alberta Press, Edmonton, Canada, 1983.
2. Gaut, D: Philosophical analysis as research method. In Leininger, M (ed): Qualitative Research Methods in Nursing. Grune and Stratton, New York, 1985, pp 73–80.
3. Heidegger, M: Being and time (Macquarrie, J, and Robinson, E, trans). In Kell, D (ed): Martin Heidegger: Basic Writings. Harper and Row, New York, 1977, pp 41–89.
4. Cohen, M: A historical overview of the phenomenological movement. Image J Nurs Schol 19:31, 1987.
5. Speigelberg, H: The Phenomenological Movement: A Historical Introduction (vols. I & II). Martinus Nijhoff, The Hague, Netherlands, 1960.
6. Lauer, Q: The Triumph of Subjectivity. Fordham University Press, New York, 1958.
7. Heidegger, M: On Being and Time (Stambaugh, J, trans). Harper Torchbooks, New York, 1972.
8. Allen, D: Hermeneutics: Philosophical Traditions and Nursing Practice Research. Nurs Sci Q 6:174, 1995.
9. Merleau-Ponty, M: The Primacy of Perception. Northwestern University Press, Evanston, IL, 1964.
10. Sartre, J: Search for a Method. Vintage Books, New York, 1963.
11. Van Manen, M: Researching the Lived Experience. State University of New York Press, Buffalo, NY, 1990.
12. Lunenberg, J: Interpretive research methodology: Broadening the dialogue. Adv Nurs Sci 16:57, 1993.
13. Mitchell, G, and Cody, W: The role of theory in qualitative research. Nurs Sci Q 6:170, 1993.
14. Mariano, C: Qualitative research: Instructional strategies and curricular considerations. Nurs Health Care 11:354, 1990.
15. Munhall, P: Theoretical considerations in qualitative research. In Munhall, P, and Boyd, C (eds): Nursing Research: A Qualitative Perspective, ed 2. National League for Nursing, New York, 1993, pp 424–453.

16. Van Kaam, A: Existential Foundation of Psychology. Doubleday, New York, 1984.

17. Guba, E, and Lincoln, Y: Effective Evaluation. Jossey-Bass, San Francisco, 1981.

18. Giorgi, A: Psychology as a Human Science: A Phenomenologically Based Approach. Harper and Row, New York, 1970.

19. Patterson, J, and Zderad, L: Humanistic Nursing. Wiley and Sons, New York, 1976.

20. Colaizzi, P: Psychological research as a phenomenologist views it. In Vaille, R, and King, M (eds): Existential Phenomenological Alternatives for Psychology. Oxford University Press, New York, 1978.

21. Parse, R: Parse's research methodology with an illustration of the lived experience of hope. Nurs Sci Q 3:9, 1990.

22. Boyd, C, and Munhall, P: Qualitative research proposals and reports. In Munhall, P, and Boyd, C (eds): Nursing Research: A Qualitative Perspective, ed 2. National League for Nursing, New York, 1993, pp 424–453.

# 13

# Ethnographic Research: Focusing on Culture

Donna Schwartz-Barcott, PhD, RN

## LEARNING OBJECTIVES

*At the end of this chapter, you will be able to:*
1. Identify a historical overview of an ethnography and its use in nursing.
2. Describe major characteristics of ethnographic research.
3. Outline three stages of an ethnographic research study.
4. Delineate major findings from an ethnography in relation to a specific culture or subculture.
5. Identify potential applications of ethnographic research for nursing practice.

## GLOSSARY OF KEY TERMS

**Ethnography.** A qualitative research approach developed by anthropologists, involving the study of individuals, artifacts, or documents in the natural setting. The researcher is intimately involved in the data collection process and seeks to understand fully how life unfolds for the individual or group under study.

**Fieldwork.** An anthropological research approach that involves prolonged resi-

dence with members of the culture that is being studied. Field notes are written as detailed descriptions of researchers' observations, experiences, and conversations in the "field" (research setting).

**Participant observer.** A technique in anthropological fieldwork. It involves direct observation of everyday life in study participants' natural settings and participation in their lifestyle and activities to the greatest extent possible.

Ethnographic research as a qualitative approach to inquiry provides the opportunity for researchers to conduct studies that attend to the need for intimacy with members of a culture. Researchers play a significant role in identifying, interpreting, and analyzing the culture under study. More than just observing, the researcher often becomes a participant in the cultural scene. Excerpts from ethnographies of three very different cultures are illustrated in Excerpts 13.1 to 13.3.

Anthropologist Colin Turnbull focused on the small homogeneous culture of a tribe of nomads in Africa in the early 1950s. Nurse anthropologist Antoinette

## ETHNOGRAPHY: CULTURE OF A TRIBE OF NOMADS ON THE AFRICAN CONTINENT

The Ituri rain forest in the middle of Africa is "a vast expanse of dense, damp, and inhospitable looking darkness." For the BaMbuti Pygmies it is home, "a cool, restful, shady world with light filtering lazily through the tree tops that meet high overhead and shut out the direct sunlight. The BaMbuti roam the forest at will in small isolated bands or hunting groups. For them there is little hardship, so they have no need for belief in evil spirits. For them it is a good world."

*Source: Turnbull, CM: The Forest People: A study of the Pygmies of the Congo. Simon and Schuster, 1962, pp 11, 12, 14.*

Ragucci looked at the Italian subculture in an urban environment in the United States between 1968 and 1969. Nurse researcher Bonnie Farmer focused on the organizational culture of owners, managers, staff, and residents of a nursing home. In all three examples, the researchers immersed themselves in the way of life of a group of people in order to describe and understand their culture from the vantage point of those who lived the experience. These excerpts reflect the hallmarks of cultural ethnography and doing fieldwork.

This chapter examines ethnography as a qualitative research method. A brief historic overview of its emergence in anthropology and nursing is provided, with a discussion of its major characteristics and stages. The intent is to provide a better sense of what to expect from this kind of approach and suggest how nurses might begin to think about and possibly apply the findings to nursing practice.

## ETHNOGRAPHY: ITALIAN SUBCULTURE IN AN URBAN ENVIRONMENT IN THE UNITED STATES

The North End has remained essentially Italian for the last 40 to 50 years. The sounds and scenes in the narrow, winding streets remind one more of the cities of Palermo and Naples than of Boston, with its colonial past. From the outside there is a sense of tradition and homogeneity in this Italian enclave, but from within one can see that traditional cultural values and practices are changing, as each succeeding generation appears to take on more and more of the values of the mainstream culture; like the women in the younger generation who speak of genes, chromes, or vitamins while their elders mention the value of blood, herbs and foods as curing agents and sometimes look to mystical or supernatural phenomena as etiological agents.

*Source: Ragucci, AT: Generational continuity and change in concepts of health, curing practices, and ritual expressions of the women of an Italian-American enclave. Doctoral dissertation, Boston University, 1971.*

EXCERPT 13.3

## ETHNOGRAPHY: ORGANIZATIONAL CULTURE OF A SKILLED NURSING FACILITY IN NEW ENGLAND

The Meadows, an 86-bed skilled nursing facility in New England, is a nice place and probably among the best of its kind. It appears much like a hotel with a reputation for fine service. Here, there is no wavering in the driving force of service, the absolute importance of appearances, or the influence of residents' rights. Within the Meadows of Madison, these values are common, shared and expected. Staff, residents, and family are clear in their expectations of how life should be at the Meadows even though everyday life does not always match expectations. Service may sporadically falter, appearances may temporarily be unappealing, and residents' rights may be threatened but the commonly shared belief of these values for the Meadows is constant.

*Source: Farmer, B: A Nursing Home and its Organizational Climate: An Ethnography. Auburn House, Westport, CT, 1994.*

## HISTORICAL OVERVIEW

**Ethnography** literally means "study and description of a culture of a particular group of people." It is the oldest qualitative research method in use today, having originated in the mid-1800s. The case study method in sociology (later called participant observation) represents another qualitative research method with a long and distinctive tradition.[1] It is used to describe and understand social life, mainly in urban settings of Western societies. Over the last 15 years, numerous qualitative research methods have emerged from this tradition, some of which have been called ethnography.[2,3] In fact, ethnography has become such a popular term that at least one sociologist has actually suggested that all qualitative research be labeled as such.[4]

Anthropologists developed ethnography as a way to study foreign cultures at a time when they were frustrated with existing methods. They had been relying on data gathered by travelers, explorers, missionaries, and foreign residents. The data were often superficial, haphazard, and ethnocentric (i.e., interpreting behaviors in light of one's own culture). Even when anthropologists were able to provide direction on what and how to observe the thoughts, feelings, and behaviors of another group of people, the accounts were often misleading. It was hard for the outsider not to reinterpret strange behavior in familiar terms because it is easier to understand something familiar.[5] The notion of anthropologists going to the field to collect their own data was a highly innovative, almost revolutionary, idea in 1885. Today, **fieldwork** is the essence of conducting an ethnography. Fieldwork is an approach that involves prolonged residence with members of the culture being studied.

Anthropologists in the 1800s were also concerned about the potential disappearance of primitive (meaning nonliterate) peoples and their cultures. As Margaret Mead, a renowned anthropologist, described in her autobiography, "in remote parts of the world ways of life about which nothing was known were vanishing before the onslaught of modern civilization. The work of recording these unknown ways of life had to be done now or they would be lost forever. Other things could wait but not this most urgent task."[6] This concern and sense of urgency also included cultures closer to home. "Among many American Indian groups, the last old women who spoke a language that had developed over thousands of years were already senile ... the last man who had ever been on a buffalo hunt would soon die."[6]

Ethnography became a way of "getting the whole configuration of culture down correctly before it disappeared" and dealing with cultural problems, such as deciphering what are the most stable and enduring cultural traits (e.g., the kind of tools a people used and the techniques for making them, the form of the family, or a people's beliefs about healing and the supernatural world).[6] Currently, ethnography remains central to the study of culture within anthropology, although it has been refined and explicated more fully over time, and a variety of other types of cultural research have emerged.

## CULTURE, ETHNOGRAPHY, AND NURSING

Nurses first became interested in ethnography as a source of information and as a research method for better understanding patients from diverse cultures in the mid-1950s. Madeline Leininger, one of the first nurse anthropologists, wrote that her interest in culture began to emerge when she was working as a child psychiatric mental health nurse. Excerpt 13.4 provides a piece of Leininger's writing on the subject of culture within mental health.

This initial interest in different cultures "at home" was fueled in 1961 with the formation of the Peace Corps and the direct involvement of nurses in diverse cultures abroad. Dorothy Sutherland, a nurse adviser for the Peace Corps, wrote that more than 300 nurses volunteered and lived in 33 developing countries, ranging

---

**EXCERPT 13.4**

### ETHNOGRAPHY: CULTURE WITHIN MENTAL HEALTH

The behavior and nursing care needs of African, Jewish, Appalachian, German, and Anglo-American children were clearly different except for some physical care needs. In a way, I experienced cultural shock and I felt helpless to assist children who so clearly expressed different cultural patterns and ways they wanted care. These cultural differences were related to playing, eating, sleeping, interaction, and many other areas of daily care. The children were so expressive and persistent in what they wanted or needed, yet I was unable to respond appropriately to them—I did not understand their behavior. Later, I came to learn that their behavior was culturally constituted and influenced their mental health. Even though I was knowledgeable about psychotherapy and mental health nursing, this was not sufficient to understand and help these children. In addition, the available psychotherapies seemed inappropriate for them.

*Source: Leininger, MM: Culture Care Diversity and Universality: A Theory of Nursing. National League for Nursing Press, New York, 1991, p 14.*

from Pakistan and India in Asia to Tanganyika and Togo in Africa. At the time, she described their experiences in the following way. "All Peace Corps volunteer nurses are working under conditions far more difficult than those they have known at home. This they anticipated when they volunteered to play a part in their country's effort to help the peoples in the emerging nations. From their sustained efforts to learn another language and understand the host country's culture, history and customs, and to live and work successfully with the members of another community, they are gaining far more in knowledge and increased skills than most believe they will ever be able to give to those they have come to help."[7]

For many nurses, this immersion in another country gave them first-hand experience with how exciting, challenging, frustrating, and rewarding it can be to learn a new culture. They also learned that there may not be only one right way of doing something and that one needs to guard against ethnocentrism because it can so easily lead to judging all groups except your own as inferior.[8]

A host of new questions emerged about how cultures influence people's experiences with health and illness and with the nature of "helping" itself.

The interest in culture was further augmented by the general movement of nurses into doctoral education, some of whom pursued their doctorates in anthropology under the nurse scientist program. Graduates of these programs began writing about how ethnography and its findings could enhance nursing practice and be a useful method for nursing research.[9-11]

In the 1980s, writings on ethnography and nursing studies using the method gained considerable momentum. By 1995, the term seems to have emerged everywhere in nursing, although not always conveying much meaning and adding considerably to the cross-disciplinary confusion of the term. More than 360 articles were identified from a computer search of the Cumulative Index to Nursing and Allied Health Literature under the term "ethnography," from 1982 to mid-1995. In these articles, the term was used more often to refer to a particular type of computer software ("ethnograph"), a specific style of interview ("ethnographic interview"), or other types of field research (e.g., participant observation unrelated to culture) than to depict fieldwork aimed at the study of a culture of a particular group of people.

## MAJOR CHARACTERISTICS OF ETHNOGRAPHY

Whether in a remote forest in Venezuela or an Italian enclave in the United States, the essence of ethnography is doing fieldwork aimed at describing and understanding a specific culture. The researcher lives for an extended time among a given group of people who share a common culture. As a **participant observer,** the researcher enters into the everyday life and activities of the people of the culture being studied. By watching what goes on, talking with individuals, and participating in activities, the researcher comes to know the culture shared by this group of people. Researchers may supplement their observations (which are recorded as field notes) with a wide variety of additional data collection tools (e.g., key informant interviewing, collections of life histories, structured interviewing, questionnaires, documents, photographs). They usually publish their findings in a book or monograph and, like the process itself, these are often referred to as an ethnography. Later they may select certain findings with relevance to a particular subject (e.g., health beliefs), theoretical debate (e.g., the generalizability of a particular theory of cultural change), or methodological issue (e.g., the use of deception in fieldwork) and publish these in various journal articles.

Traditionally, anthropologists selected a tribe or village in a relatively distinct, clearly bounded small-scale society as the field for studying a culture. Most American anthropologists in the mid-1800s selected a field that was in or near U.S. borders, such as the Kwakiuti Indians living on Vancouver Island off the coast of British Columbia[12] or the Winnebago Indians of the eastern central states.[13] This changed after World War II, when researchers shifted their attention to more foreign and remote cultures, such as the Paharis in the peasant and mountain village of Sirkanda in the lower Himalayas of northern India,[14] the Yanomamo Indians of southern Venezuela,[15] or the Nyoro in a rural community in Buyoro, Africa.[16] World War II changed the position of the United States in world affairs and brought with it new opportunities for foreign travel. At the same time, the number of universities in the United States expanded dramatically and, with them, the number of anthropology departments. It became the norm for dissertation research to include intensive fieldwork in a single culture, often exotic and remote.[17]

During the last 20 years, an increasing number of anthropologists have turned their attention to studying mainstream culture and ethnicity in the United States.[18,19] Here, the field is most often a rural community, urban neighborhood, or small city. The newest type of ethnography is emerging in organizational settings such as schools, neighborhood health centers, and hospitals. Nurse researchers doing ethnography have selected a diversity of "fields," from the foreign and remote to ethnic groups in the United States[20–22] to institutional settings to professional subcultures.[23–25]

In ethnography, "entering the field" almost always means entering as a stranger into an unfamiliar setting, even when that setting is in the researcher's own society. The researcher uses this position of stranger to learn how it is to think, feel, and act like the people around him or her. It is the difference between the researcher's own culture and that of the people being studied that helps in identifying the distinctive behaviors, thoughts, and emotions, as well as the rules influencing these in the culture under study.

Researchers tend to reside in the field for about a year, although the exact time has varied from as little as 8 months for Edmund Leache's famous study of the Pul Eliya of Ceylon to as long as 5 years for Frank Cushing's work with the Zuni.[17] Germain,[26] a nurse researcher at the University of Pennsylvania, summarizes reasons why a long residence (1 year, in this case) is so important. Generally, 1 year has been considered a reasonable time to be accepted by persons in the subculture and to learn the subculture's manifest and latent aspects, to attend to a wide variety of the subculture's activities, to see members in various contexts, and to follow certain events to their conclusions. More time or less time in the field may be required, depending on the research questions and the complexity of the subculture. The goal is in-depth knowledge of the subculture rather than surface familiarity.

## ETHNOGRAPHIC STYLES

Over the years, a number of variations of ethnography have emerged in anthropology. However, scholars have only recently tried to identify and classify these.[17,19,27,28] A major point of distinction across types relates to the definition of culture being used. Sanday's[27] identification of holistic and semiotic styles is the most characteristic of what is used in nursing today. Holistic ethnography incorporates the broadest definition of culture, with its focus on culture as a way of life. Semiotic ethnography focuses more narrowly on an ideational definition: culture as encompassing values, beliefs, and attitudes. In the following discussion of stages in an ethnographic study, examples are drawn primarily, but not solely, from holistic ethnography, the oldest style of ethnography. For an overall orientation to semiotic ethnography, see Sanday[27]; for an example of its usage in nursing, see Aamodt.[29]

## STAGES IN AN ETHNOGRAPHIC RESEARCH STUDY

The planning and implementing of an ethnographic research study takes place in three stages: pre-fieldwork, fieldwork, and post-fieldwork (Table 13.1).

---

TABLE 13.1 STAGES OF IMPLEMENTING AN ETHNOGRAPHIC RESEARCH STUDY

**Pre-Fieldwork**
- Choosing a people, field, problem
- Searching the literature and gathering information on the people and the problem
- Formulating a systematic plan of investigation
- Making preparations

**Fieldwork Phase I**
- Making contacts and gaining experience
- Settling in and establishing a role
- Beginning to gather information and mapping out visible features of culture

**Phase II**
- Working with informants
- Identifying major themes
- Focusing on gathering information on selected problem
- Doing some sampling
- Selecting additional techniques for further data collection

**Phase III**
- Continuing with participant observation—now raising more sensitive questions
- Double-checking data
- Obtaining large volumes of information

**Post-Fieldwork**
- Finalizing the analysis and findings
- Writing up the study (selecting an audience, a voice, and data for presentation)

## Pre-Fieldwork

The researcher usually starts by choosing a group of people, a field, and/or a problem. Table 13.2 illustrates examples of some choices nurse researchers have made.

Five of the most frequently cited scholarly reasons researchers use in making their selections are listed here:

1. A particular group of people is known to exist but has never been ethnographically put on record (e.g., Mbumti pygmies of Africa).
2. A certain topic or aspect of culture has not been described among a given group of people (e.g., children's acquisition of a culture's perspectives on health and healing).
3. A specific theoretical problem needs investigating (e.g., cultural conflict in health beliefs and practices).
4. A practical problem needs some possible solutions (e.g., low usage of family planning methods among Cambodian refugee women despite verbalization that small families are desirable).

TABLE 13.2 EXAMPLES OF PEOPLE, FIELDS, AND PROBLEMS STUDIED BY NURSE RESEARCHERS

| People | Field | Problem | Researcher |
|---|---|---|---|
| Italian | A neighborhood in Boston | Culture change, health beliefs, and practices in three generations of Italian immigrants | Ragucci, A. |
| Papago | A village on the Papago Indian Reservation, Southern Arizona | Enculturation: how children acquire the Papago perspectives on health and healing | Aamodt, A.M. |
| Polish | Arizona Polish Club, Tucson, AZ | The meaning of caring among second-generation Polish elders | Rempusheski, V.F. |
| Cambodian | East Bay Area of San Francisco, CA | Impact of role and status change on use of family planning among Cambodian refugee women | Kulig, J. |
| American (culture of rural life) | A small farming town in the Great Plains | What is the culture of rural community life and in what ways and how does it affect health of elderly residents? | Craig, C.E.[30] |

5. A society, previously studied, needs to be restudied to see what changes have occurred in the interim (e.g., Samoa after colonialization).

However, in reality, researchers base their final choices on a combination of reasons, including one or more of those in the preceding list, along with personal interests and abilities and practical considerations. For example, Ragucci[21] combined the need for information on the current health beliefs and practices of Italian immigrants in the United States (#2) and the need to examine the speed and direction of change in this area among different generations (#3) with her interest in Italian immigrant patients, knowledge of the Italian language, and general familiarity with the culture as a second-generation Italian herself and her physical proximity to a well-established Italian immigrant neighborhood.

Having made the aforementioned decisions, the researcher seeks more specific and detailed knowledge about the people and culture under study as well as the problem to be examined. Researchers draw on a wide range of scholarly and lay sources (e.g., regional, historical, ethnographic, geographical, and journalistic) and often go to great lengths to secure any existing information. Excerpt 13.5 is an example of how Ragucci identified more specific and detailed knowledge.

It is this type of preparation that enhances the researcher's flexibility in the field. It helps in understanding the context and orientation of the people in the culture being studied. It alerts the researcher to the kinds of beliefs and practices that might be encountered later. It also helps the researcher in formulating a more specific and systematic plan of investigation for the fieldwork stage. This plan is looser than the "research designs" you see in more quantitative research. It usually includes three phases. In the first phase, the researcher focuses on gaining entry, establishing relationships, and beginning to describe the culture (or some major aspect of it). In the second phase, the researcher usually concentrates more directly on the specific

## EXCERPT 13.5

### EXAMPLE OF MORE SPECIFIC AND DETAILED KNOWLEDGE ABOUT THE PEOPLE AND CULTURE

Ragucci, in preparation for her study of Italian immigrants in the North End, searched through historical, anthropological and folklore studies, as well as journalistic accounts (much of which was in Italian) reflecting daily life in Italy and linguistic and cultural traditions including health beliefs and practices of Italians in Italy. She also looked for any variations in these practices across the three provinces (Abruzzese, Camparia, and Sicily) from which most of the Italian immigrants in the North End had emigrated. Additionally, Ragucci drew on any existing information on Italian immigrants in the U.S. in general and then turned specifically to anthropological work on the folklore of health—the area out of which her focus on the "problem" of changing health beliefs and practices across generations in the Italian enclave would be drawn.

*Source: Ragucci, AT: Generational continuity and change in concepts of health, curing practices, and ritual expressions of the women of an Italian-American enclave. Doctoral dissertation, Boston University, 1971.*

problem. In the third phase, the researcher often spends considerable time double-checking and validating analyses and interpretations emerging from the first two phases. The amount of time devoted to any of these phases, but particularly the first two, varies widely across researchers. In the past, when the primary focus was on describing an unrecorded culture, the greatest amount of time was spent in the first phase. More recently, researchers have focused more attention and time on a specific problem under study (phase two) and used the initial phase only to gain entry, establish contacts, and obtain an overall sense of the culture, more as a backdrop than as the central focus of investigation.

As final preparation for the field, the researcher also has to give thought to a host of practical considerations (e.g., training in the language; arranging for funding; locating a specific site and planning for residence in a new location, one in which there may be potential political, social, or other deterrents to overcome). For most researchers, this preparatory period can take up to a year, especially when clearances from foreign governments are involved and national funding is sought. Sometimes, one can actually enter the field ahead of time to prepare for a longer stay, especially if the field site is near home. Aamodt,[20] in her study of the Papago Indians in Arizona, arranged for an initial 3 $1/2$-week visit 7 months before beginning fieldwork. During this initial visit, she "helped out" at a local Catholic mission and lived with one of the parishioners: a mother, "Conchita," and her three children. Conchita, who spoke some English and had a new home, albeit without indoor plumbing, gave Aamodt a place to stay, fed her, and guided her during an initial introduction to the community and helped her gain facility with the Papago language. In the ensuing 7 months, Aamodt secured funding from three sources: the American Nurses Foundation, the U.S. Division of Nursing, and the University of Arizona, College of Nursing.

Even with all this preparation and preplanning, the researcher needs to remain open-minded and ready to "shift gears," as it is often the unexpected that leads to the most important discoveries in the field. As one author of the most detailed research text on ethnography argues, "speculative ability, freedom of imagination, intuition, adaptability, flexibility, resourcefulness and ingenuity count as much in the field as the most meticulous planning."[17]

## Fieldwork

### Phase I

The researcher's main overall approach in the field is participant observation. Participant observation and taking field notes begin immediately as the researcher enters the field and settles in. During this phase, the researcher focuses on making contacts, developing trust, and gaining acceptance as well as establishing a consistent role and becoming familiar with daily routines. For most researchers, this is a period of considerable personal adjustment.

Researchers give much thought to what role to take and how to introduce themselves. Whatever role is chosen, it enhances the researcher's exposure to certain people, activities, and events and decreases the chances of seeing or participating in others. Because every role has a particular vantage point, the researcher tries to find one that allows maximum exposure to the culture as a whole and the specific problem of interest. In Excerpt 13.6, the anthropologist Ferraro[31] talks about how he decided on what role he would take in his work with the Kikuyu in Kenya.

For nurse researchers, the struggle is often over whether to take the primary role of nurse, to not disclose that role, or to play it down. Ragucci[21] describes this situation in Excerpt 11.7.

However, even with the care and forethought devoted to defining the role, people may not always believe the nurse researcher, especially during the initial phase of fieldwork. Ragucci describes in Excerpt 13.8 some of the reactions she received. It usually takes the researcher much of the first phase to establish the trust and acceptance of the people being studied. For Ragucci, entry into the social life of the North End came about slowly. It was 4 months before she began feeling accepted as a neighbor and friend by those families living in proximity.

Also during this initial period of adjustment, the researcher develops a daily set of activities to provide some sense of order and begins to collect data on those features of the new environment that can be recorded without much assistance. These tend to include the less personal and socially intense elements of the setting and culture. For the researcher in a tropical climate, the daily activities may

---

**EXCERPT 13.6**

## ROLE OF FERRARO (ANTHROPOLOGIST) IN HIS WORK IN KENYA

There are any number of ways ... to answer the question, Who are you? (a question, incidentally, that will be asked frequently and requires an honest and straightforward answer). In my own case ... I could have said, with total honesty, that I was a student (I was finishing my PhD), an anthropologist (my research was funded by NIMH), a visiting research associate at the University of Nairobi, and a teacher. Yet, many of these roles, while accurate, were not particularly understandable to the people asking the question. Even though the reason for my being there was that I was an anthropologist, that particular role has little meaning to people with little or no education. So I selected a role that was comprehensible—the role of teacher, a role that was both well-known and, much to my advantage, well-respected. Even though I wasn't teaching at the time, I had taught professionally prior to doing fieldwork, and I had planned on a career in college teaching upon returning to the States. So, when asked who I was and what was I doing there, I always said that I was a teacher collecting information about Kikuyu culture so that I could teach my students about it. Had I not standardized my introductions, but instead told one person that I was an anthropologist, another that I was a student, and still another that I was a teacher, the local people would have thought that either I was lying or, perhaps equally as bad, that I didn't know who I was.

*Source: Ferraro, G: Cultural Anthropology: An Applied Perspective, ed 2. West Publishing, New York, 1995, p 91.*

> **EXCERPT 13.7**
>
> **EXAMPLE OF RAGUCCI'S WRITING DEPICTING HER STRUGGLE OVER THE ROLE OF BEING A NURSE**
>
> The problems arising out of the dual role of the participant-observer was compounded by the fact that I had functioned at one time in the capacity of a staff nurse and clinical nursing professor in Boston area hospitals. Since the perception of the researcher as a health professional might have introduced an element of bias it was decided not to emphasize this role and yet, at the same time, not to deny it. Too, if the nursing role was categorically denied, it might have aroused suspicions because I might be recognized by persons who may have been patients or visitors at the institutions where I had functioned. It was decided that the most plausible explanation for my presence in the North End would be that of "a graduate student interested in making a study of health, particularly the old customs and ways of treating illness." The assumption of a graduate student identity appeared to be an adequate explanation. This was further reinforced by the fact that, in recent years, large numbers of impecunious graduate students were living in the North End because of the availability of low rent apartments.
>
> *Source: Ragucci, AT: Generational continuity and change in concepts of health, curing practices, and ritual expressions of the women of an Italian-American enclave. Doctoral dissertation, Boston University, 1971.*

commence shortly after dawn, with a period of relaxation when the sun is at its peak, followed by evenings spent writing up information collected during the day.

In Boston, Ragucci used this initial phase of fieldwork to concentrate on learning about the formal community organizations and the general ecological and demographic features of the Italian enclave of the North End. She set up unstructured interviews with representatives of health, social, and spiritual agencies, observed meetings of the North End Neighborhood Council (made up of middle-class professionals), and attended meetings of the North End Rehabilitation and Conservation Committee (made up of neighbors concerned with problems of the North End).

*Phase II*

During the middle phase of the fieldwork, the researcher augments his or her continuing participant observation by working closely with a small number of informants: individuals who are willing and able to express cultural information verbally. Researchers tend to form close long-term social relationships with their informants. These relationships do not have the formality associated with interviewing but are more like conversations between friends or didactic transactions between an uninformed, eager student (the researcher) and the teacher (the informant). In this kind of relationship, researchers can do the following:

1. Clarify and obtain additional information about what they are observing in the field
2. Probe for the cultural meanings behind these observations

## EXAMPLE OF HOW RAGUCCI WAS PERCEIVED

The North End women and men viewed my presence in their midst in a variety of ways. Some neighbors had difficulty in comprehending my identity as a graduate student because I did not adhere to the routine schedule which they associated with class attendance. Others did not understand my seeming abundance of leisure time. When I met them in the neighborhood during the day, they would invariably ask the question, "Aren't you working today?" This query proved to be most difficult to answer to the satisfaction of a working class group oriented to regular working hours. I found that the most satisfactory responses to this question were: "I don't have any classes today (or during the summer)" or the more facetious but truthful "I'm working all the time."

Later, feedback from my neighbors revealed that, at different times and in different contexts, I was perceived in a variety of roles and occupations according to their own frame of reference. I was told that neighbors who had watched my furniture being moved into the apartment had speculated that I was "a bride because my furniture looked new." During the initial weeks in the field the question of my ethnic identity was evidently a topic for discussion in the small groups. Some insisted that I was not Italian "because I did not look Italian." Others thought I was either a Jewish or Armenian social worker. . . . One neighbor, believing I was a teacher, prevailed upon me to tutor her 8-year-old daughter in mathematics. A reciprocal arrangement was made—I helped the child master the intricacies of the "new math" and at the same time I had an opportunity to learn the dialect of the mother's *paese*.

*Source: Ragucci, AT: Generational continuity and change in concepts of health, curing practices, and ritual expressions of the women of an Italian-American enclave. Doctoral dissertation, Boston University, 1971.*

3. Confirm the validity of the ways in which they are beginning to make sense of their data
4. Gain information on ways of living that ceased to exist or have been sharply modified before their arrival

In her study of Italian women of the North End, Ragucci worked with small groups of informants who were part of the established neighborhood social system. In Excerpt 13.9, she discusses her association with one group of third-generation women and some of the kinds of data and insights she gained from her informal neighborhood gatherings with these women.

During this phase, researchers begin to identify emerging themes and categorize and analyze general features of the culture. For example, Ragucci organized her data according to a scheme used in the Human Relations Area Files for coding data from ethnographies from around the world and as a basis for making cross-cultural comparisons. The scheme contains 70 major topics and more than 700 subject categories, ranging from settlement patterns and technology to kinship, law, and social problems; also included are topics concerning human biology, clothing, behavioral

EXCERPT 13.9

## EXAMPLE OF INFORMANTS

During the summer months we sat in front of the tenement and in the winter we moved to the warmth of the kitchen. Current ailments, deaths, or hospitalization of neighbors and friends would invariably appear as topics for discussion. Some visits were specifically oriented to fulfill one's obligations to the sick and ailing. The neighbors customarily gathered at the homes of hospitalized persons when family members returned from the afternoon or evening hospital visiting hours. A veritable mine of data was collected on these occasions. The family members would report their perceptions of the progress of the hospitalized person, the perceived rationale of the prescribed treatment and very often, their perception of the quality of medical and nursing care administered to the relative ... wakes and picnics yielded a wealth of pertinent data. Wakes provide a setting where folk or laymen's theories about the etiology of disease and cause of death are more likely to be expressed. An opportunity to assess the current usages of herbal remedies by members of the first and second generation occurred during a combined picnic and pilgrimage to a religious shrine located in a rural area. Elderly women used this occasion to replenish their supply of herbs and the researcher was able to elicit the people's beliefs about the curing properties of these substances.

*Source: Ragucci, AT: Generational continuity and change in concepts of health, curing practices, and ritual expressions of the women of an Italian-American enclave. Doctoral dissertation, Boston University, 1971.*

processes, and personality. Table 13.3 illustrates some of the topics and subcategories that Ragucci probably used to code her field notes related to the general features of the culture as a whole and the specific health beliefs and practices of the Italian immigrant group of the North End.

The nature of the researcher's specific problem or area of interest points to ways of organizing data. Ragucci constructed a typology on "traditional folk medicine" and "contemporary folk medicine" as a device for organizing and analyzing data in order to address her interest in changes in health beliefs and practices across different generations of the Italian immigrant women.

A researcher may analyze field notes in several ways. Bernard[32] talks about one of the most traditional inductive approaches, referred to as the "ocular scan" or simply "eyeballing." Researchers use this approach when trying to discern themes and patterns of interest. The researcher lays out his or her notes in piles on the floor, lives with them, handles them, reads them over and over again, tacks bunches of them to a bulletin board, and eventually gets a feel for what is in them. "This may not seem like a very scientific way of doing things, but it works. Some researchers have advocated the use of computers for storing field notes and for reading them. This is certainly an important new option, especially for very large, multidisciplinary projects, with multiple investigators, multiple field sites, and perhaps 10,000 pages or more of field notes."

TABLE 13.3 CATEGORIES USED TO CODE FIELD NOTES

**16 Demography**

161 Population
162 Composition of Population
163 Birth Statistics
164 Morbidity
165 Mortality
166 Internal Migration
167 Immigration and Emigration
168 Population Policy

**57 Interpersonal Relations**

571 Social Relationships and Groups
572 Friendships
573 Cliques
574 Viking and Hospitality
575 Sodalities
576 Etiquette
577 Ethics
578 Ingroup Antagonisms

**74 Health and Welfare**

741 Philanthropic Foundation
742 Medical Research
743 Hospitals and Clinics
744 Public Health and Sanitation
745 Social Insurance
746 Public Assistance
747 Private Welfare Agencies
748 Social Work

**75 Sickness**

751 Preventive Medicine
752 Bodily Injuries
753 Theory of Disease
754 Sorcery
755 Magic and Mental Therapy
756 Psychotherapists
757 Medical Therapy
758 Medical Care
759 Medical Personnel

**77 Religious Beliefs**

771 General Character of Religion
772 Cosmology
773 Mythology
774 Animism
775 Eschatology and God
776 Spirits and God

Like most fieldworkers, Ragucci reviewed her field notes at frequent, usually daily, intervals. It was probably somewhere near or in the middle of phase II that Ragucci discovered she was actually seeing evidence of culture change in health beliefs and healing practices of women in the Italian enclave (from traditional to contemporary folk medicine) across four, rather than three, generational groups: first generation, older second generation (those over age 50 years), young second generation, and third generation.

During this second phase, researchers often use additional techniques for collecting data, although some methods (e.g., mapping and census taking) are frequently begun in phase I. The techniques selected may range from highly qualitative (e.g., use of the Rorschach ink-blot test to identify culture-based personality traits) to quantitative (e.g., use of the household survey to enumerate family structure and values). Researchers usually do not decide on what additional techniques to use until they have been in the field for quite awhile. They like to closely fit and refine selected techniques to the particular language and practices of the people being studied and the specific problem of interest. Table 13.4 lists some of the more frequently used techniques.

Ragucci interplayed participant observation with four of the techniques in Table 13.4. She did the following:

- Analyzed government documents to identify demographic features (e.g., population's size and density, morbidity, and mortality) and general social and health problems of members of the Italian enclave
- Mapped out the physical features and buildings of the Italian community in the North End
- Analyzed the Patron Saint Ceremonial of St. Anthony of Padua to examine

---

TABLE 13.4 ADDITIONAL TECHNIQUES USED FOR DATA COLLECTION

1. Census Taking: Collection of basic demographic data (e.g., age, occupation, marital status, household composition) about the people being studied.
2. Mapping: Identifying the location of people, material culture, and environmental features in space in order to understand how people interact with their physical environment.
3. Document Analysis: Examination of data such as vital statistics records, newspapers, or personal diaries to supplement information collected through interviewing and participant observation.
4. Collecting Genealogies: A system of written notation of all of the kin relationships of informants, in order to study the kinship system.
5. Life Histories: Comprehensive biography of an informant's life, which often provides a vivid example of the way in which general cultural patterns are integrated in a person's life.
6. Event Analysis: Detailed written and photographic documentation of such events as weddings, funerals, and festivals in the culture under investigation.
7. Interviewing: A face-to-face encounter in which a respondent is asked a set of questions designed to obtain information central to the aims of the researcher.
8. Questionnaires and Surveys: A method for systematically obtaining standardized information about the attitudes, behavior, and other characteristics of a population.

---

the persistence of traditional religious beliefs and practices and to see if these paralleled the same generational changes she had seen in the health sphere

*Phase III*

In the final fieldwork phase, the researcher can raise more sensitive questions and obtain an increasingly large volume of information. Phase III is when researchers concentrate on double-checking and monitoring field information to do the following:

1. Support and further refine central themes identified earlier
2. Evaluate data gathered by specialized techniques
3. Broaden understanding of how representative the research findings are of members of the culture as a whole

**Post-Fieldwork**

The researcher returns home during this stage to finalize and write up the findings of the field research, although this will have already been started in the field. In writing up the findings, the researcher makes several major choices related to what audience to address, which voice to use, what data to present, and how to organize the findings. These choices are reflected in the various formats you might see in published ethnographies.

Most researchers choose to write for a scholarly audience, take an authoritative voice (as though they were neutral observers), and begin with the findings. This is followed by a presentation of selected data to support those findings. This "classic" ethnography is usually begun with a brief overview of the setting and the people being studied, followed by a review of the specific problem being addressed and a discussion of the fieldwork phase. The description of the researcher and his or her relationship to the subjects is usually provided in this section of the write-up. The bulk of the text follows, consisting of impersonally written, monologic descriptions of the culture that analyze the specific problem. The actual presentation is usually rich in detail and well ordered, first with regard to the culture as a whole and second with regard to the specific cultural problem being addressed. In this classic format, the researcher is intent on capturing the culture as a whole and tries to avoid depicting any one individual in too much detail for fear of confusing individual personality characteristics with attributes of the culture as a whole. At the same time these presentations vary somewhat, according to the specific theories, interpretations, or styles of analysis used by the researcher.

**QUESTIONS TO CONSIDER WHEN CRITIQUING ETHNOGRAPHIC RESEARCH**

Identify an ethnographic research study to critique. Read the study to see if you recognize any key terms discussed in this chapter. Remember that all studies may not contain all key terms. The following questions serve as a guide in critiquing ethnographic research:

1. *Has the researcher clearly identified the culture to be studied?* Ethnography as a qualitative approach provides an opportunity for intimacy with members of a culture. Identify if the researcher has focused on a particular culture and described the culture in detail.
2. *Was the study conducted in the field? fieldwork performed?* A characteristic of ethnographic research is the participant's cultural immersion. This requires researchers "living" among the people being studied, making contacts, and establishing a role. Has the researcher provided evidence that cultural immersion occurred?
3. *Does the researcher clearly describe his or her role in the study?* Researchers must understand the role they play in the discovery of cultural knowledge. Because the researcher becomes the "instrument", he or she is required to participate in the culture, observe the participants, document observations, interview members of the cultural group, examine documents, possibly collect artifacts, and report the findings. Is there evidence that the researcher has participated in various activities to discover the cultural knowledge needed to organize and interpret a variety of experiences?
4. *Were multiple sources of data (i.e., participant observations, document analysis, life histories, analysis) used?* After identifying the type of culture being studied, identify if data sources were appropriate.
5. *Was time in the field adequate to meet the purpose of the study?* The length of time spent in the field varies among studies and depends on the research question, complexity of the culture, time required to build relationships, and access to data. Fieldwork requires complete commitment through constant observation and participation in various cultural activities. Look to see if the researcher has identified time spent in cultural immersion and if it makes sense.

## SUMMARY OF KEY IDEAS

1. Ethnographic research includes both anthropological and historical research strategies.
2. In ethnographic studies, the researcher becomes immersed in the subjects and their way of life in order to understand the cultural forces that shape behavior.
3. The aim of the ethnographer is to learn from (rather than to study) members of cultural groups to understand their worldviews as they define it.
4. The planning and implementing of an ethnographic study takes place in three stages: pre-fieldwork, fieldwork, and post-fieldwork.

## LEARNING ACTIVITIES

1. Identify one article from these research-oriented journals within the last 5 years that describes an ethnographic study: *Applied Nursing Research,*

*Nursing Research, Research in Nursing and Health, and Western Journal of Nursing Research.*

a. Did the article follow the definition of ethnographic research as defined by this chapter? Why or why not?

b. Describe how the researcher was immersed in the subject's way of life.

2. Identify an area of study that would be amenable to the ethnographic approach. Discuss:

a. The purpose of the study.

b. The setting for data collection.

c. The timeline associated with data collection.

d. How the researcher might function to obtain data.

## References

1. Emerson, RM: Contemporary Field Research: A Collection of Readings. Little, Brown, Boston, 1983.
2. Denzin, NK, and Lincoln, YS: Handbook of a Qualitative Research. Sage Publications, Thousand Oaks, CA, 1994.
3. Oftand, J: Analytic ethnography: Features, failings and futures. J Contemp Ethnography 24:30, 1995.
4. Hammersicy, M: What's Wrong with Ethnography: Methodological Explorations. Routhledge, New York, 1992.

5. Honigmann, JJ: The Development of Anthropological Ideas. The Dorsey Press, Homewood, IL, 1976.
6. Mead, M: Blackberry Winter: My Earlier Years. Pocket Books, New York, 1972.
7. Sutherland, DJ: Nursing in the Peace Corps. Nurs Outlook 11:888, 1963.
8. Bruno, P, and Shanahah, M: Teaching Peace Corps volunteers. Am J Nurs 65:96, 1965.
9. Leininger, M: Nursing and Anthropology: Two Worlds to Blend. John Wiley and Sons, New York, 1970.
10. Ragucci, AT: The ethnographic approach and nursing research. Nurs Res 21:485, 1972.
11. Aamodt, AM: The child view of health and healing. Communicating Nurs Res 5:38, 1972.
12. Boas, F: Kwakiutl Ethnography. University of Chicago Press, Chicago, 1966.
13. Radin, P: Crashing Thunder: The Autiobiography of an American Indian. Appleton, New York, 1922.
14. Berreman, GD: Behind Many Masks (Monograph 4). Society for Applied Anthropology, New York, 1962.
15. Chagnon, NA: Yanomamo: The Fierce People. Holt, Rinehart and Winston, New York, 1968.
16. Beattie, J: Bunyoro: An African Kingdom. Holt, Rinehart and Winston, New York, 1965.
17. Ellen, RF: Ethnographic Research: A Guide to General Conduct. Academic Press, New York, 1984.
18. Messerschmidt, DA: Anthropologists at Home in North America: Methods and Issues in the Study of One's Own Society. Cambridge University Press, New York, 1981.
19. Moffatt, M: Ethnographic writing about American culture. Ann Rev Anthropology 21:205, 1992.
20. Aamodt, AM: Enculturation process and the Papago child: An inquiry into the acquisition of perspectives on health and healing. Doctoral dissertation, University of Washington, 1971.
21. Ragucci, AT: Generational continuity and change in concepts of health, curing practices, and ritual expressions of the women of an Italian-American enclave. Doctoral dissertation, Boston University, 1971.
22. Rempusheski, VF: Exploration and description of caring for self and others with second generation Polish American elders. Doctoral dissertation, University of Arizona, 1985.
23. Farmer, B: The Meadows of Madison: An ethnographic study of the organizational climate of a nursing home. Doctoral dissertation, University of Rhode Island, 1995.
24. Stuhler-Schlag, MK: An ethnography of hospice home care. Doctoral dissertation, Rutgers University, 1985.
25. Wolf, ZR: Nurses' Work: The Sacred and the Profane. Pennsylvania Press, Philadelphia, 1988.
26. Germain, C: Ethnography: The method. In Munhall, PL, and Oiler, CJ (eds): Nursing Research: A Qualitative Perspective. Appleton-Century-Crofts, Norwalk, CT, 1986, p 147.
27. Sanday, PR: The ethnographic paradigm. In Van Maanen, J (ed): Qualitative Methodology. Sage Publications, Thousand Oaks, CA, 1983.
28. Werner, O, and Schoepfle, MG: Systematic Fieldwork: Foundations of Ethnography and Interviewing. Sage Publications, Thousand Oaks, CA, 1987.
29. Aamodt, AM: Discovering the child's view of alopecia: Doing ethnography. In Munhall, PL, and Oiler, CJ (eds): Nursing Research: A Qualitative Perspective. Appleton-Century-Crofts, Norwalk, CT, 1986, p 163.
30. Craig, CE: Down home: An ethnography about community process and health of older persons in a rural setting. Doctoral dissertation, University of Colorado Health Science Center, 1991.

31. Ferraro, G: Cultural Anthropology: An Applied Perspective, ed 2. West Publishing, New York, 1995.

32. Bernard, RH: Research Methods in Cultural Anthropology. Sage Publications, Thousand Oaks, CA, 1988.

## Suggested Readings

*Ethnographies of Ethnic Groups in the United States*

*Cambodians*

Kulig, JC: Role status changes and family planning use among Cambodian refugee women. Doctoral dissertation, University of California at San Francisco, 1991.

*Chicanos*

Zavella, P: Women's work and Chicano families: Cannery workers of the Santa Clara Valley. Cornell University Press, Ithaca, 1987.

*Franco-Americans*

Drew, JC: A nursing study of health and illness beliefs, explanatory models and help-seeking patterns among Franco-Americans. Doctoral dissertation, University of Texas at Austin, 1990.

*Haitians*

Laguerre, MS: American Odyssey: Haitians in New York City. Cornell University Press, Ithaca, 1984.

*Italians*

diLeonardo, M: The Varieties of Ethnic Experience: Kinship, Class and Gender among Italian Americans. Cornell University Press, Ithaca, 1984.

Tricarico, D: The Italians of Greenwich Village: The Social Structure and Transformation of an Ethnic Community. Center for Migration Studies, New York, 1984.

*Jews*

Kugelmass, J: The Miracle of Intervale Avenue: The Story of a Jewish Congregation in the South Bronx. Schocken, New York, 1986.

Shokeid, M: Children of Circumstances: Israeli Emigrants in New York. Cornell University Press, Ithaca, 1988.

*Punjabi Sikh of Pakistan*

Gibson, MS: Accommodation Without Assimilation: Sikh Immigrants in an American High School. Cornell University Press, Ithaca, 1988.

*Taiwanese*

Hsiang-Shui C: Chinatown No More: Taiwan Immigrants in Contemporary New York. Cornell University Press, Ithaca, 1992.

# 14

# Grounded Theory Research

Cheryl Tatano Beck, DNSc, RN, CNM, FAAN

## LEARNING OBJECTIVES

*At the end of this chapter, you will be able to:*

1. Discuss symbolic interactionism as the theoretical framework of grounded theory.
2. Describe the steps in the research process for grounded theory.
3. Compare and contrast theoretical sampling with statistical sampling.
4. Explain the constant comparative method of data analysis.
5. Describe the difference between substantive and theoretical coding.
6. List criteria that can help a researcher decide on a core category.
7. Identify at least six families of theoretical codes.
8. Discuss criteria for judging grounded theory.
9. Distinguish between a core category and a basic social process.

## GLOSSARY OF KEY TERMS

**Basic social process.** Type of core category that has two or more clear emergent stages.

**Category.** Type of concept that is usually used for a higher level of abstraction.

**Coding.** Process by which data are conceptualized.

**Constant comparative method of data analysis.** Form of qualitative data analysis that categorizes units of meaning through a process of comparing incident to incident until concepts emerge.

**Core category.** Pattern of behavior that is relevant and/or problematic for persons in a study.

**Formal theory.** Theory developed for a conceptual or formal area of inquiry.

**Grounded theory.** Discovery of a theory from data that have been systematically obtained through research.

**Memos.** Write-up of ideas about codes and their relationships as they occur to the researcher while coding.

**Open coding.** First phase of substantive coding, which occurs before core variables emerge; initial discovery of categories.

**Selective coding.** Process of selecting core variables.

**Substantive codes.** Conceptual meanings given by generating categories and their properties. These meanings conceptualize the empirical substance of the area of research.

**Substantive theory.** Theory developed for

an empirical or substantive area of research.

**Symbolic interactionism.** Theoretical orientation to qualitative research; focus is on the nature of social interaction among individuals.

**Theoretical codes.** Conceptual models of how substantive codes may relate to each other as hypotheses to be included in the theory.

**Theoretical sampling.** Process used in data collection that is controlled by the emerging theory; researcher collects, codes, and analyzes the data.

## GROUNDED THEORY

Grounded theory is a qualitative research method based on the symbolic interactionist perspective of human behavior. In the 1960s, two sociologists at the University of California, San Francisco, Barney Glaser and Anselm Strauss, developed this method. Glaser received his training at Columbia University and Strauss came from the University of Chicago. **Grounded theory** is the discovery of theory from data that have been systematically obtained through research. It is theory generated from data collected about an area of study.[1] Grounded theory differs from quantitative research. In quantitative research, the investigator identifies a research problem, selects a theory or conceptual framework, and deduces hypotheses to test. Grounded theory does not start with an existing theory; it generates a theory to explain a substantive area. The research product ends with a theoretical formulation or integrated set of conceptual hypotheses.[1]

Grounded theory combines both inductive and deductive research methods. With the use of inductive processes, the theory emerges from the data. Deduction is then used to test the theory empirically. The two types of theory that are generated through an inductive approach are substantive theory and formal theory. **Substantive theory** is developed for an empirical area of inquiry such as patient care, whereas **formal theory** is developed for a conceptual area of inquiry.[2] An example of a substantive theory is displayed in Excerpt 14.1. This study described health problems among homeless women with children living in a transitional shelter. Categories or patterns of behavior were present among participants (homeless women) and are described in the article.

## SYMBOLIC INTERACTION

**Symbolic interaction** provides the theoretical underpinnings of grounded theory. This social psychological theory is traced back to two sociologists from the University of Chicago, George Herbert Mead[3] and his student, Herbert Blumer.[4] Symbolic interaction focuses on the nature of social interaction among individuals. Basic principles central to symbolic interaction include the fact that human beings act in relation to one another, take each other's acts into account as they themselves act, and provide meaning to specific symbols in their lives.[4]

In summarizing symbolic interactionism, Charon[5] identified several central ideas. Symbolic interaction is an active, dynamic image of human beings when the focus

## EXAMPLE OF SUBSTANTIVE THEORY DERIVED FROM DATA

### Findings

When asked to describe their health, study participants often described their mental health concerns. They reported alcohol and other drug use, bipolar disorders, depression, suicidal behaviors, self-mutilation, and anxiety related to repeated physical and emotional abuse from male partners. These women pushed physical health into the background of their lives and frequently had difficulty articulating physical health concerns. Moreover, many ailments that a health care clinician would consider serious and warranting treatment, these women considered mundane. Such ailments included cystitis, otitis media, and sexually transmitted diseases.

As for managing their health problems, data analysis revealed four conditions as most salient: shame, fear, lack of information, and lack of eligibility. These conditions and the fragmented health care system had consequences for how a woman typically cared for her health problems: overcoming it alone. A description of these conditions, actions, and interactions follows.

**Shame.** Participants reported experiencing shame under many different circumstances. For some residents, shame was linked to years of drug and alcohol use. One respondent recounted a lengthy story about how she had "got off drugs by herself" because she was "too embarrassed to seek help from someone else." She confided that she had not told the shelter staff about her history of drug use.

**Fear.** Still other circumstances exacerbated problems associated with shame. It was not uncommon for a woman to have one or more children living in foster care because of charges of child abuse and neglect. Some women actively pursued regaining custody of children no longer living with them. These women, who struggled to control a variety of problems including psychiatric illness and substance abuse while parenting, feared they would be unable to retain custody of their children.

**Lack of information.** In addition to shame and fear, the women in this study had limited information about their own health and that of their children. They were unfamiliar about the need for Pap tests for themselves and immunizations for their children. Moreover, they had limited information about health care services available in the community.

**Eligibility.** Some of the study participants were ineligible to receive publicly-funded health care services such as Medicaid. One resident, who was attempting to regain custody of her newborn son by living in the shelter and attending a drug recovery program, lost her Medicaid eligibility because she had lost her Aid to Families with Dependent Children (AFDC) benefits. She said that she could not afford treatment for other health related problems. Another resident, also ineligible for Medicaid, reported that she did not have enough money to purchase prescribed digoxin for a cardiac problem present since childhood.

*Source: Hatton, DC: Managing health problems among homeless women with children in a transitional shelter. Image J Nurs Schol 29:33, 1997, with permission.*

is on the interaction rather than the individual. This is in contrast to viewing human beings as passive individuals responding to others and the environment. Interaction refers to individuals acting in relation to one another. Likewise, individuals act according to the way a situation is defined. The focus of symbolic interactionism is the present, not the past. Blumer[6] posits that human interaction is a positive shaping process. Participants have to build up their own lines of conduct by constant interpretation of others' ongoing action. This complex interrelationship between what the participant or actor brings to the situation and what occurs in social interaction is diagrammed by Charon[5] (Fig. 14.1).

Implications for research activity can be derived from symbolic interactionism.[7] To understand human behavior, one must examine the nature of social interaction. Within natural settings, social behavior is examined from an individual and group perspective. The researcher examines the world from an individual's perspective and discovers how to interpret himself or herself in the context of others. As an observer, the researcher translates the meaning obtained from interactions into a language understood by others.

## Research Problem/Questions

In grounded theory, the research problem is discovered, as is the process that resolves it.[1] The grounded theorist moves into an area of interest with no specific problem in mind. Researchers should be careful not to force the data with the grounded theorist's own preconceived problem, keeping an open mind to the emergence of the participant's problem.

The question is asked: "What is the chief concern or problem of the people in the substantive area, and what accounts for most of the variation in processing the problem?"[1] Excerpt 14.2 displays two research questions that guided a grounded theory study about postpartum depression.[8]

## Data Collection

Grounded theorists must go into the field, or natural world, to view the environment as informants do and focus on the interaction under study. Participant observation,

---

**EXCERPT 14.2**

### RESEARCH QUESTIONS FROM GROUNDED THEORY STUDY ON POSTPARTUM DEPRESSION

1. What is the specific social psychological problem that women experience during postpartum depression?
2. What social psychological process do postpartum depressed women use to resolve this fundamental problem?

*Source: Beck, CT: Teetering on the edge: A substantive theory of postpartum depression. Nurs Res 42:42, 1993, with permission.*

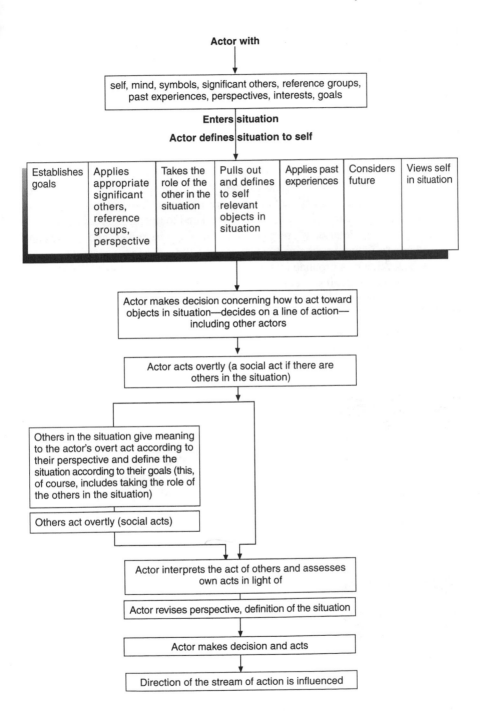

**FIGURE 14.1** Interaction of participant (actor) with social environment.

informal interviewing, and formal interviewing are the three main sources of data generation. Unstructured observational data are gathered by participant observation. While participating in the functioning of a social group, the researcher is observing and is recording data. Participant observation is combined with informal interviewing. Like everyday conversations, informal interviewing can last from a few minutes to more than an hour. The grounded theorist writes field notes to record data obtained through participant observation and interviewing. An example of field notes written during the postpartum depression study is given in Excerpt 14.3.

Formal interviewing is also used, when the researcher wishes more in-depth information. Unstructured formal interviews are used most frequently to obtain detailed information in the participant's own words. Formal interviews are audiotaped to capture the participant's interview word-for-word. A researcher may use an interview guide consisting of several questions related to the topic. A time and place for conducting the interview are agreed to by the researcher and participant. Informed consent must be obtained before starting the interview.

At the beginning of a grounded theory study, the researcher asks general research questions. As theory begins to emerge, the researcher asks more specific questions to elicit information needed to saturate developing codes and categories. Based on the evolving theory, the grounded theorist asks different participants different questions. Excerpt 14.4 addresses the data-gathering techniques and interview questions used in the postpartum depression study.

---

## EXCERPT 14.3

### EXAMPLE OF FIELDNOTES

During today's support group meeting the group leader, myself, and three mothers attended the meeting. Two of these mothers were attending the support group for the first time. B. has a teenage handicapped daughter and a 3-month-old daughter. Postpartum depression hit B. about 6 weeks postpartum "like a ton of bricks." She experienced anxiety to the point of being nauseated. She cannot concentrate to even write one check. At first she thought someone should drop the baby. Later on it was B. thinking she should drop the baby. She told her husband, if need be, just lock her up so she won't harm the baby. Loss of control is the worst thing for B. She says she is always used to being in control. J., the second new mother to the support group today, has four children. Her baby is 2 weeks old. With all four children J. suffered postpartum depression. With each of her first three children, postpartum depression lasted about 6 months. J. just suffered in silence with the first three children. J. is breast feeding and her husband doesn't want her to stop because formula is too expensive. Therefore, she can't be on any antidepressives. J. has no medical insurance so she can't afford to see a psychiatrist. J.'s postpartum depression began as soon as she walked out of the hospital. She said it was like a veil came over her. She has no energy or interest in anything.

*Source: Beck, CT: Teetering on the edge: A substantive theory of postpartum depression. Nurs Res 42:42, 1993, with permission.*

**EXCERPT 14.4**

## EXAMPLE OF DATA-GATHERING TECHNIQUES AND INTERVIEW QUESTIONS

Participant observation, and both informal and formal interviews, were methods of data collection used. Data collection took place over an 18-month period. The researcher assisted in facilitating a postpartum depression support group, which met twice a month throughout this time. During the group meetings, the researcher's role was one of nursing consultant to the mothers by answering questions, providing suggestions, and helping to facilitate the group meetings. After each support group meeting, the researcher immediately wrote fieldnotes on the interactions that had occurred during the meeting.

Twelve mothers who had attended the support group were interviewed in-depth. The interviews took place in private at either the women's homes or in the facility where the support group was held. These mothers were asked to describe their experiences with postpartum depression starting with the onset of symptoms and continuing through the recovery period. All interviews were audiotaped, transcribed, and reviewed to detect errors or omissions that may have occurred during the transcribing.

**Initial Interview Questions**

1. Would you please share with me your story of postpartum depression from the beginning of your symptoms and continue through your recovery (or until the present time if you are still experiencing it)?
2. Would you please describe your interactions with your baby, family, friends, and health care professional during your postpartum depression?
3. When you were suffering through postpartum depression, what was a typical day like for you?

**Focused Interview Questions**

1. Did you experience any loss of control during your postpartum depression? If so, in what specific aspects of your life did you experience this loss of control?
2. Were there any specific strategies you used to try and cope with your loss of control?

*Source: Beck, CT: Teetering on the edge: A substantive theory of postpartum depression. Nurs Res 42:42, 1993, with permission.*

## Theoretical Sampling

**Theoretical sampling** is the process of data collection for generating theory, whereby the researcher jointly collects, codes, and analyzes data and then decides what data to collect next in order to develop the grounded theory. This process of data collection is controlled by the emerging theory.[9] The grounded theorist uses theoretical sampling for emergence to fill in thin areas and extend the substantive theory. This is the process by which data collection is continually guided.

Theoretical sampling is done to discover categories and their properties. Unlike statistical sampling, used in quantitative research, a predetermined sample size is not calculated. In theoretical sampling, sample size is determined by generated data and analyses. Theoretical sampling is continued until the categories are saturated. Saturation indicates repetition of data when nothing new is found. Excerpt 14.5 displays a memo written while conducting the grounded theory study on postpartum depression. It illustrates the process of theoretical sampling.

## Coding

From the first day of fieldwork, the grounded theorist is simultaneously collecting, coding, and analyzing data. **Coding** is a process to conceptualize data into patterns called concepts. The **constant comparative method of data analysis** is a form of qualitative data analysis that makes sense of data by constantly comparing incidents until categories and concepts emerge. A **category** is a higher level of abstraction. A property is a characteristic of a category.[1]

Two types of coding are used in grounded theory: substantive and theoretical. **Substantive coding** is the first stage of constant comparative data analysis, in which the initial discovery of categories and their properties occurs. Substantive coding consists of open and selective coding. The grounded theorist starts without any preconceived codes. During **open coding,** data are broken down into incidents and examined for similarities and differences. When coding each incident, the grounded theorist asks the neutral question, "What category or property of a category does this incident indicate?"[1] Open coding ends when it yields a core category. Excerpt 14.6 provides an example of substantive coding from one of the interviews in the postpartum depression study. **Selective coding** beings only after the researcher is sure the core variable has emerged. For the grounded theorist, to code selectively for a core variable means to delineate only variables that relate to the core variable.

Glaser[2] also suggests constructing a typology as one approach to examining data. Typologies are based on differentiating criteria associated with the concept. The researcher constructs a typology when the dimensions of a concept can be cross-tabulated. Each cell within the table must make a difference in its relation to other categories; otherwise the typology is not useful to the theory being generated.

Figure 14.2 illustrates an example of the typology, "Battling the System," and some of its dimensions from the grounded theory study on postpartum depression.

<hr>

**EXCERPT 14.5**

## EXAMPLE OF THEORETICAL SAMPLING MEMO

Two younger primiparas in their early twenties who I have interviewed seem quite emphatic about never having another baby because they refuse to gamble on having postpartum depression again. There is a pregnant woman in her thirties who just started attending the support group. This is her fourth pregnancy and she had postpartum depression after each of her first three pregnancies! I will approach her after the next support group meeting to ask if she would be willing to be interviewed.

*Source: Beck, CT: Teetering on the edge: A substantive theory of postpartum depression. Nurs Res 42:42, 1993, with permission.*

EXCERPT 14.6

## EXAMPLE OF SUBSTANTIVE CODING

| | |
|---|---|
| It's like you're just not real. You're there and you're not there. You don't feel anything good. You just feel full of guilt. I felt like the worst person in the world. The worst mother, and I had failed. I couldn't understand why I wasn't enjoying holding my son or taking care of him. I didn't want to do anything that I liked to do before. I was living in these thoughts that I was a horrible person, a horrible mother, and what's wrong with me? What's wrong with me? I was just obsessed on this all day long. That was where I was all day in my mind. At that point I would scream and have thoughts about hurting myself because I just couldn't get out of the pain. I just wanted to get out of the world. Everything was black. | Feeling unreal. Lacking positive emotions. Consuming guilt. Not understanding. Lacking interest. Obsessive thinking.  Questioning.   Contemplating death. |

*Source: Beck, CT: Teetering on the edge: A substantive theory of postpartum depression. Nurs Res 42:42, 1993, with permission.*

A typology was created based on criteria of how much the mothers and the health-care professionals knew about postpartum depression. How rapidly a mother was correctly diagnosed as suffering from postpartum depression and received effective treatment depended on the amount of knowledge both parties had about this mood disorder.

Hutchinson[10] identified three levels of coding that are used in grounded theory. Level I coding involves in vivo or substantive codes, using participants' words. Level II coding is used to move data to a more abstract level; codes at this level are called categories. Some of the in vivo codes can be collapsed into Level II codes. Level III coding involves developing theoretical constructs. These constructs add

**Mother's Postpartum Depression Knowledge**

| | | + | − |
|---|---|---|---|
| **Health-Care Professional's Postpartum Depression Knowledge** | + | Rapid, correct diagnosis | Delayed, correct diagnosis |
| | − | Misdiagnosis Mother continues search | Postpartum depression undetected or misdiagnosed |

FIGURE 14.2 Typology of battling the system.

theoretical meaning and scope to the substantive theory.[2] Figure 14.3 illustrates these three levels of coding and how they were collapsed to generate one construct in the postpartum depression study.

**Theoretical coding,** which focuses on how substantive codes relate to each other, weaves the fractured pieces of the story back together again. The grounded theorist needs to be familiar with many theoretical codes in order to be alert to the subtleties of the relationships in the data. Glaser[2] lists 18 families of theoretical codes (Table 14.1). These coding families are not mutually exclusive; they overlap considerably. Figure 14.4 highlights theoretical coding in the postpartum depression study. Horrifying anxiety attacks, relentless obsessive thinking, and enveloping fogginess were three conditions of postpartum depression. These conditions caused alarming unrealness, isolating oneself, and contemplating and attempting self-destruction. Mothers used the strategies of battling the system, praying for relief, and seeking solace at support groups to cope. As a result of these strategies, mothers experienced unpredictable transitioning, mourning lost time, and guarded recovery.

The goal of grounded theory is to generate a theory around a core category. A **core category** represents a pattern of behavior that is relevant and/or problematic for persons involved in a study.[2] Glaser[2] identified the following criteria to help a researcher decide on a core category:

1. It must be central. It can be related to as many other categories as possible.
2. It must recur frequently in the data.
3. It takes more time to saturate the core variable than other categories.

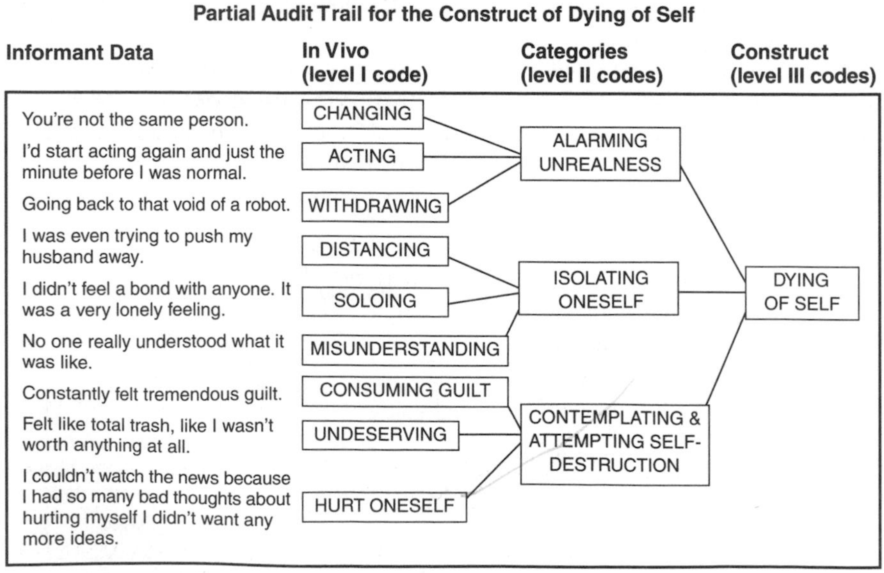

**Partial Audit Trail for the Construct of Dying of Self**

FIGURE 14.3 Partial audit trail for the construct of dying of self.

TABLE 14.1  CODING FAMILIES

1. The Six C's: Causes, contexts, contingencies, consequences, covariance, conditions
2. Process: Stages, phases, progressions, passages, graduations, transitions. A process must have at least two stages
3. Degree Family: Limit, range, intensity, extent, amount, grades, continuum, probability, level, cutting points
4. Dimension Family: Dimensions, elements, division, piece, properties, facet, slice, sector, portion, segments, part, aspect, section
5. Type Family: Type, form, kinds, styles, classes, genre
6. Strategy Family: Strategies, tactics, mechanisms, manipulation, maneuvering, dealing with, handling, techniques, ploys, means, goals
7. Interactive Family: Mutual effects, reciprocity, mutual trajectory, mutual depending, interdependence, interaction of effects, covariance
8. Identity—Self Family: Self-image, self-concept, self-worth, self-evaluation, identity, social worth
9. Cutting Point Family: Boundary, critical juncture, cutting point, turning point, breaking point
10. Means—Goal Family: End, purpose, goal, anticipated consequences, products
11. Cultural Family: Social norms, social values, social beliefs, social sentiments
12. Consensus Family: Clusters, agreements, contracts, uniformities, opinions
13. Mainline Family: Social control, recruitment, socialization, stratification, status passage, social organization, social order, social institutions, social interaction, social worlds, social mobility
14. Theoretical Family: Parsimony, scope, integration, density, conceptual level, relationship to data, relationship to other theory, clarity, fit, relevance, modifiability, utility, condensibility, inductive-deductive balance, use of theoretical codes, interpretive, explanatory, predictive power
15. Ordering or Elaboration Family: Structural, temporal, generality
16. Unit Family: Collective, group, notion, organization, aggregate, situation, context, arena, social world, behavioral pattern, territorial units, society, family and positional units: status, role, role relationship
17. Reading Family: Concepts, problems, hypotheses
18. Models: Model the theory pictorially by either a linear model or a property space

4. It relates meaningfully and easily to other categories.
5. It has clear and grabbing implication for formal theory.
6. It has considerable carry-through in relation to the analysis of the processes the analyst is working on.
7. It is completely variable.
8. It accounts for variation in the problematic behavior and is a dimension of the problem.
9. It can be any kind of theoretical code: a process, a condition, a consequence. When it is a process, additional criteria also apply.

**Basic social processes** (BSPs) are core categories that depict social processes as they continue over time, regardless of varying conditions. All BSPs are core variables, but not all core categories are BSPs. BSPs must have two or more clear

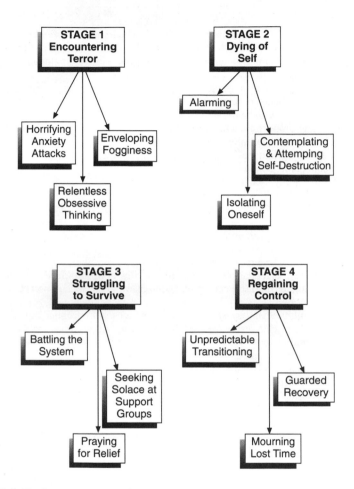

**The Four-Stage Process of Teetering on the Edge**

FIGURE 14.4 The four-stage process of teetering on the edge.

emergent stages. A core category is always present in grounded theory, but a BSP may not be. Stages are the prime property of BSPs. BSPs are labeled using a gerund ("-ing"). Figure 14.4 summarizes the BSP called "teetering on the edge," which emerged from the grounded theory on postpartum depression. This BSP is a four-stage process mothers used to resolve the basic social psychological problem of loss of control. This central problem of loss of control emerged from the data just as the BSP did. The four stages of teetering on the edge included encountering terror, dying of self, struggling to survive, and regaining control. The title, "Teetering on the Edge" described how mothers walked a fine line between sanity and insanity.

## Review of the Literature

In a grounded theory study, the review of literature does not occur at the start. The grounded theorist begins by collecting data in the field and generating a theory. When the theory appears to be sufficiently grounded and developed, the literature is reviewed and related to the developing theory.[2] By waiting to complete a literature review, the researcher avoids contaminating the data with preconceived concepts that may or may not be relevant. Grounded theory discovers concepts and hypotheses rather than tests or replicates hypotheses.

Excerpts 14.7 to 14.9 are examples of related lay literature validating the emerging grounded theory of "teetering on the edge."[8] One mother's poem on postpartum depression, published in the newsletter *Depression After Delivery*,[11] is in Excerpt 14.7. The poem was analyzed to examine which substantive codes from the developing grounded theory were validated. Excerpt 14.8 is another article recounting a mother's story of postpartum depression, published in the journal *Mothering*.[12] Her personal account of the benefits she received by attending a support group validated one of the mothers' strategies that emerged in phase 3 of "teetering on the edge":[8] seeking solace at support groups. The last example of related lay literature is an excerpt from an anonymous article entitled "Postpartum Illness Feels Like A Thief,"[13] which was published in *Depression After Delivery* (Excerpt 14.9). Two consequences that emerged in the fourth phase of "teetering on the edge," mourning lost time and guarded recovery, are clearly highlighted in this story.

## Memos

**Memos** are the write-up of ideas as they emerge while the grounded theorist is coding for categories, properties, and their relationships. Memos are written up as ideas occur to the grounded theorist while he or she is comparing, coding, and analyzing the data. The length of a memo can be a sentence, a paragraph, or even several pages. The researcher is not constrained by having to "write correctly" at all times. The purpose of memos is to record the researcher's ideas and get them on paper. Sorting memos in a theoretical outline is an essential step in grounded theory research. Excerpt 14.10 shows one memo written while conducting the postpartum depression study. The end product of sorting memos can be found in the outline presented in Table 14.2.[8]

## Criteria for Judging Grounded Theory

Glaser[2] identified four criteria for judging grounded theory: fit, work, relevance, and modifiability. Fit refers to categories identified by the emerging theory corresponding to the data collected. Data should not be forced to fit preconceived categories or be discarded in favor of keeping an existing theory intact. Work involves indicating that the grounded theory explains what happens, predicts what will occur, and interprets an area of substantive or formal inquiry. Grounded theory must also achieve relevance. An area of study must be relevant and comprehensible

**EXCERPT 14.7**

## UNTITLED POEM ON POSTPARTUM DEPRESSION

| | |
|---|---|
| Loneliness | Feeling lonely |
| Emptiness | Devoid of feeling |
| Waking from a restless, near-sleepless night | Sleeplessness |
| To a tearful, hopeless morning | |
| Overwhelmed by the thoughts of the new day | Overwhelming |
| Devastation | |
| Confusion | Fogginess |
| Wondering why such a happy time has become one | Questioning |
|    of such despair feeling betrayed by life and its promises | |
| Hopelessness | Lacking hope |
| Worthlessness | Undeserving |
| Doubting that things ever change | |
| Questioning that a second chance at life | Undeserving |
| Is even deserved | |
| What has happened to me? | Questioning |
| Why am I so unhappy? | |
| Who is this person I've become? | |
| Why can't I be myself again? | |
| Isolation | Isolating |
| Resignation | Lacking hope |
| Living in the depths of a bottomless pit | Living hell |
| Wanting to reach beyond it to others | Feeling immobilized |
| But remaining incapable of stretching across the abyss | |
| Will someone reach to me? | Questioning |
| I'm just so tired of it all! | Exhausting |

*Reprinted with permission: Buchanan, P: Untitled poem on postpartum depression. Heartstrings: The National Newsletter of Depression After Delivery 1, 1990, p 3.*

to individuals in the setting. The final criteria for judging grounded theory is modifiability. Theory is always being modified. A grounded theory can never be more correct than its ability to work the data. As new data reveal themselves in research, the theory is modified.

## APPLICATION OF GROUNDED THEORY IN NURSING

Grounded theory is especially suited to knowledge development in nursing because nursing is a practice discipline whose essence lies in processes.[14] Through grounded theory, the processes that underlie social experience are discovered and become the

## CONTACT WITH OTHER MOTHERS

Barring extreme cases, one of the most effective and surely the safest means of combating PPD is through contact with other women who have experienced it or are at least sympathetic to it. Getting in touch with other mothers is wonderfully therapeutic because it solves so many problems associated with PPD: it validates the reality of the condition: it counters the isolation and loneliness with some degree of levity and companionship: it gives hope—hope that PPD will be overcome, and that life will regain its luster and even take on more beauty and meaning.

Seeking solace at support groups

*Source: Leathe, M: Postpartum depression. Mothering 72–77, 1987.*

basis for nursing interventions. As emphasized by Glaser,[2] one of the best arguments for use of grounded theory is that it frees the researcher to discover what *is* going on rather than assume what *should* be going on. Because grounded theory involves an emerging substantive theory from data, the main problem or concern for people in a social setting also must emerge from the data. The researcher remains sensitive to how participants in the social setting interpret and give meaning to their situation. Discovering the problem or focus of the study and what processes account for its solution helps ensure the clinical relevance of the emerging theory. The crucial point of grounded theory for nursing resides in its practical application. Nursing interventions are designed and implemented based on substantive theory grounded in the data.

## Clinical Research Examples

Four clinical research studies are presented, illustrating the applicability of grounded theory in different clinical situations.

### Study 1

The process that occurs in a spinal cord injury (SCI) unit was investigated using grounded theory. For 5 months, Nelson[15] was a participant observer in a 30-bed SCI unit. Effective SCI rehabilitation involved a basic social process of reintegration. Four phases of reintegration emerged: buffering, transcending, toughening, and launching. Buffering involved a nurturing and protective process to lessen and absorb the recently injured SCI patient's shock of injury and the indignities of being

**EXCERPT 14.9**

## POSTPARTUM ILLNESS FEELS LIKE A THIEF

Postpartum illness feels like a thief to those involved with the illness. To the new mother, it steals away her sense of motherhood. She is not the mother she had hoped to become and she is robbed of the joy that she has expected for so long. To her partner, the illness quietly steals away his partner's zest for life—the woman he has loved and with whom he has wanted to establish a family. It steals away their loving time together since the new mother is so preoccupied by her depression or psychosis.

*Mourning lost time*

When one is robbed, one feels violated. What in life is more valuable than experiencing a birth and the joy of a new child?

*Mourning lost time*

The thief lingers in the minds of women once they have suffered the illness. Suppose the thief strikes again? What if I have another baby?

*Guarded recovery*

"Ten years ago I went through postpartum depression. That time of my life still haunts me. I never had any more children for fear that I could go through that again."

*Guarded memory*

"To this day, I have almost no recall of my son's first 6 months of life. It makes me sad that I seem to have missed out on what is supposed to be a happy time.

*Mourning lost time*

*Source: Anonymous: Postpartum illness feels like a thief. Depression After Delivery Newsletter 1:3, 1989.*

a patient. During transcending, SCI patients were helped to recognize and rise above culturally imposed limitations and negative beliefs about persons with disabilities. The toughening phase involved compensating for physical limitations, gaining independence, and maintaining social interactions "without using the disability"— meaning that patients did not con people into helping them with things the patients are capable of doing but do not want to do. Launching focused on exposing SCI patients to the real world, exploring options for living in the community, promoting

TABLE 14.2 SORTING MEMOS TO PRODUCE AN OUTLINE

**Loss of Control: Basic Social Psychological Problem**

Teetering on the edge: Basic social process
  I. Encountering terror
      A. Horrifying anxiety attacks
      B. Relentless obsessive thinking
      C. Enveloping fogginess
  II. Dying of self
      A. Alarming unrealness
      B. Isolating oneself
      C. Contemplating and attempting self-destruction
  III. Struggling to survive
      A. Battling the system
      B. Praying for relief
      C. Seeking solace at support groups
  IV. Regaining Control
      A. Unpredictable transitioning
      B. Mourning lost time
      C. Guarded recovery

the patient's autonomy and decision making, and facilitating discharge from the rehabilitation program.

*Study 2*

Mishel and Murdaugh[16] investigated the processes used by family members of heart transplant recipients to cope with the unpredictability brought on by the need for and receipt of heart transplantation. Twenty family members who attended three separate support groups participated in the study. "Redesigning the dream" was the basic social process families used to adjust to heart transplantation. Their initial dream that life would return to normal after the patient received a new heart had to be revised to fit the reality of the medical-technological treatment. The three phases of this process were immersion, passage, and negotiation. Immersion occurred while waiting for a donor. In this phase, a family member (usually the partner)

**EXCERPT 14.10**

EXAMPLE OF MEMOING

When talking about their recovery from postpartum depression, women repeatedly qualify their recovery with terms such as vulnerable, wary, fragile, cautious, and susceptible. In labeling the category for recovery I need to qualify it and use the term "guarded recovery."

*Source: Beck, CT: Teetering on the edge: A substantive theory of postpartum depression. Nurs Res 42:42, 1993, with permission.*

pledges himself or herself to the patient's welfare. Three categories of immersion occur during this stage: freeing self, symbiosis, and trading places. The family member frees himself or herself from tasks in the home, at work, and from social commitments. All attention is devoted to the patient. Symbiosis refers to the benefits received by patients, owing to the close union with the family member while partners suffer from a sense of loss. Trading places also occurs during this stage, as the partner takes on many of the roles the patient performed before the cardiac illness.

After transplant surgery, the second stage of passage begins. This stage consists of three categories: catharsis, vacillation, and awareness. In catharsis, the family member expresses and relives stressful events to help discharge the tension that accumulated during immersion. Vacillation refers to the ebb and flow in the belief of a return to normal life. Gradually, the partner becomes aware of the need to redefine "normal."

The third and final stage in redesigning the dream is negotiation, which occurs during recovery. In the negotiation stage, a dynamic interaction takes place between the patient and family member. Four negotiation passages were identified: recognizing the risks versus second chance, back to normal versus recognizing the risk, "smelling the roses" versus life as it used to be, and life together versus time for self.

## Study 3

Swanson and Chenitz[17] described the psychosocial process that young adults used to adapt to living with genital herpes. Seventy young adults who had a history of genital lesions for at least 6 months were interviewed. The basic social process of regaining a valued self had three phases. The first phase, protecting oneself, focused on guarding and defending the self against a tainted identity and a perceived sense of loss during the time of diagnosis. In the second phase, renewing oneself, the young adult took action to reappraise the self by reaching out and striving to balance his or her life. Preserving oneself, the third phase, included adopting a management style that permitted the individual to live with genital herpes in accordance with his or her sense of self.

## Study 4

A grounded theory of the healing process of female adult incest survivors was generated by Draucker.[18] Eleven survivors, ranging in age from 20 to 64 years, participated in the study. The core variable that emerged was labeled "constructing a personal residence." This process of constructing a residence consisted of three phases: building a new relationship with the self, regulating boundaries, and influencing the community in a meaningful way. Constructing a new relationship with the self involved abdicating responsibility for the abuse, moving to self-acceptance, and providing a structure within which to provide for one's self-care and safety. In the second stage, regulating boundaries, the women limited access to oneself (building walls), allowed entrance of supportive others (building doors), redefined interpersonal relationships, and maintained control in interpersonal relationships (building gates). Influencing one's community, the third phase, involved assisting other survivors and becoming involved in abuse prevention.

These four examples of clinical research are only the "tip of the iceberg" with regard to the applicability of grounded theory in nursing. Nurse researchers have conducted grounded theory studies on a variety of clinical topics, including alcoholic denial,[19] mothering twins during the first year of life,[20] premature menopause in women with early-stage breast cancer,[21] psychosocial needs of intensive care unit patients,[22] change process among women at risk for HIV who engage in survival sex,[23] vulnerability of clients with diabetes and hypertension,[24] preventing fatigue associated with lung and colorectal cancer,[25] support for spouse caregivers in the context of prostate cancer,[26] HIV-positive Mexican and Puerto Rican women,[27] and loneliness in female adolescents.[28]

## QUESTIONS TO CONSIDER WHEN CRITIQUING GROUNDED THEORY RESEARCH

Identify a grounded theory research study to critique. Read the study to see if you recognize any key terms discussed in this chapter. Remember that all studies may not contain all key terms. The following questions serve as a guide in critiqing grounded theory research:

1. *Does the question lend itself to be researched in a social setting?* Grounded theory research is an interactionist perspective and is appropriately used when the phenomena of interest can be examined through social interaction. The research question should lead to data collection from multiple sources of data as well as from a range of people in the social setting, focusing on how they perceive themselves and others.

2. *Were multiple data sources used to collect data?* When evaluating grounded theory research, it is important to pay particular attention to data collection techniques. Identify data collection strategies used in the study (i.e., observation, interview, document analysis, participant observation). Interview data should be backed up with observational data whenever possible. Likewise, a wide range of subjects should be contacted to ensure that the researcher is seeing as much diversity as possible in responses.

3. *What is the nature and scope of the literature review?* One of the most important functions of the literature review is to allow the reader to "see" the phenomenon of interest as the research did at the beginning of the study. The literature review does not dictate the focus of the research. Thus, there is usually no conceptual or theoretical framework presented in a grounded theory research report. The purpose of grounded theory is to generate theory, not test it. However, the literature may suggest directions for early fieldwork and add depth to the theoretical scheme once it is developed.

4. *Does the theory make sense?* Evaluating the theory is the most important step. Does the integration of categories and constructs make sense? Do the concepts hang together logically? Is there sufficient evidence (data) to

support the concepts? One of the most time-consuming aspects of conducting grounded theory research is coding and the ability to coin terms that are meaningful to others. Reseachers are constantly coming up with drafts and asking colleagues to review their coding structures to be sure the terms and jargon used is understandable as the theoretical scheme is presented.

## SUMMARY OF KEY IDEAS

1. The goal of grounded theory is to generate a theory around a core variable that accounts for a pattern of behavior that is relevant and problematic for those persons involved.
2. Symbolic interaction is the theoretical underpinning of grounded theory.
3. In grounded theory the research problem is as much discovered as the process that resolves it.
4. Literature review is delayed until the theory is grounded in the data to avoid contaminating the researcher's efforts to generate concepts from the data with preconceived concepts that may not fit or be relevant.
5. In theoretical sampling the process of data collection is controlled by the emerging theory.
6. The grounded theorist simultaneously collects, codes, and analyzes data.
7. Theoretical sampling is continued until the categories are saturated.
8. Substantive coding and theoretical coding are the two main types of coding in grounded theory.
9. All basic social processes are core variables, but not all core variables are basic social processes.
10. Sorting memos in a theoretical outline is an essential step.
11. Criteria for judging grounded theory include fit, work, relevance, and modifiability.

## LEARNING ACTIVITIES

1. Identify a couple of research studies that use grounded theory methodology, and answer the following questions:
   a. Describe how the social situation being studied was identified by the researcher.

   b. What were the data-gathering techniques used by the researcher?

c. How long was data collection?

d. How were subjects and sites determined?

e. How did the researcher attempt to develop a theory about the social situation that was based on observation/interviewing and literature review?

f. How were the researcher's opinions and thoughts about the topic addressed?

## References

1. Glaser, B: Basics of Grounded Theory Analysis. Sociology Press, Mill Valley, CA, 1992.
2. Glaser, B: Theoretical Sensitivity. Sociology Press, Mill Valley, CA, 1978.
3. Mead, GH: Mind, Self, and Society. University of Chicago Press, Chicago, 1934.
4. Blumer, H: Symbolic Interactionism: Perspectives and Method. Prentice Hall, Englewood Cliffs, NJ, 1969.
5. Charon, J: Symbolic Interactionism: An Introduction, An Interpretation, An Integration. Prentice Hall, Englewood Cliffs, NJ, 1992.
6. Blumer, H: Sociological implications of the thought of George Herbert Mead. Am J Soc 71:535, 1966.
7. Chenitz, W, and Swanson, J: From Practice to Grounded Theory. Addison-Wesley, Menlo Park, CA, 1986.
8. Beck, CT: Teetering on the edge: A substantive theory of post-partum depression. Nurs Res 42:42, 1993.
9. Glaser, B, and Strauss, A: The Discovery of Grounded Theory: Strategies for Qualitative Research. Aldine de Gruyter, New York, 1967, p 45.
10. Hutchinson, S: Grounded theory: The method. In Munhall, P, and Oiler, C (eds): Nursing Research: A Qualitative Perspective. Appleton-Century-Crofts, Norwalk, CT, 1986, pp 111–130.

11. Buchanan, P: Untitled poem on postpartum depression. Heartstrings: National Newsletter of Depression After Delivery 1:3, 1990.
12. Leathe, M: Postpartum depression. Mothering 72–77, 1987.
13. Anonymous: Postpartum illness feels like a thief. Heartstrings: National Newsletter of Depression After Delivery Newsletter 1:3, 1989.
14. Stern, P, and Pyles, S: Using grounded theory methodology to study women's culturally based decisions about health. In Stern, P (ed): Women, Health, and Culture. Hemisphere Publishing, Washington, DC, 1986, pp 1–24.
15. Nelson, A: Patients' perspectives of a spinal cord injury unit. SCI Nurs 7:44, 1990.
16. Mishel, M, and Murdaugh, C: Family adjustment to heart transplantation: Redesigning the dream. Nurs Res 36:332, 1987.
17. Swanson, J, and Chenitz, W: Regaining a valued self: The process of adaptation to living with genital herpes. Qualitative Health Res 3:270, 1993.
18. Draucker, C: The healing process of female adult incest survivors: Constructing a personal residence. Image J Nurs Schol 24:4, 1992.
19. Wing, D: Transcending alcoholic denial. Image J Nurs Schol 27:121, 1995.
20. Beck, CT: Releasing the pause button: Mothering twins during the first year of life. Qualitative Health Res 12:593, 2002.
21. Knopf, MT: Carrying on: The experience of premature menopause in women with early stage breast cancer. Nursing Res 51:9, 2002.
22. Hupcey, JE: Feeling safe: The psychosocial nees of ICU patients. Image J Nurs Schol 32:361, 2000.
23. Mallory, C, and Stern, PN. Awakening as a change process among women at risk for HIV who engage in survival sex. Qualitative Health Res 10:581, 2000.
24. Weiss, J, and Hutchinson, SA: Warnings about vulnerability in clients with diabetes and hypertension. Qualitative Health Res 10:521, 2000.
25. Olson, K, et al: Evolving routines: Preventing fatigue associated with lung and colorectal cancer. Qualitative Health Res 12:655, 2002.
26. Fergus, KD, et al: Active consideration: Conceptualizing patient-provided support for spouse caregivers in the context of prostate cancer. Qualitative Health Res 12:492, 2002.
27. Valdez, M: A metaphor for HIV-positive Mexican and Puerto Rican women. Qualitative Health Res 13:517, 2001.
28. Davidson, P: The process of loneliness for female adolescents: A feminist perspective. Health Care for Women International 16:1, 1995.

# part 3

# Utilization of
# Nursing Research

# Interpreting and Reporting Research Findings

Courtney Lyder, ND, APRN, CS, GPN

## LEARNING OBJECTIVES

*At the end of this chapter, you will be able to:*
1. List factors to consider when interpreting research findings.
2. Explain how to interpret results and discuss findings of a study.
3. Distinguish between statistical and clinical significance.
4. Describe a logical sequence for writing a research report.
5. Identify methods of disseminating research findings.

## GLOSSARY OF KEY TERMS

**Abstract.** A brief summary of a research study; usually includes the purpose, methods, and findings of a study.

**Clinical significance.** Findings that have meaning for patient care in the absence or presence of statistical significance.

**Generalizability.** Extent to which research findings can be generalized beyond the given research situation to other settings and subjects; also called external validity.

**Refereed journal.** A journal that uses expert peers in specified fields to review and determine whether a particular manuscript will be published.

**Research report.** A document that summarizes the key aspects of a research study; usually includes the purpose, methods, and findings of a study.

**Statistical significance.** The extent to which the results of an analysis are unlikely to be the effect of chance.

Writing their interpretation of research findings is important and challenging for researchers. In this final stage of the research process, results are to be conveyed clearly, with accurate interpretations. Research findings are interpreted and discussed based on research question(s) and/or hypotheses cited in a study. In addition, results are discussed in relation to the broader significance or lack thereof for nursing practice. This chapter reviews important factors to be considered when evaluating conclusions and interpreting findings from a research study. In addition, it discusses aspects of preparing a research report and how to disseminate findings.

## INTERPRETING RESEARCH FINDINGS

Once research data have been collected and analyzed, the researcher proceeds to interpret the results. Interpreted results become findings for others to evaluate. Interpreting research findings involves organizing and explaining the meaning of data. Interpretation of findings is usually found toward the end of a research report, under the heading of results, conclusions, or discussion.

The results section of a research report contains only a report of results. In conducting a study, a researcher gains considerable amounts of information. Unless this information specifically relates to the research question(s) and/or hypotheses, such information is not included in the results. Interpreting the research results includes examining the meaning of results, considering the significance of the findings, generalizing the findings, drawing conclusions, and suggesting implications for practice and/or further study.[1]

### Examining the Meaning of Results

In quantitative studies, outcomes of statistical tests are included to show or support the statement of results. Although the inclusion of calculated values, degrees of freedom, and the significance level is important, the narrative portion of the results section should emphasize the variables of interest rather than just statistics. The researcher should provide meaning when reporting the results. For example, in a study of adolescents with diabetes who have a history of hypoglycemia-related seizures or loss of consciousness, the statement "the differences in generalized worry about diabetes and fear of hypoglycemia were significant ($t = 6.21$, $df = 35$, $p < .05$)," is not as meaningful to the reader as what is displayed in Excerpt 15.1. In this excerpt, authors discuss the type of statistical analysis (t-tests) performed and define the two groups of adolescents and how they differ on several variables. Readers are also referred to several tables in which descriptive statistics associated with the t-test (e.g., means and standard deviations) are displayed. Information provided in the text and tables is not redundant but complementary.

Research findings are to be reported as objectively as possible. Quite often, the researcher extrapolates more meaning than is present. Some call this tendency going beyond the data.[1] For example, a researcher conducts a study to investigate the efficacy of a hydrocolloid dressing in healing a stage 2 pressure sore (dermis is exposed). Results indicate that the use of hydrocolloid dressings healed a stage 2 pressure sore by 50 percent in 2 days versus 5 days for 4 × 4 gauze dressings ($p < .0001$). The researcher interprets the result to mean that hydrocolloid dressings can be used to heal all stages of pressure sores by 50 percent within 2 days. Is this interpretation correct? The finding that hydrocolloid dressings healed stage 2 pressure sores by 50 percent within 2 days is correct. However, the data indicate that only stage 2 pressure sores were studied. Additionally, because the researcher did not include other stages of pressure sores, taking only 2 days to heal 50 percent of the pressure sores is probably unrealistic. This is an example of the researcher going beyond the data. Situations like this are not always this obvious. Researchers

EXCERPT 15.1

## DESCRIBING MEANINGFUL RESULTS OF A STUDY IN THE TEXT OF AN ARTICLE

**Results**

T-tests were conducted with adolescent subject data to assess differences between adolescents with and without a SLC experience ever (Table 5). Adolescents who had experienced a SLC episode since diagnosis had a lower percentage of glucose values within the desired target range (p = .009) and a tendency to keep their glucose values above the target range (p = .08) compared with adolescents with no history of hypoglycemic seizures. Adolescents who reported having had a seizure within the past year indicated greater overall fear of hypoglycemia (p = .005), which was due mainly to the difference in HFS worry scale scores (p = .004), a greater negative impact of diabetes upon their lives (p = .05), and greater generalized worry (p = .02) than those who had not had a SLC experience within the past year (Table 6).

*Source: Marrero, DG, et al: Fear of hypoglycemia in the parents of children and adolescents with diabetes: Maladaptive or healthy response? Diabetes Educ 23:281, 1997, with permission.*

should take a more conservative approach when interpreting and discussing research findings.

## Considering the Significance of Findings

Another important factor to consider when interpreting research findings is clinical significance. Research findings that have meaning for patient care in the absence or presence of statistical significance are called **clinically significant.** Achieving statistical significance, however, does not automatically mean that the study has value for the discipline of nursing. **Statistical significance** indicates that the findings from an analysis are unlikely to be the result of chance. Interpretation of findings must make logical sense. For example, results of a study indicate a significant difference between the ages of men and women (M = 57.5 and F = 51.5, respectively). Can you reasonably conclude that this represents clinical significance? Statistical significance can be achieved if there is an adequate sample size. However, is it a clinically significant difference? The word "significant" should be used when reporting statistical results and clarified when describing clinical results. Likewise, a study that is clinically significant does not need to be statistically significant. The reader of research must not only base evaluation of a study on its rigor but also on its clinical significance.

## Generalizing the Findings

An essential feature of results of a study is **generalizability,** the extent to which research findings can be generalized beyond the given research situation to other settings and subjects. This is also termed external validity. When interpreting the findings of a study, the researcher examines risks to validity that may have been introduced at various stages of the research process, one of which involves selecting the sample. The intent of random sampling is to produce a representative sample. The focus is on the extent to which the sample represents the target population (see Chapter 7) so the results can be applied to the entire target population. If the sample is not representative, researchers can describe only what was found in the sample.

In conducting a study, the researcher needs to consider whether sample size is too small to allow generalization of findings. For example, 10 subjects were recruited into a study to test the efficacy of a nursing intervention to promote somnolence within 30 minutes. Results indicated that 2 subjects became somnolent after 10 minutes, 3 subjects after 25 minutes, and the remaining 5 subjects after 40 minutes. The researcher could interpret the data by averaging the mean time until somnolence for all 10 subjects to support the effectiveness of the protocol. However, if the sample size had been 100 and the results indicated 2 subjects became somnolent after 10 minutes, 3 subjects after 25 minutes, with the remaining 95 subjects becoming somnolent after 40 minutes, the protocol would not be considered effective.

## Drawing Conclusions

Conclusions are derived from research findings. In order to draw conclusions, the researcher must interpret the results within the context of the study (e.g., organizing framework, literature review, research design). Phrases like "the results of this study indicate" and "the study findings demonstrate" link the summary of results and the meaning of those results. In forming conclusions, it is important to remember that research never proves anything but instead offers *support* for a position.[1]

## Limitations

Limitations are aspects of a study that are potentially confounding to the main study variables. For example, a limitation is created if the time of day a treatment is administered can influence the level of subjects' responses. Additional study limitations include sample deficiencies, design problems, weakness in data collection procedures, and use of unreliable measures. Limitations are generally reported in the discussion section of an article so that the interpretation of results is made with knowledge of the potential impact on the limiting factors.

## Suggesting Implications for Practice, Further Study, or Both

Implications are based on conclusions from a study and provide specific suggestions for practice, further research, or both.

## RESEARCH REPORT

Preparing a **research report** is an essential component of the research process. A research report summarizes key aspects of a study and includes the following elements: title, abstract, introduction (purpose of study and review of literature), methods (sample, setting, data collection), results, discussion, and conclusions. Most research reports consist of 15 to 20 pages. However, theses (required for some master's degree programs) or dissertations (required for most doctoral degrees) are significantly longer (50 to 200 pages). The difference in length is in the amount of detail given to specific sections of the research report.

## Title

The title of a study captures the essence of the study. It is written to attract readers and inform them of the purpose of the study. Most titles tend to be no longer than 15 words and identify key words from the study. Key words are often used by indexing services to categorize the study's contents. A title such as "Diabetes Mellitus" is somewhat vague. A reader is likely to say, "what about diabetes?" Expanded, this title could be "Diabetes Mellitus and School-Aged Children." This is better, but does not suggest a possible research focus. With a few more words, the following title captures the essence of the study: "Coping Strategies of School-Aged Children with Diabetes Mellitus." The title section may also include the author name(s), credentials, and academic and/or clinical affiliations, with addresses.

## Abstract

The **abstract** is a brief, succinct summary of a research study. Although abstracts usually consist of only 100 to 300 words, readers are able to decide whether the study meets their needs or interests. A well-written comprehensive abstract provides the reader with an overview of the remaining sections of the report. Excerpt 15.2 gives an example of an abstract in which the authors highlight the purposes of the study and a brief summary of important findings.

## Introduction

The introduction section of a research report includes the purpose of the study and literature review. After reading the first one or two paragraphs of the introduction, the reader should have an understanding of the problem being studied and why the problem is important. Information on the incidence and/or prevalence associated with the problem is usually presented here. The purpose of the study is usually included at the beginning or at the end of the introduction section. Some researchers believe that by placing the purpose at the beginning of the introduction section, it quickly draws the attention of the reader. Other researchers end the introduction with a statement of purpose, identifying variables to be investigated. Regardless of

## EXCERPT 15.2

### EXAMPLE OF AN ABSTRACT

The purposes of this study were to describe the health-promoting lifestyle behaviors of 397 employed Mexican American women and to compare them with women in other published reports that used the Health-Promoting Lifestyle Profile (HPLP). Mexican American women had the highest HPLP total scores of all minority groups, but lower scores than all predominantly white groups. HPLP self-actualization and interpersonal support were the highest subscale scores. The exercise subscale was the lowest for all groups, including minorities. Canonical analysis revealed two significant canonical variate pairs explaining 88% variance. Age, education, self-efficacy, health locus of control (internal and powerful others), and current health status made statistically significant contributions to all HPLP subscale scores. Study results support previous research findings and make an important contribution to understanding the factors that influence Mexican American women's health-promoting lifestyle behaviors.

*Source: Duffy, ME, Rossow, R, and Hernandez, M: Correlates of health-promotion activities in employed Mexican American women. Nurs Res 45:18, 1996, with permission.*

where the researcher places the purpose statement, the statement must be clear and understandable. As seen in many journal articles, the statement of purpose is not always identified under a separate heading, nor is it always found under the general heading "Introduction." In Excerpt 15.3 the opening paragraph contains the purpose statement and serves as an introduction for the study.

## EXCERPT 15.3

### PLACEMENT OF STATEMENT OF PURPOSE IN OPENING PARAGRAPH OF RESEARCH REPORT

For the past few decades, public health efforts have been directed at reducing the prevalence of smoking. Although these efforts have some success among adults, teen smoking prevalence has changed significantly. Currently, about 3000 minors begin smoking in the United States each day, and teen smoking accounts for approximately 85% to 90% of new smokers (Houston et al, 1994). Moreover, data from the 1992 Monitoring the Future Study showed that the 30-day prevalence of cigarette use among females in 8th and 10th grades was 1% to 2% higher than the use among males (Johnston, O'Malley, & Bachman, 1993). The purpose of this study was to evaluate the empirical adequacy of models based on the Theory of Planned Behavior to predict cigarette-smoking intention in three culturally diverse groups of teenage females, specifically African-Americans, Puerto Ricans, and non-Hispanic whites.

*Source: Hanson, MJ: The theory of planned behavior applied to cigarette smoking in African-American, Puerto Ricans, and non-Hispanic white teenage females. Nurs Res 46:155, 1997, with permission.*

## Literature Review

The literature review identifies what is currently known about the subject under study and reflects relevant background information necessary to support justification for the study. An updated literature review is extremely important to validate the need for a study. Limitations in current thought regarding the problem may be identified in this section. The literature review section usually gives the reader background information on a theoretical/conceptual framework, which helps guide the study. An example of a literature review within the context of a theoretical framework (e.g., Ajzen's Theory of Planned Behavior) is displayed in Excerpt 15.4.

---

### EXCERPT 15.4

### EXAMPLE OF THEORETICAL FRAMEWORK AND RELATED LITERATURE SECTION OF RESEARCH REPORT

The Theory of Planned Behavior (Ajzen, 1985, 1991), designed to predict behavior and enhance understanding of its psychological determinants, provided the framework within which to study cigarette smoking (Table 1). According to the theory, intention to perform or not to perform a behavior is the immediate determinant of the behavior. Intention, in turn, is a direct function of three independent variables—attitude, subjective norm, and perceived behavioral control. Specifically, an individual's intention to smoke cigarettes is a function of attitude toward smoking, perception of what significant others would think about her smoking, and perception about self-control over smoking behavior. In addition, Ajzen and Madden (1986) postulated that perceived behavioral control, together with the influence of intention, can also directly predict behavior in some cases where behavior is not under an individual's total control.

A few investigators have studied cigarette smoking intention and behavior using some of the concepts of the Theory of Planned Behavior. In a longitudinal study of Canadian adult males and females, Godin, Valois, Lepage, and Desharnais (1992) demonstrated that attitude, subjective norm, and perceived behavioral control were significant predictors of intention to smoke, predicting 54% of the variance in smoking intention among smokers. Furthermore, the investigators found that intention predicted actual smoking behavior 6 months later.

Godin and Lepage (1988) studied the intention of pregnant women to not smoke after childbirth and found that both attitude and perceived behavioral control, which the investigators called perceived self-efficacy, contributed significantly to the prediction of smoking intention. The correlation between perceived behavior control and intention was .84; between attitude and intention was .75. However, Boissonneault and Godin (1990), who studied 71 cigarette smokers to identify psychosocial factors influencing intention to smoke in the work-site areas designated for smoking, found that only perceived behavioral control significantly predicted smoking intention.

*Source: Hanson, MJ: The theory of planned behavior applied to cigarette smoking in African-American, Puerto Ricans, and non-Hispanic white teenage females. Nurs Res 46:155, 1997, with permission.*

## Methods

The methods section of the research report is written to inform the reader about the research design, sample, setting, and data collection procedures/instruments. The researcher may also include information on the reliability and validity of instruments. The researcher should outline procedures used in data collection and address any modifications to the original plan. The methods section ends with a discussion of how data will be analyzed, including specific statistical techniques. Depending on the intended audience for the research report, the methods section may vary in length. Research-based nursing journals (e.g., *Applied Nursing Research, Journal of Nursing Scholarship, Nursing Research, Research in Nursing and Health, Western Journal of Nursing Research*) tend to have much lengthier methodology sections than do clinical journals (e.g., *Journal of Gerontological Nursing; Journal of Wound, Ostomy and Continence Nursing; Public Health Nursing; The Diabetes Educator*).

Excerpt 15.5 displays the methods section of a research report describing risky drug and sexual behavior in a sample of homeless or drug-recovering women as well as these women's immediate sources of social support. Enough information was provided to enable others to replicate the study. The researchers described the subjects participating in the study, type of data collected, data collection procedures, and analysis of data.

## Results

The results section of a research report focuses on pertinent findings and answers the research question(s) or tests hypotheses. Data are presented objectively, with little discussion. Tables, graphs, and/or figures are usually presented. The advantage of using tables and graphs is the ability to simplify large amounts of research findings succinctly and logically. Information provided in tables or graphs should not duplicate what is in the text. For example, if the reader reports means in a table, there is no need to repeat them in the text. Instead, tables, graphs, and figures are used to enhance the text.[3,4]

Excerpt 15.6 provides an illustration of a results section of a research report. To provide a more complete understanding of the results, the researchers presented the results in the text and summarized the results in a table. Two research questions were asked:

1. One year after diagnosis with human papillomavirus (HPV), what advice and information do affected persons give to newly diagnosed individuals?
2. Are there gender differences in the advice and information given by affected persons? Note how the results focused directly on the research questions.

In addition, frequencies and percentages presented in the table are not repeated in the text.

## EXAMPLE OF METHODS SECTION OF RESEARCH REPORT

**Method**

*Subjects and Setting.* The study was conducted in 9 homeless shelters and 11 residential drug recovery programs in Los Angeles with 240 women and their closest source of social support (e.g., closest supportive person). All participants were interviewed independently and compensated with $5. Women were eligible for the study if they met all the following criteria:

1. They were 18 to 69 years of age;
2. They were considered at risk for AIDS as a result of being an IDU or other drug user, a sexual partner of an IDU, diagnosed with an STD, or reporting unprotected sex with multiple partners; and
3. They had a supportive person willing to participate. Of the 255 women approached for the study, 240 (94%) agreed to participate.

All designated supportive persons of the subjects also agreed to participate.

*Instruments.* The questionnaires were available in English and translated to written Spanish. Semantic validity of the instruments translated into Spanish was well established. Sociodemographic characteristics, including age, years of education, race, marital status, employment, birth country, religion, and history of STD, were assessed with a structured questionnaire. AIDS risk behavior was assessed in terms of sexual activity and drug use in the past six months. Sexual activity was measured by items that inquired about risky activities engaged in during the past six months. These included number of sexual partners, engaging in sex for money, having a sex partner who was shooting drugs, and engaging in sex without using a condom with a regular partner or with a nonregular partner.

Drug use was measured by the Drug Use Questionnaire, which has been revise from the AIDS Initial Assessment Questionnaire (AIA) (Myers, Snyder, Bryant, & Young, 1990) and tested on a population with a history of drug addiction, prostitution, and homelessness. Psychological well-being was measured by the 5-item Mental Health Index (MHI-5). For each item, responses on a 6-point scale range from "all of the time" to "none of the time." The MHI-5 has well established reliability and validity and has been shown to detect significant psychological disorders, including major depression, general affective disorders, and anxiety disorders. Cronbach's alpha for this sample was .75.

*Procedure.* The study was approved by the Human Subjects Protection Committee of the University of California, Los Angeles. Homeless shelters and drug recovery programs were recruited through letters sent to their directors. All interested women met with African-American or Latino nurses and outreach workers who were extensively trained in working with homeless and drug addicted women, particularly in areas related to HIV/AIDS.

*(continued)*

**EXCERPT 15.5**

## EXAMPLE OF METHODS SECTION OF RESEARCH REPORT *(continued)*

*Analysis.* Women and their supportive persons (SPs) were contrasted on the categorical study variables by McNemar's test of symmetry and on continuous variables by paired t-tests. The psychological well-being score on the MHI-5 was dichotomized at 66. Individuals may be at high risk for mental health problems if they score less than 66 out of 100. To partially compensate for the large number of tests and focus on differences that are more likely to be meaningful, only results that were significant at the .01 level are reported.

*Source: Nyamathi, A, Flaserud, J, and Leake, B: HIV-risk behaviors and mental health characteristics among homeless or drug-recovering women and their closest sources of social support. Nurs Res 46:133, 1997, with permission.*

**EXCERPT 15.6**

## EXAMPLE OF RESULTS SECTION OF RESEARCH REPORT

**Results**

The first research question focused on the advice and information persons with HPV would give others at time of diagnosis. A total of 19 advice and information categories in six general areas were identified: maintaining a balanced perspective, treatment, sexual behavior, knowledge, self-care, and other.

Under the general area titled "maintaining a balanced perspective" were four categories. The first concerned advice to avoid blaming oneself for getting HPV and to guard against letting HPV affect self-esteem. Others advised, "Don't feel badly about yourself or blame yourself." The second category included responses advising newly diagnosed persons to recognize that their disease and their feelings will improve over time. A third category contained responses advising newly diagnosed persons to maintain a positive outlook and move forward with their lives. The final category included responses advising newly diagnosed persons to remember that they are not alone and that millions of other people have HPV also.

Table 1 shows frequencies for each of the types of responses. Participants gave a range of one to four responses; all were coded. The general area of advice given most frequently focused on maintaining a balanced perspective about living with HPV. The second research question addressed gender differences in the advice and information affected persons would give to newly diagnosed persons. Frequencies of responses by gender are also in Table 1. Statistical tests of the gender differences were not possible because of the small number of men in the sample. However, examination of percentages suggest a number of interesting similarities and differences.

*Source: Taylor, CA, Keller, ML, and Egan, JJ: Advice from affected persons about living with human papillomavirus infection. Image J Nurs Schol 29:27, 1997, with permission.*

## Discussion

The discussion section focuses on a nontechnical interpretation of the results. Researchers use the discussion section to explain what the results mean in relation to the purpose of the study. In addition to telling the reader what the results mean, many authors use this section to explain why they think the results turned out as they did. Although such a discussion is occasionally found in articles where the data support the researcher's hunches, authors are much more inclined to point out possible reasons for the obtained results when those results are inconsistent with their expectations.[5] Limitations of a study are also addressed. "Conclusion" is used interchangeably with "Discussion." It is unusual, therefore, to find research reports that contain both a discussion and a conclusion section.[5] Excerpt 15.7 displays a discussion section of a research report that draws some conclusions, refers to implications for practice, and discusses limitations and generalizability of findings.

## References

The reference list is very important to the research report. This section provides the reader with additional literature related to the particular topic. Information in the reference list also provides the reader with a clearer understanding as to why and how the researcher conducted the particular study. When possible, primary data sources should be used instead of secondary data sources (see Chapter 3). References for the study should be current. However, sometimes older references, or "classics," may be used if they form the foundation for the problem under study.

## DISSEMINATING RESEARCH FINDINGS

Communicating research findings is the final stage in the research process. By presenting and publishing research findings, researchers advance the body of knowledge unique to the discipline of nursing. Communicating research findings also promotes the critique and replication of studies, identification of additional research problems, and use of findings in practice. Nursing research is of little value if the results are never presented to other nurses.

## Publication

One method of communicating research findings is through publication. Publishing a research report has the advantage of reaching a larger audience, based on the circulation of a particular journal. The disadvantage of publishing a research report is the delay in receiving feedback and potential delay in the actual publication of the report. It is not uncommon to have a research report published 6 months to 1 year after it is originally submitted.

There are currently more than 100 nursing journals in the United States.[6,7] However, nurse researchers are not limited to publishing nursing research strictly in

**EXCERPT 15.7**

## EXAMPLE OF DISCUSSION SECTION OF A RESEARCH REPORT

**Discussion**

Many participants gave advice in the general area of "keeping a balanced perspective on life." Newly diagnosed persons were encouraged to maintain a positive outlook, remember that many others are affected by the virus, and avoid letting HPV influence their self-evaluations. Such responses demonstrate a belief that this virus can have a powerful effect on one's self-concept and self-definition. Hence, participants were warning others to keep the disease in perspective.

Half the participants also advised newly diagnosed persons to obtain treatment and monitoring of their infection. One might expect that all of the respondents would advise people to seek treatment and monitoring. However, treatment of HPV can be frustrating and warts often recur despite many efforts to control them. Participants who did not advise people to seek treatment might have been expressing their frustration about the lack of effective interventions and pessimism about the extent to which treatment and monitoring is helpful.

**Implications for Practice**

The variety of advice given indicates that responses to HPV can range from feelings of complete devastation to the rare perception that the diagnosis has no effect at all. In working with clients, practitioners can make no assumptions about the impact of HPV. Instead, a careful exploration of the client's reaction to this diagnosis is needed. It is critical for practitioners to pay attention to clients' self-evaluations and self-esteem. For some, the disease may begin to define the person. Social isolation, avoidance of intimacy, and depression can occur. The sense of isolation and stigma might be eased if clients are given information about the HPV newsletter of the American Social Health Association.

**Summary and Limitations**

Because of the nature of the sample, the findings should be interpreted with caution. Respondents were two-thirds women and mostly white, young adults who were fairly well educated. The low average income of the sample is probably a reflection of the large number of college students and not a true indication of economic status. All of these factors limit generalizability of findings. As with any open-ended questions, there is the possibility of memory bias and researcher bias in conducting the content analysis. Despite these limitations, the study provides important information about clients' perspectives about the advice and information needed by persons newly diagnosed with HPV.

*Source: Taylor, CA, Keller, ML, and Egan, JJ: Advice from affected persons about living with human papillomavirus infection. Image J Nurs Schol 29:27, 1997, with permission.*

nursing journals. Nursing research can be found in several medical, health, and lay journals. The decision whether to publish in a research- or clinically-based journal is left to the researcher. There are, however, similarities in writing the research report for publication.

The preparation of a research report or manuscript for publication differs little among journals. However, depending on the focus of the journal, a researcher may expand a specific section of the research report. For example, a researcher might spend more time (pages) in discussing findings in relation to nursing practice in clinical journals. On the other hand, if journals are research-based, the researcher might spend more time (pages) developing the methodology section of the manuscript.

## Query Letter

A query letter is written to an editor to determine the level of interest the editor has regarding publishing a research report. Although all journals do not require query letters, these letters can save the researcher a lot of time. A query letter should include the title and purpose of the study, name(s) and credentials of investigator(s), and a contact person to whom the editor may respond. In addition, the study should be described or an abstract submitted. If an editor is interested in the manuscript, he or she will ask the researcher to submit the entire manuscript. A response usually occurs within several weeks.

## Manuscript Guidelines

Journals provide Information for Authors, giving instructions on manuscript preparation. In some journals the information is in every issue; other journals may publish the information only twice a year. Information for Authors provides the following information: journal's mission statement, type of articles the journal accepts, readership, and manuscript format (e.g., type of referencing, page limitation, specific instructions on preparing tables and figures, copyright). It is imperative that the researcher follow these directions.

## Review Process

Once the researcher submits the manuscript, the review process begins. A peer-reviewed, or **refereed, journal** is one that has expert peers in specified fields to review and determine whether a particular manuscript will be published. Most peer-reviewed journals assign from two to four reviewers to critique the manuscript. In most instances, the author is blinded to the reviewers of the manuscript. The review process may last from a month to a year. Along with the reviewers, the editorial staff may also critique the manuscript, based on its originality, timeliness of the problem, objectivity, honesty, completeness, readability, and rigor of the study.

## ORAL PRESENTATIONS

Presentations are another method of communicating a research report. Presentations can be done formally at local, regional, or national levels, as well as informally between peers. Oral presentations have several advantages over publishing. One is the ability to disseminate findings much more quickly. Another advantage is the ability to get feedback from participants either during or after the presentation. This direct feedback can be an invaluable experience and help the researcher rethink the research findings. The disadvantage of using presentation format to communicate research results is a limited amount of people will get the information. Many nursing journals or organizations will send out a Call for Papers to present at a conference. Often they identify a theme or specialty focus for the conference and request abstracts to be related to the topic.

The format for presenting a research report is very similar to that for presenting a published report. Most presentations are done in a specified amount of time. Conferences allow from 20 minutes to an hour for the researcher to present the report. Thus, the challenge for the researcher is to limit the report to only the essential points of the study. Extraneous explanations of insignificant findings are often avoided. Nurse researchers often use slides, overheads, or handouts to further communicate their findings at presentations.

## POSTER PRESENTATION

Poster presentations are another method for communicating a research report. Most conferences have poster sessions concurrently with oral presentations. Poster presentations have become increasingly popular in the past 10 years. The advantage of this method derives from the ability of the researcher to engage in an active dialogue with other researchers. The disadvantage is that only a limited number of people will read the poster and only a limited amount of information can be presented.

The goal of the poster presentation is to present the research report visually. Thus, the poster must be presented in a manner that is succinct and easily understood. Often, several people might be reading the poster at the same time. The research report format is also followed for the poster presentation; however, only significant information is provided on the poster. Graphs and photographs are often used to enhance the results. Most researchers supplement the poster presentation with written handouts.

The organization sponsoring the conference gives the nurse researcher guidelines in regard to the size of the poster display. Most often, conferences require that a poster be 4 feet × 6 feet for mounting board and 3 feet × 6 feet for an easel. There are no standard methods for arranging a poster. Figure 15.1 illustrates a suggested layout for a poster presentation.

## QUESTIONS TO CONSIDER WHEN CRITIQUING THE INTERPRETATION OF RESEARCH FINDINGS

Identify a research study to critique. Read the study to see if you recognize any key terms discussed in this chapter. Remember that all studies may not contain all key terms. The following questions[1] serve as a guide in critiquing interpretation of research results:

1. *Have the results of the study been interpreted appropriately?* Begin by reviewing the methods and results section to judge the validity of the study

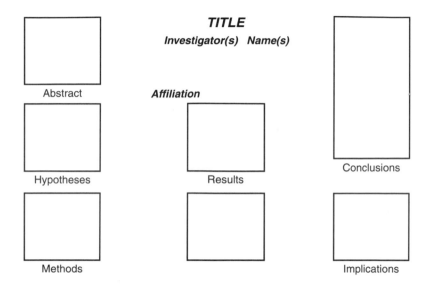

**FIGURE 15.1** Suggested layout for poster presentations.

and to have the necessary information to answer the research questions or test the hypotheses. Look to see if there is a clear statement of the author's major conclusions based on his or her interpretation of the results.

2. *Has the author identified limitations to the study?* Limitations of the study should be identified and explained. Some of these factors may have been identified before the study began, and others will become evident during the course of data collection. Consider the importance of limitations with respect to the interpretation of study results.

3. *Were the results clinically significant?* Findings may or may not have statistical significance; however, they may still have significance for nursing practice. For example, use of a certain sedative in combination with an analgesic consistently reduces the perception of pain in a variety of postoperative conditions. Although difference between groups may not be statistically significant, the trend consistently favors the use of the sedative in combination with the analgesic; therefore, the results have clinical significance.[8]

4. *Did the author discuss how the results of the study apply to practice, education, theory, and research? Were suggestions for further study presented?* Read over the discussion section. The importance of the study should be highlighted in terms of the potential contributions to practice, education, theory, and research, as appropriate. This is particularly true if the results are to be used to inform practice or identify new and challenging research questions.

## SUMMARY OF KEY IDEAS

1. Research findings are discussed in relation to the purpose, research question(s), and hypotheses of the study.
2. The discussion section of a research report explains the results of a study.
3. Discussion of research findings should not go beyond the data presented.
4. Discussion of research findings should identify any threats to internal or external validity and reliability that might explain the findings.
5. Studies should be clinically significant even though statistical significance has not been achieved.
6. A research report summarizes a research study.
7. Publication, oral presentation, and poster presentation are effective methods of communicating research reports.

## LEARNING ACTIVITY

1. Select a nursing research study and identify whether all hypotheses and/or research question(s) have been addressed in the results and discussion sections.

2. In the same nursing research study, identify the strengths and limitations of the authors' results and discussion sections. Do the research findings relate to nursing practice, education, and/or policy?

3. Lyder et al[9] completed a study to evaluate the effect of condom catheters in controlling incontinence odor. The entire nursing staff in a Veterans Administration unit (n = 16) independently rated environmental odor in four rooms before and 1 week after condom catheter removal. Odor was rated on a 4-point scale, from no smell (1) to extreme smell (4). The results indicated that there were statistically significant differences for the factors of room ($p = .03$) and time ($p = .001$). Mean odor ratings were 2.10 (little smell) before and 3.07 (extreme smell) after condom catheter removal. The interpretation and discussion section concluded that although the nurse raters were aware of the intervention, removal of condom catheters from urofecal incontinent men resulted in increased unpleasant odor. Additionally, the increased smell was offensive to residents, families, and nursing staff. The

study also suggested that the use of condom catheters for separation of incontinent urinary and fecal streams may have protective effects on the skin. Based on the purpose of the study, does the interpretation and discussion section correspond with the purpose of the study? Do the authors go beyond the data? Explain your answer. Based on the interpretation and discussion presented, rewrite this section.

4. Select a conference, and attend both an oral and a poster presentation. Identify the components of the research process, and delineate the advantages and disadvantages of both presentations. Were the presentations clinically significant?

5. Select a nursing research study from a research-based nursing journal, and construct a poster.

## References

1. Burns, N, and Grove, SK: The Practice of Nursing Research: Conduct, Critique, and Utilization, ed 4. WB Saunders, Philadelphia, 2001, pp 623–633.
2. Polit, DF, Beck, CT, and Hungler, BP: Essentials of Nursing Research: Methods, Appraisal, and Utilization, ed 5. Lippincott Williams & Wilkins, Philadelphia, 2001, p 60.
3. Teel, C: Completing the research process: Presentations and publications. Neurosci Nurs 22:125, 1990.
4. Tornquist, EF: Strategies for publishing research. Nurs Outlook 31:180, 1983.
5. Huck, SW, and Cormier, WH: Reading Statistics and Research, ed 2. HarperCollins, New York, 2000, pp 13–14.
6. Knapp, T: Supply (of journal space)

and demand (by assistant professors).
Image J Nurs Schol 26:247,
1994.

7. Swanson, E, McCloskey, J, and
Bodensteiner, A: Publishing
opportunities for nurses: A
comparison of 92 U.S. journals.
Image J Nurs Schol 23:33, 1991.

8. Gillis, A, and Jackson, W: Research
for nurses: Methods and
interpretation. FA Davis, Philadelphia,
2002, p 590.

9. Lyder, C, Mccray, G, and Kutty-
Singh, M: Efficacy of condom
catheters in controlling incontinence
odor. Appl Nurs Res 5:188, 1992.

# 16

# Critiquing Research Reports

James A. Fain, PhD, RN, BC-ADM, FAAN

## LEARNING OBJECTIVES

*At the end of this chapter, you will be able to:*

1. Distinguish between a research critique and research review.
2. Apply principles that make a critique constructive rather than destructive.
3. Incorporate a set of guidelines in the critique of research reports.

## GLOSSARY OF KEY TERMS

**Research critique.** Critical evaluation of a piece of reported research.

**Research review.** Identification and summary of major findings and characteristics of a study.

Nurses are expected to participate in research activities by evaluating and interpreting research reports for applicability to nursing practice. Nurses must decide the appropriateness and adequacy of research findings for use in practice. Publication of research reports in no way guarantees quality, value, or relative worth. Deciding the overall usefulness of a research report requires systematic review and critical appraisal. Failing to critique a research report adequately may adversely affect the outcomes of entire populations of patients. This chapter focuses on conducting a comprehensive evaluation of a research report. Specific attention is directed to providing general critique guidelines. Included are evaluation components for both quantitative and qualitative research.

## RESEARCH CRITIQUES VERSUS RESEARCH REVIEWS

A **research critique** is a critical appraisal of the strengths and weaknesses of a research report.[1,2] Critiquing a research report involves evaluating aspects of the research process. All research studies have strengths and weaknesses; by weighing them, the overall applicability of findings is determined.

Research reports are evaluated based on how well the research process was executed. Using specific criteria and guidelines, the evaluator makes precise and objective judgments about the research study, weighing its strengths and weaknesses. Critiquing research reports does not mean correcting grammar and writing style. However, clarity in writing is essential. A good research critique is two or three pages long and evaluates major aspects of the research process. Outlining the critical components of the research process helps in writing the report in a knowledgeable and professional manner. Inadequate organization is perhaps the most common presentation flaw in research reports. The written evaluation of a study emerges as a research critique.

A distinction is made between research critiques and research reviews. In a **research review** the study is described by focusing on major aspects of the study and summarizing the most important points.[1,2] One such example is the publication by the American Association of Critical-Care Nurses, *Nursing Scan in Critical Care*. In this publication, a reviewer gives a synopsis of a recently published research study, pointing out major characteristics of the study. A commentary follows, highlighting important features, usually followed by implications for practice.

Research critiques are often difficult to complete because of feelings of insecurity as a beginning researcher. How then do you develop a feeling of competence? Individuals believe that they either can or cannot make scholarly comments, but it is unrealistic to expect to be an expert at any skill without practice. Constructive criticism is a skill and requires practice.

Use of certain words or phrases in a research critique can be important features of sensitive criticism. Use positive terms whenever possible, and begin by commenting on a study's overall strengths. Avoid such terms as "good," "nice," or "bad," as they do not communicate specific information. For example, the statement, "the study contained a good review of literature" does not convey any meaning. Instead, the following brief statement contains more information and meaning: "The cited review of literature identified the major published studies related to diabetes education and empowerment." Wilson[3] provides several do's and don't's in critiquing research reports, which are summarized in Table 16.1.

## GUIDELINES FOR A CRITIQUE OF A RESEARCH REPORT

Critique guidelines are key components to consider when evaluating research reports. Table 16.2 lists critical components of the research process to be evaluated. Although each component is equally important in determining a study's worth, researchers need to consider overall strengths and weaknesses as the ultimate determinants. Detailed guidelines and questions associated with critiquing research reports can be found in many nursing research textbooks.[1,2] A simple list of suggested questions is listed here:

A. Title of the Research Report
   1. Does the title accurately describe the type of study? major variables? population to which the study applies?
B. Problem Statement
   1. Is the problem clearly stated with pertinent background information?
   2. Is there justification for the study?

TABLE 16.1 Do's AND Don't's FOR SENSITIVE CRITIQUES

| Do | Don't |
|---|---|
| 1. Try to convey a sincere interest in the study you are critiquing. | 1. Nitpick or find fault on trivial details. |
| 2. Be sure to emphasize the points of excellence that you discover. | 2. Ridicule or demean an investigator personally. |
| 3. Choose clear, concise statements to communicate your observations rather than ambiguous ones. | 3. Try to include flattery that is designed merely to boost a researcher's self-esteem. |
| 4. When pointing out a study's weakness, provide explanations that justify your comments. | 4. Base your summary and include recommendations about the study on some loose and perhaps biased attitude toward the state of all science in a particular discipline or on a particular topic. |
| 5. Include supportive and encouraging comments when they are warranted. | 5. Write your critique in condescending, patronizing, or condemning language. |
| 6. Be aware of your own negative attitude toward a particular approach to science or any personal hostilities that could distort your ability to judge a study on its own merits. | 6. Forget that your purpose is to advise the researcher and to improve the work. |
| 7. Offer practical suggestions that are not overly esoteric or unrealistic. | |
| 8. Remember that empathy for the researcher is often crucial to being an effective critic. | |

TABLE 16.2 CRITICAL COMPONENTS OF THE RESEARCH PROCESS TO BE EVALUATED

A. Problem Statement
  Clarity of problem
  Significance of problem for nursing
  Purpose of study
  Conceptual/theoretical framework
  Literature review
  Hypotheses/research questions
B. Research Methodology
  Research design
  Sample/setting
  Data collection procedures
  Data collection instruments
  Data analysis
C. Results, Conclusions, and Interpretations
  Results of data analysis
  Discussion of findings
  Recommendations/implications for further study in practice, education, research

  3. Is the problem significant to nursing?

  4. Is the problem researchable (can data be collected and analyzed)?

C. Conceptual/Theoretical Framework

  1. Is there a conceptual model or framework identified?

  2. If not specifically identified, is a model or framework implied?

  3. Is the conceptual model/framework clearly developed?

  4. Is the conceptual model/framework applicable to the research?

D. Review of Literature

  1. Is the literature cited reviewed critically?

  2. Are classic as well as current citations used?

  3. Does the researcher cite supporting as well as opposing, studies?

  4. Is the literature review organized logically? Are there appropriate subheadings?

  5. Are most primary sources included?

  6. Does the literature review conclude with a brief summary?

E. Purpose of the Study

  1. Is there a purpose statement?

  2. Is the purpose statement appropriate for the study (declarative statement, research question, hypothesis)?

F. Research Questions/Hypotheses

  1. Are the research questions/hypotheses clearly stated?

G. Operational Definitions

  1. Are relevant variables defined operationally?

H. Research Design

  1. Is the type of research design identified?

  2. Does the research design fit appropriately according to the variables studied and purpose of the study?

I. Sample

  1. Are the target and accessible populations described clearly?

  2. Was the method of choosing the sample (probability versus nonprobability) appropriate?

  3. Were inclusion and exclusion criteria used to select subjects for the study?

  4. Based on the sampling procedures, were there any threats to external validity (generalizability of findings)? If so, does the author acknowledge these threats?

J. Data Collection Procedures

  1. Are the steps in collecting data described clearly and concisely?

K. Data Collection Instruments

  1. Are the instruments/scales used to collect data appropriate for the problem and method?

  2. Are these instruments/scales reliable? valid?

  3. Are the means of establishing reliability/validity discussed?

  4. Is each instrument described as to how it was scored? range of possible scores? What does a high/low score mean?

L. Human Subjects
  1. Is evidence of human subject review and approval discussed?
  2. Are issues of subject anonymity or confidentiality addressed?
M. Data Analysis
  1. Is the choice of statistical procedures appropriate for the methodology proposed?
N. Results
  1. Are the characteristics of the sample described?
  2. Are the research questions/hypotheses answered separately?
  3. Do the results limited to data reflect the research questions/hypotheses?
  4. Are generalizations made that are not warranted on the basis of the sample used?
  5. Are tables, charts, and/or graphs used to present data? If so, are they labeled clearly and discussed in the text?
O. Discussion
  1. Are limitations of the study described?
  2. Does the researcher relate findings to the problem and purpose of the study?
  3. Does the researcher state whether study results support or refute previous studies?
  4. Are there any unexpected (serendipitous) findings?
P. Implications and Recommendations
  1. Are generalizations made beyond the sample identified in the study?
  2. Are suggestions/recommendations made by the researcher for nursing practice, education, and/or further research?
  3. Are these suggestions/recommendations based on the findings of this study?

## RESEARCH APPRAISAL CHECKLIST

Duffy[4] proposes a research appraisal checklist for evaluating research reports. The purpose of the checklist is to facilitate students' evaluation of aspects of research reports. The checklist does not provide criteria with which to judge a research report. However, the statements associated with each category represent commonly accepted statements used by researchers when critically appraising strengths and limitations of a research report.

The research appraisal checklist consists of 51 statements that are important to consider. Statements are grouped into eight categories, which are title, abstract, problem, review of literature, methodology, data analysis, discussion, and form and style. Statements are anchored by a rating scale that ranges from "1," "Not Met," to "6," "Completely Met." A rating of "NA" is used when a statement is not applicable. Comments summarizing reasons why a statement is rated low can be particularly helpful. Use of the research appraisal checklist may be helpful as a way of introducing and identifying steps of the research process that are essential to critique. The checklist provides a set of statements in an easy-to-use format that allows students an opportunity to appraise research reports efficiently and compare their results with others.

## RESEARCH CRITIQUE OF A QUANTITATIVE STUDY

The following is an example of an author's research critique of several sections of a quantitative research report.

### Title

Patient Empowerment Program for People with Diabetes

> C R I T I Q U E .    The title is brief but conveys to the reader one of the major variables under study. The sample is implied by the phrase, "people with diabetes." However, the reader cannot ascertain whether the sample being studied refers to those with type 1 or type 2 diabetes.

### Problem Statement

Diabetes patient education has long been viewed as a process designed to provide patients with the knowledge, skills, and motivation to manage their diabetes. A compliance-adherence approach regarding the philosophy and practice of diabetes patient education has prevailed for the past two decades. Within this model of care, behavioral strategies were used to increase compliance with recommended treatments. To more adequately understand and improve diabetes self-management, different models of care are needed that improve upon previous research. Recently, patient empowerment has been offered as an alternative to the compliance-adherence approach to diabetes management and patient education. The purpose of this proposed clinical study is to test the feasibility of a patient empowerment program. The program was designed by Feste (1991) and does not focus on the provision of information. Instead, the program helps individuals with diabetes develop skills and self-awareness in the areas of goal-setting, problem-solving, stress management, coping, social support, and motivation.

> C R I T I Q U E .    The statement of the problem is clearly stated and constitutes an effort to improve patients' diabetes management. This is a very important issue, particularly in the current health-care management cost-containment environment. The problem is researchable and provides direction for specifying the research design and methodology. The purpose statement is clear in stating what the study hopes to accomplish.

### Review of Literature

Type 2 diabetes is the most common form of diabetes and accounts for 90 percent of all diabetes in the United States. However, many cases go undiagnosed.

RESEARCH APPRAISAL CHECKLIST

| Criteria | Appraisal Rating | | | | | | | Comment |
|---|---|---|---|---|---|---|---|---|

TITLE

| | | | | | | | | |
|---|---|---|---|---|---|---|---|---|
| 1. The title is readily understood | 1 | 2 | 3 | 4 | 5 | 6 | NA | |
| 2. The title is clear | 1 | 2 | 3 | 4 | 5 | 6 | NA | |
| 3. The title is clearly related to content | 1 | 2 | 3 | 4 | 5 | 6 | NA | |

Category Score:

ABSTRACT

| | | | | | | | | |
|---|---|---|---|---|---|---|---|---|
| 4. The abstract states problem and, where appropriate, hypotheses clearly and concisely | 1 | 2 | 3 | 4 | 5 | 6 | NA | |
| 5. Methodology is identified and described briefly | 1 | 2 | 3 | 4 | 5 | 6 | NA | |
| 6. Results are summarized | 1 | 2 | 3 | 4 | 5 | 6 | NA | |
| 7. Findings and/or conclusions are stated | 1 | 2 | 3 | 4 | 5 | 6 | NA | |

Category Score:

PROBLEM

| | | | | | | | | |
|---|---|---|---|---|---|---|---|---|
| 8. The general problem of the study is introduced early in the report | 1 | 2 | 3 | 4 | 5 | 6 | NA | |
| 9. Questions to be answered are stated precisely | 1 | 2 | 3 | 4 | 5 | 6 | NA | |
| 10. Problem statement is clear | 1 | 2 | 3 | 4 | 5 | 6 | NA | |
| 11. Hypotheses to be tested are stated precisely in a form that permits them to be tested | 1 | 2 | 3 | 4 | 5 | 6 | NA | |
| 12. Limitations of the study can be identified | 1 | 2 | 3 | 4 | 5 | 6 | NA | |
| 13. Assumptions of the study can be identified | 1 | 2 | 3 | 4 | 5 | 6 | NA | |
| 14. Pertinent terms are/can be operationally defined | 1 | 2 | 3 | 4 | 5 | 6 | NA | |
| 15. Significance of the problem is discussed | 1 | 2 | 3 | 4 | 5 | 6 | NA | |
| 16. Research is justified | 1 | 2 | 3 | 4 | 5 | 6 | NA | |

Category Score:

REVIEW OF LITERATURE

| | | | | | | | | |
|---|---|---|---|---|---|---|---|---|
| 17. Cited literature is pertinent to research problems | 1 | 2 | 3 | 4 | 5 | 6 | NA | |
| 18. Cited literature provides rationale for the research | 1 | 2 | 3 | 4 | 5 | 6 | NA | |
| 19. Studies are critically examined | 1 | 2 | 3 | 4 | 5 | 6 | NA | |
| 20. Relationship of problem to previous research is made clear | 1 | 2 | 3 | 4 | 5 | 6 | NA | |
| 21. A conceptual framework/theoretical rationale is clearly stated | 1 | 2 | 3 | 4 | 5 | 6 | NA | |

*(continued)*

RESEARCH APPRAISAL CHECKLIST *(continued)*

| Criteria | Appraisal Rating | | | | | | | Comment |
|---|---|---|---|---|---|---|---|---|
| **REVIEW OF LITERATURE** *(continued)* | | | | | | | | |
| 22. Review concludes with a brief summary of relevant literature and its implications to the research problem under study<br>Category Score: | 1 | 2 | 3 | 4 | 5 | 6 | NA | |
| **METHODOLOGY** | | | | | | | | |
| A.  Subjects | | | | | | | | |
| 23. Subject population (sampling frame) is described | 1 | 2 | 3 | 4 | 5 | 6 | NA | |
| 24. Sampling method is described | 1 | 2 | 3 | 4 | 5 | 6 | NA | |
| 25. Sampling method is justified (especially for non-probability sampling) | 1 | 2 | 3 | 4 | 5 | 6 | NA | |
| 26. Sample size is sufficient to reduce type 2 error | 1 | 2 | 3 | 4 | 5 | 6 | NA | |
| 27. Possible sources of sampling error can be identified | 1 | 2 | 3 | 4 | 5 | 6 | NA | |
| 28. Standards for protection of subjects are discussed<br>Category Score: | 1 | 2 | 3 | 4 | 5 | 6 | NA | |
| B.  Instruments | | | | | | | | |
| 29. Relevant reliability data from previous research are presented | 1 | 2 | 3 | 4 | 5 | 6 | NA | |
| 30. Reliability data pertinent to the present study are reported | 1 | 2 | 3 | 4 | 5 | 6 | NA | |
| 31. Relevant previous validity data from previous research are presented | 1 | 2 | 3 | 4 | 5 | 6 | NA | |
| 32. Validity data pertinent to present study are reported | 1 | 2 | 3 | 4 | 5 | 6 | NA | |
| 33. Methods of data collection are sufficiently described to permit judgment of their appropriateness to the present study<br>Category Score: | 1 | 2 | 3 | 4 | 5 | 6 | NA | |
| C.  Design | | | | | | | | |
| 34. Design is appropriate to study questions and/or hypotheses | 1 | 2 | 3 | 4 | 5 | 6 | NA | |
| 35. Proper controls are included where appropriate | 1 | 2 | 3 | 4 | 5 | 6 | NA | |
| 36. Confounding/moderating variables are/can be identified | 1 | 2 | 3 | 4 | 5 | 6 | NA | |
| 37. Description of design is explicit enough to permit replication<br>Category Score: | 1 | 2 | 3 | 4 | 5 | 6 | NA | |

RESEARCH APPRAISAL CHECKLIST *(continued)*

| Criteria | Appraisal Rating | Comment |
|---|---|---|
| **DATA ANALYSIS** | | |
| 38. Information presented is sufficient to answer research questions | 1  2  3  4  5  6  NA | |
| 39. Statistical tests are identified and obtained values are reported | 1  2  3  4  5  6  NA | |
| 40. Reported statistics are appropriate for hypothesis/research questions | 1  2  3  4  5  6  NA | |
| 41. Tables and figures are presented in an easy-to-understand, informative way | 1  2  3  4  5  6  NA | |
| Category Score: | | |
| | | |
| **DISCUSSION** | | |
| 42. Conclusions are clearly stated | 1  2  3  4  5  6  NA | |
| 43. Conclusions are substantiated by the evidence presented | 1  2  3  4  5  6  NA | |
| 44. Methodological problems in the study are identified and discussed | 1  2  3  4  5  6  NA | |
| 45. Findings of the study are specifically related to conceptual/theoretical basis of the study | 1  2  3  4  5  6  NA | |
| 46. Implications of the findings are discussed | 1  2  3  4  5  6  NA | |
| 47. Results are generalized only to population on which study is based | 1  2  3  4  5  6  NA | |
| 48. Recommendations are made for further research | 1  2  3  4  5  6  NA | |
| Category Score: | | |
| | | |
| **FORM AND STYLE** | | |
| 49. The report is clearly written | 1  2  3  4  5  6  NA | |
| 50. The report is logically organized | 1  2  3  4  5  6  NA | |
| 51. The tone of the report displays an unbiased, impartial, scientific attitude | 1  2  3  4  5  6  NA | |
| Category Score: | | |

GRAND TOTAL:

In the United States, the prevalence of type 2 diabetes is lowest in Caucasians (non-Hispanic whites) and elevated in African-American, Hispanic-American, and Native-American populations. Regardless of its prevalence in different populations, type 2 diabetes is a serious disease that warrants the same comprehensive treatment as that given to individuals with type 1 diabetes. There is scientific evidence that early detection, treatment, and rigorous attention to self-care, facilitated by quality diabetes education, can significantly reduce the incidence and progression of diabetes (DCCT Research Group, 1993). Results of the Diabetes Control and

Complications Trial (DCCT) led to reevaluation of the team concept and definition of team members' roles. The burden of diabetes can have a negative effect on the life satisfaction of individuals and their families. Individuals with type 2 diabetes need to take personal responsibility for their own disease management.

Patient empowerment has been offered as an alternative to the knowledge model approach to diabetes management and patient education (Anderson, Funnell, Barr, Dedrick, & Davis, 1991; Funnell, Anderson, Arnold, Barr, Donnelly, Johnson, Taylor-Moon, & White, 1992). Whereas it had been common to speak of noncompliance, behavior modification, and glucose control, the empowerment model refers to self-awareness, personal responsibility, informed choices, and quality of life (Feste, 1992). The notion of empowerment is appealing because of its association with such concepts as coping, social support, personal efficacy, and self-esteem (Kieffer, 1984). Rubin and Peyrot (1992) argue that new models of care need to be explored which incorporate psychosocial education as a routine and significant component of diabetes care and education.

CRITIQUE. The literature review focuses on the compliance-adherence approach to diabetes education and an empowerment approach to diabetes management. As noted by the researcher, the incidence of diabetes and the severity of complications warrant special attention of efforts to improve health and quality of life. However, references in support of expectations that DCCT results apply to type 2 diabetes patients should be provided.

The effectiveness (or lack) of the compliance-adherence approach used for the past two decades is not clearly described. If this approach has been shown to have an impact on the proposed dependent variables, it would make sense to compare the empowerment approach to the compliance-adherence approach to establish whether the empowerment approach has an effect over and above that of "usual care." Likewise, the researcher does not review studies that have used other diabetes management approaches tailored to individual patients. Primary sources are used with references complete and integrated into the development of the study.

## Hypotheses

Diabetes education that focuses on self-management, self-efficacy, and empowerment issues significantly:

- Increases positive attitudes and self-efficacy as measured by selective subscales of these testing instruments: Diabetes Attitude Scale, Self-Efficacy, and Diabetes Care Profile.
- Decreases negative attitudes as measured by appropriate DCP subscales.
- Improves glycemic control, as measured by a decrease in glycosylated hemoglobin ($HbA_{1c}$).

CRITIQUE. The researcher clearly identifies the study hypotheses with appropriate operational definitions of how variables will be measured.

## Methodology: Research Design

The proposed study is an experimental design. Patients will be randomly assigned to either an intervention or a control group. The intervention will be organized as six 2-hour group sessions held weekly. Each session will be presented by the diabetes nurse educator and dietitian to promote consistency of the intervention. At the end of 6 weeks, all subjects (intervention and control) will complete the set of questionnaires a second time. The second set of questionnaires will serve as a post-program test for the intervention group. The control group will then complete the six-session program. At the end of 12 weeks, all subjects will complete the questionnaires for a third time and provide another blood sample. This data will serve as the post-program data for the control group and as 6-week follow-up for the intervention group. The control group will return for its follow-up 6 weeks later, completing the questionnaires another time along with a blood sample.

CRITIQUE.    A strength of the proposed study is the experimental design. Criteria for study inclusion and exclusion were described appropriately. The research design describes a 6-week waiting period for control subjects, after which they receive the empowerment program. This design does not offer an uncontaminated control group for the baseline to 12 weeks pre- to post-comparison of major outcome variables. This is a flaw in the design that could be removed by not offering the empowerment program to the control group. If the protocol is followed as written, the experimental group would have a lag of 12 weeks between baseline and follow-up measures of outcome variables, and the control group would have 18 weeks. The times should be equal.

## Methodology: Sample

Criteria for inclusion in the clinical study are as follows. All subjects who are diagnosed with type 2 diabetes followed by the Diabetes Clinic will be asked to participate in the study. Type 2 is very different from type 1 diabetes. Type 2 develops classically in an older population and may or may not require use of therapeutic insulin. Individuals are usually controlled by diet, exercise, and an oral hypoglycemic agent. A small percentage of individuals will be on combination therapy (use of insulin and oral hypoglycemic). Criteria for enrollment includes English- or Spanish-speaking adults; diagnosis of diabetes for a minimum of 1 year; and no major complications associated with diabetes. The existence of serious illness or major complication, such as visual impairment, end-stage renal disease, or lower extremity amputation, will be reason for study exclusion.

CRITIQUE.    The study sample is not adequately defined. For example, there is no information regarding age, gender, or educational levels and how these will be controlled. Likewise, although subjects must have been diagnosed with diabetes for a minimum of 1 year, there is no stated restriction for length of time since first diagnosed. How will this variable be treated? Although both English- and Spanish-speaking patients will be recruited, there is no indication in the study that the intervention group leaders need to speak Spanish. It is also not clear whether separate Spanish-speaking groups will be formed. The researcher does not specify if the target population is truly representative of the entire diabetic population. Are all subjects at the institution referred to and seen at the Diabetes Clinic? If not, how are referred subjects different from subjects not referred?

## Methodology: Data Collection Procedures

The diabetes clinical nurse specialist employed by the institution will help identify eligible subjects from those who attend the Diabetes Clinic. All patients will receive a letter from the principal investigator inviting them to participate in the study. Interested patients will be asked to attend an orientation session, where a discussion about empowerment along with a sample worksheet will be discussed. All patients who choose to participate will sign an informed consent form, complete a set of questionnaires, and have a blood sample drawn for glycosylated hemoglobin ($HbA_{1c}$). Patients will be randomly assigned to either the intervention or control group.

---

C R I T I Q U E .   The researcher proposes to invite subjects to an orientation session where issues of empowerment will be discussed. The purpose of this discussion with all patients is not clear (motivational?). One wonders what the impact of such a session will be on those who are later randomized to the control group. If this session had a positive/motivational impact on control subjects, then the effect of the intervention would be more difficult to detect.

## Methodology: Data Collection Instruments

*Diabetes Attitude Scale (DAS).* Diabetes patients' attitudes will be measured with selected subscales of the DAS and selected subscales of the Diabetes Care Profile (DCP). The DAS subscale measures (1) patients' attitudes toward compliance; (2) impact of diabetes on their quality of life; and (3) views about patient autonomy. The two DCP subscales measure (1) overall positive and (2) overall negative attitudes about living with diabetes. Both the DAS and DCP are self-administered paper-and-pencil questionnaires composed of several subscales. Patients are asked to read each statement and place a check mark next to the word or phrase that is closest to their opinion about each statement. Items are scored by assigning five points to "strongly agree," four points to "agree," three points to "neutral," two to "disagree," and one point to "strongly disagree." Internal consistency for each subscale has been determined through the use of Cronbach's alpha coefficients for each subscale and ranges from 0.69 to 0.86 (Anderson, Donnelly & Dedrick, 1990). Self-efficacy measures were developed for the specific content areas of the patient empowerment program. The self-efficacy subscales measured the subject's perceived ability to identify areas of satisfaction related to living with diabetes;

identify and achieve personally meaningful goals; cope with emotional aspects of living with diabetes; manage stress; attain appropriate social support; be self-motivated; and make cost/benefit decisions about making behavior changes related to living with diabetes. Glycosylated hemoglobin is a biological marker for diabetes control. It is a routine measure of the average blood glucose control for a previous 3-month period. Subjects in good control will have an $HgbA_{1c}$ value of $<8.0\%$.

CRITIQUE.    The outcome measures selected are well described and related to the hypotheses under study. There is, however, no validity information for selected subscales. Only some of the DAS and DCP subscales will be used without explanation as to whether it is appropriate to do so. Why were these subscales selected? What do the scores mean? The description of the self-efficacy measures was equally lacking sufficient psychometric properties. Likewise, the blood glucose control measure needs more discussion. Who, for example, will draw the blood? Who will analyze it? Who will pay for it?

## Methodology: Data Analysis

The sample will be described using descriptive statistics. Sociodemographic variables will be described using frequency distributions and appropriate measures of central tendency and variability. Hypotheses 1 and 2 will be analyzed by student t-tests. The t-test will be used to determine if there are differences between mean scores of attitudes and self-efficacy pre-program and post-program (6 weeks).

CRITIQUE.    The plan of analysis is appropriate but needs to be clearer in terms of detail. Although not described, the t-tests are presumed to compare mean pre- to post-test change scores for the two groups. In addition, does this mean all self-efficacy subscales will be combined with the subscales from the DAS and DCP for analysis or that separate analysis will be performed for each subscale?

## Results and Findings

Demographic characteristics of the sample are displayed. The majority of subjects were older-aged, men, and overweight. All three hypotheses were supported. Those individuals in the intervention group had significantly higher scores on the following self-efficacy subscales: setting goals, managing stress, obtaining support, and making decisions when compared with those subjects in the control group. Likewise, subjects in the intervention group had a more positive attitude toward diabetes and improvement in glycosylated hemoglobin levels. Findings were consistent with Anderson's (1995) study.

CRITIQUE.    Findings were clearly stated and substantiated by the data presented. The researcher failed to discuss study limitations.

OVERALL STRENGTHS.    With only about one-half of all patients with chronic diseases actually staying on their treatment regimens, new approaches to diabetes education must be tested. Patient empowerment is one approach that seems relevant to diabetes self-management. The cited literature identified major published studies related to empowerment and diabetes education. The background and experience of the researcher and consultants are strong.

OVERALL WEAKNESSES.    The overall lack of detail, unfortunately, makes it difficult to evaluate the likelihood that this study will yield new and useful data. The question of how the proposed empowerment program is different from other educational programs designed for people with diabetes has not been adequately addressed nor has the question of whether the program actually "empowers" people to change.

## RESEARCH CRITIQUE OF A QUALITATIVE STUDY

The following is an example of a research critique of several sections of a qualitative research report.[5]

### Purpose

The diagnosis of diabetes brings with it a regimen that has a major impact on an individual's daily practices and lifestyle. The purpose of this grounded theory study was to investigate the experience of living with insulin-dependent diabetes mellitus.

CRITIQUE.    The purpose of this qualitative grounded theory study is clearly articulated.

### Identified Problem for Study

At the beginning of this study, I was deeply committed to the value of diabetes education programs, the need for knowledge for clients with diabetes, and the importance of diabetes control for positive health outcomes. However, I had an aversion to the word "compliance" and had begun to doubt the value of compliance/adherence relationships between diabetes clients and their educators. A review of the literature convinced me that the compliance/adherence educational framework typical of current diabetes education programs does not accurately describe, account for, or explain the experience of living with diabetes. Despite extensive research in diabetes education and social learning interventions, neither adherence nor glycemic control has been achieved. Also, a causal relationship link has not been established between these educational approaches and the desired metabolic outcomes. Consequently, a strong rationale exists for taking a new look at diabetes from the perspective of the client rather than from that of the health professional.

CRITIQUE. In grounded theory, the research problem is as much discovered as the process that resolves it. The researcher moved into an area of interest with no specific problem in mind as evidenced by the type of question asked, "What is the experience of living with insulin-dependent diabetes mellitus (type 1 diabetes)?

Study subjects were recruited through two endocrinologists who had been informed of the study methodology and asked to refer only adults with type 1 diabetes who were in good control. Two females and two males agreed to participate in the study.

CRITIQUE. There is insufficient detail about the sampling procedure and study participants. In grounded theory, a predetermined sample size is not calculated. Theoretical sampling is continued until the categories are saturated.

## Methodology

Grounded theory was selected as a research methodology. Each participant was seen several times. The purpose of the first meeting was to establish rapport, explain the study, allow opportunity for questions, and obtain written consent. At the next session, an interview was conducted using open-ended questions; this interview was audiotaped and transcribed verbatim. At the end of the interview, instructions were given for writing a personal paper about diabetes and completing a 3- to 5-day journal.

CRITIQUE. The qualitative method is clearly stated. Additional information regarding assumptions associated with grounded theory would be helpful to the reader.

## Data Collection Procedures

A comprehensive and accurate picture of the diabetes experience for the participants was obtained by triangulation from three data sources: interviews and two written tasks. The written tasks included preparing a paper about their personal diabetes stories and keeping a 3- to 5-page journal to document thoughts related to diabetes. Each participant was seen several times, twice for formal interviews and one or more times for more informal meetings.

CRITIQUE. A more detailed discussion of data collection procedures is warranted. Overall, how long was data collection for the entire study? How long were the individual interviews? Were they all audiotaped?

## Data Analysis: Organizing/Categorizing/Summarizing

Transcriptions of interviews, diabetes papers, and journals were examined and coded line by line to identify underlying processes. Coded data that seemed related were grouped into categories. Throughout the coding, data collected through interviews, diabetes papers, and journals were constantly compared for similarities and differences. As data collection and analysis continued, categories were collapsed into more general categories until the underlying theory of "becoming diabetic" emerged, a theory of integration.

CRITIQUE.    The researcher speaks about coding data after the interviews. How many original categories were identified? Very little information is provided on how the data were summarized for ease in theme identification. Reference is made to the underlying theory of "becoming diabetic." However, there is no literature review, which would have facilitated the reader's understanding of how the categories were recognized and accepted. In a grounded theory study, the review of literature does not take place until after problem identification. The grounded theorist begins by collecting data in the field and generating a theory. As the theory becomes sufficiently grounded and developed, the literature in the field is reviewed and related to the developing theory.

## Scientific Integrity: Credibility/Transferability/Dependability/Confirmability

CRITIQUE.    The researcher does not mention how scientific integrity was addressed in this study. As a qualitative study, several factors are important in establishing worthiness of findings: triangulation of data, participant observation, and prolonged engagement with participants. The researcher speaks to triangulation of three data sources with little discussion of how he/she became involved with participants in order to understand the problem. A more detailed description of the sample would have made it easier to determine credibility and transferability (external validity) of findings.

## Results of the Study

The following themes emerged: a new view of empathy, the diabetes education focuses, and the client-educator relationship. Study participants had a different view of the educator's ability to understand and empathize with them. Laura expressed her opinion about the diabetes educator who does not have diabetes. During the research process I came to a new understanding of empathy as a way of knowing, not merely a way of being. Empathy is a way of knowing of the individual, not of a group, because diabetes cannot be considered a collective experience. In other words, one person's perspective on diabetes cannot be assumed or generalized from others who also have diabetes.

Early in the education of individuals with diabetes, educators promote the notion of the "normalcy" of living with diabetes. Focusing on normalcy may only prolong the integration or becoming process or may make clients feel guilty because they do not feel guilty. Diabetes educators need to view their practice objectively, to become informed by clients' experiences, and to critique their actions. Living with diabetes cannot be defined rigidly within a generalized science of diabetes. Laura succinctly summarized this point, "You can't live the textbook." Laura, Matthew, Mike, and Sandra helped me to understand the inaccuracies of my own assumptions.

CRITIQUE.    The process of obtaining results was clear and appropriate to a grounded theory approach. The researcher was likewise aware of his/her own knowledge and assumptions regarding the research problem so as to minimize unnecessary bias.

## Discussion of Findings

The findings of this grounded theory study provide insight into the experience of living with diabetes, the focus of diabetes education, and the client/education relationships. The recommendations derived from this study represent a significant move away from conventional diabetes education practice. Early in the study I recognized a difference in perspective about diabetes between myself as diabetes educator and the participants. A memo I wrote exemplifies my recognition of these differences: "I am struck by the difference in the way in which Matthew looks at diabetes and the way in which I as a diabetes educator perceive it. I have always seen the diabetes regimen—diet, exercise, insulin, and stress reduction—as the central focus and presumed that these must somehow be accommodated into a diabetic's lifestyle. Matthew does not talk about these aspects but, although he is involved with these, I get the feeling that he does not approach them with the same preoccupation that I do. Matthew's focus is on his body, paying attention to its needs and demands, whereas we [diabetes educators] focus on the 'regimen.' "

CRITIQUE.    Discussion of research findings were consistent with a grounded theory approach. This shows an appropriate use of memoing, where the researcher recorded his/her ideas while coding and analyzing the data.

## SUMMARY OF KEY IDEAS

1. A research critique is a critical appraisal of the strengths and weaknesses of a research report.
2. The writing of a research critique should be clear, concise, well organized, and grammatically correct.
3. A research review provides a description of the most important features of a research study.

**LEARNING** ACTIVITIES

1. Select a quantitative and qualitative research report to critique.

   a. Examine the title of the article.

   b. Critique the problem and purpose statements.

   c. Critique the conceptual/theoretical model and literature review.

   d. Evaluate the research questions/hypotheses.

   e. Critically evaluate aspects of the research methodology (i.e., design, sample, setting, data collection procedures and instruments, data analysis).

   f. Critique results.

   g. Examine study discussion/conclusions.

## References

1. Polit, DF, and Hungler, BP: Nursing Research: Principles and Methods, ed 6. Lippincott Williams & Wilkins, Philadelphia, 1999, pp 623–624.
2. Burns, N, and Groves, SK: The Practice of Nursing Research: Conduct, Critique, and Utilization, ed 4. WB Saunders, Philadelphia, 2001, pp 663–681.
3. Wilson, HS: Introduction to Research in Nursing, ed 2. Addison-Wesley Nursing, Philadelphia, 1993.
4. Duffy, ME: A research appraisal checklist for evaluating nursing research reports. In Waltz, CF, and Jenkins, LS (eds): Measurement of Nursing Outcomes, vol 1: Measuring Nursing Performance in Practice, Education, and Research, ed 2. Springer Publishing Company, New York, 2001, pp 313–323.
5. Hernandez, CA: The experience of living with insulin-dependent diabetes: Lessons for the diabetes educator. Diabetes Educator 21:33, 1995.

## Suggested Readings for Critiques

Anderson, RM, et al: Learning to empower patients: Results of professional education program for diabetes education. Diabetes Care 14:584, 1991.

Anderson, RM, et al: Patient empowerment: Results of a randomized controlled trial. Diabetes Care 18:943, 1995.

Anderson, RM, Donnelly, MB, and Dedrick, RF: Measuring the attitudes of patients toward diabetes and its treatment. Patient Educ Counseling 16:231, 1990.

Diabetes Control and Complications Trial (DCCT) Research Group: The effect of intensive treatment of diabetes on the development and progression of long-term complications in insulin dependent diabetes mellitus (IDDM). N Engl J Med 329:977, 1993.

Feste, CC: A practical look at patient empowerment. Diabetes Care 15:922, 1992.

Feste, CC: Empowerment: Facilitating a path to personal self-care. Miles Incorporated Diagnostics Division, Elkhart, IN, 1991.

Funnell, MM, et al: Empowerment: An idea whose time has come in diabetes education. Diabetes Educ 17:37, 1991.

Kieffer, C: Citizen empowerment: A developmental perspective. Prev Human Serv 3:9, 1984.

Rubin, RR, and Peyrot, M: Psychosocial problems and interventions in diabetes. Diabetes Care 15:1640, 1992.

# 17 Research Utilization

Leslie H. Nicoll, PhD, MBA, RN
Suzanne C. Beyea, PhD, RN, CS

## LEARNING OBJECTIVES

*At the end of this chapter, you will be able to:*

1. Define research utilization.
2. Describe the purpose of research utilization.
3. Identify the various models of nursing research utilization.
4. Contrast the differences between research and research utilization.
5. Describe the steps of research utilization.
6. Discuss barriers to and facilitators of research utilization.
7. Discuss strategies to promote the utilization of research in practice.

## GLOSSARY OF KEY TERMS

**Barrier.** Any factor or influence that negatively affects the utilization of research.

**Facilitator.** Any factor or influence that positively affects the utilization of research.

**Knowledge diffusion.** The process by which new information becomes part of practice and subject to evaluation.

**Research utilization.** The systematic process by which research-based knowledge becomes incorporated into practice.

Nursing research is of little value unless the knowledge generated is incorporated into practice, where it ultimately benefits patient care. Nurses who conduct research must communicate their findings in journals that are read by nurses who practice. Practicing nurses must read the research reports and discuss this knowledge with colleagues. Research utilization bridges the gap between the worlds of practicing clinicians and researchers and is the key to ensuring that nursing practice is research-based. This chapter focuses on the research utilization process and provides an overview of several nursing research utilization models. The application of the Stetler Model of research utilization is addressed.

## RESEARCH UTILIZATION

**Research utilization** is the process by which knowledge generated from research becomes incorporated in clinical practice. The process is ongoing and systematic, and it includes critical analysis of research findings along with implementation and evaluation of any resultant changes in practice. Research utilization consists of several activities that assist clinicians to incorporate research findings into practice to improve patient outcomes.

Research utilization differs from the research process. When research is conducted, a problem is identified, and a study is designed and implemented to answer research questions or test hypotheses. Findings from such a study are then utilized. Research generates new knowledge, whereas research utilization applies that knowledge to clinical practice.

Disseminating research findings helps nurses develop research-based policies, procedures, and clinical practice guidelines. Strategies to ensure research-based practice are important components of the research utilization process. These strategies promote consistent, cost-effective, quality care and improved patient outcomes. Research-based care promotes a professional practice environment in which nurses use critical thinking skills to make evidence-based patient care decisions. In today's practice settings, insurers and consumers demand evidence that specific interventions or procedures are the most appropriate, thus making research-based care a necessity.

## Purpose and Scope

The purpose of nursing research utilization is the application of available knowledge to improve patient outcomes. Specific objectives include developing an inquiring mind, asking questions, critiquing research reports, synthesizing findings, implementing a practice or policy change, and evaluating specific patient outcomes. Research utilization facilitates the processes by which nurses examine, understand, and improve clinical nursing practice.

Historically, there has been a gap between research and clinical practice. Some research findings are adopted by clinicians; other findings are never incorporated into clinical practice. Research findings are not incorporated for several reasons. Some clinicians never read about or hear of research findings; others do not feel empowered to make changes in practice. Researchers may not publish research findings or make them available to clinicians.

Several theorists have examined the process of knowledge diffusion and utilization. **Knowledge diffusion** is the process by which new information becomes part of practice and subject to evaluation. Rogers[1] describes five steps associated with knowledge diffusion (awareness of an innovation, persuasion, decision stage, implementation stage, and confirmation stage), whereas Havelock[2] suggests that linkages between researchers and clinicians are critical to knowledge diffusion and proposes six phases (generation, verification, transformation, transfer, reception, and utilization). Regardless of how many steps are involved, the process of research utilization is complex and highly variable. Factors that affect diffusion include the setting, resources, educational background, and experience of the clinician. No single reason is responsible for the gaps between research and practice. To promote research utilization, a number of models or approaches have been developed (Table 17.1).

TABLE 17.1  NURSING RESEARCH UTILIZATION MODELS

| Date | Model | Reference |
|------|-------|-----------|
| 1975–1977 | Western Interstate Commission for Higher Education | Krueger, JC: Utilization of nursing research: The planning process. J Nurs Adm 8:6, 1978. |
| 1975–1981 | Conduct and Utilization of Research in Nursing | Horsley, JA, Crane, J, and Crabtree, MK: Using Research to Improve Nursing Practice: A Guide, Grune & Stratton, New York, 1983. |
| 1976–1985 | The Nursing Child Assessment Satellite Training Project | King, D, Barnard, KE, and Hoehn, R: Disseminating the results of nursing research. Nurs Outlook 29:164, 1981. |
| 1976 | Stetler/Marram Model | Stetler, CB, and Marram, G: Evaluation of research findings for applicability in practice. Nurs Outlook 24:559, 1976. |
| 1994 | Stetler | Stetler, CB: Refinement of the Stetler/Marram model for application of research findings to practice. Nurs Outlook 42:15, 1994. |
| 1977 | Dracup-Breu | Dracup, KA, and Breu, CS: Using research findings to meet the needs of grieving spouses. Nurs Res 27:212, 1978. |
| 1987 | The Quality Assurance Model Using Research | Watson, CA, Bulechek, GM, and McCloskey, JD: QAMUR: A quality assurance model using research. J Nurs Quality Assurance 2:21, 1987. |
| 1994 | Iowa Model of Research in Practice | Titler, MO, et al: Infusing research into practice to promote quality care. Nurs Res 43:307, 1994. |
| 1989 | American Association of Critical Care Nurses | Mitchell, PH, et al: American Association of Critical-Care Nurses Demonstration Project: Profile of excellence in critical care nursing. Heart Lung 18:219, 1989. |
| 1987 | Goode Research Utilization Model | Goode, C, et al: Use of research-based knowledge in clinical practice, J Nurs Adm 17:11, 1987. |
| 1989–1994 | University of North Carolina | Funk, SG, Tournquist, EM, and Champagne, MT: A model for improving the dissemination of nursing research. West J Nurs Res 11:361, 1989. |

## NURSING RESEARCH UTILIZATION MODELS

Nursing research utilization models were developed to enable the use or dissemination of nursing research. Improving patient outcomes is the ultimate goal of nursing research utilization models. Many of these efforts were funded projects that focused on adoption of clinical innovations. Table 17.2 illustrates the target population, structure, process, and specific outcomes associated with several popular models of nursing research utilization.

The target population may be an individual nurse, educator, or researcher or a group of individuals interested in the same practice issue. The structure may be established within an institution or professional nursing organization. Research utilization projects may be influenced by available resources and support systems. Initial goals include facilitating practitioners' application of research findings or changing clinical practice. Other goals may include dissemination of research findings or development of research-based protocols and clinical practice guidelines.

Identifying the clinical problem is the first step for many research utilization models, such as the Conduct and Utilization of Research in Nursing (CURN) Project,[3] the Iowa Model of Research in Practice,[4] and the Dracup-Breu Model.[5] After identifying the problem, existing research is reviewed and critiqued. If insufficient information to change practice is found, it may be necessary to rely on expert opinion until clinical trials are conducted. If adequate research exists, a decision to use or reject the data is made. If a change in practice is recommended and implemented, measuring the expected outcome is the next step. Thus, evaluation is a continuous, ongoing process.

The University of North Carolina Model[6] for nursing research utilization focuses on dissemination of findings. This group organized annual research conferences where clinical research updates were presented. The steps of this model included a call for abstracts, research presentations, and publication of conference monographs. This model's overall goals relate to the delivery of research-based care and improving patient outcomes.

The Stetler (previously Stetler-Marram) Model[7,8] establishes an organizing framework with specific criteria to help practitioners make decisions about the applicability of research findings. The Stetler Model focuses on assisting the individual or groups of clinicians with research utilization and evaluation. The six steps in the Stetler Model are described in Table 17.3. The Stetler Model was applied among advanced practice nurses in oncology nursing when discussing problems and opportunities encountered during examination of bereavement care. Excerpts 17.1 to 17.6 illustrate applications of the Stetler Model.

Specialty-based models have emerged as a recent trend in nursing research utilization. With ever decreasing agency resources, specialty organizations have begun to recognize the need for and effectiveness of collaborating on research-related issues. The American Association of Critical Care Nurses[9] initiated a project that examined the structure, process, and outcomes valued in critical care nursing practice. The development and implementation of a demonstration project followed research utilization efforts that examined research-based literature.

TABLE 17.2  MODELS OF NURSING RESEARCH UTILIZATION: STRUCTURE, PROCESS,
AND OUTCOMES

| Model | Target Population | Structure | Process | Outcomes |
|---|---|---|---|---|
| Western Interstate Commission for Higher Education | Individual | Caregiver | 1. Problem definition<br>2. Research retrieval<br>3. Research review<br>4. Development of research-based care | Change in problem identification |
| Conduct and Utilization of Research in Nursing | Group | Institution-based | 1. Problem identification<br>2. Assessment of knowledge base<br>3. Design of practice change<br>4. Clinical trial<br>5. Adoption or rejection of change<br>6. Diffusion of innovation<br>7. Institutional change | Changes in patient outcomes |
| The Nursing Child Assessment Satellite Training Project | Individual | Nurse practitioner/ educator | 1. Recruitment<br>2. Translation of research findings<br>3. Dissemination of findings<br>4. Evaluation | Education of nurse practitioners |
| Stetler (previously Stetler/Marr-am Model) | Individual | Caregiver | 1. Preparation<br>2. Validation<br>3. Comparative findings evaluation<br>4. Decision making<br>5. Translation/ application<br>6. Evaluation | Application of research |
| Dracup-Breu | Group | Institution-based | 1. Problem identification<br>2. Selection of research for review and critique<br>3. Establishment of objectives<br>4. Analysis of setting and creation of plan<br>5. Implementation<br>6. Evaluation of outcomes | Change in practice |

*(continued)*

TABLE 17.2 MODELS OF NURSING RESEARCH UTILIZATION: STRUCTURE, PROCESS, AND OUTCOMES *(continued)*

| Model | Target Population | Structure | Process | Outcomes |
|---|---|---|---|---|
| The Quality Assurance Model Using Research | Group | Institution-based | 1. Identification of practice problem<br>2. Review of literature<br>3. Decision to use findings or conduct study<br>4. Pilot study<br>5. Evaluation<br>6. Decision to modify, use, or reject<br>7. Change in practice<br>8. Publication | 1. Change in patient outcomes<br>2. Dissemination of findings |
| Iowa Model of Research in Practice | Group | Institution-based | 1. Identification of problem or knowledge-focused triggers<br>2. Assembling relevant research literature<br>3. Critique, determination of sufficiency of research base<br>4. Pilot if knowledge base is sufficient; study if insufficient<br>5. Decision making<br>6. Practice change<br>7. Monitoring of outcomes | Change in practice |
| American Association of Critical Care Nurses | Group | Professional organization | 1. Intraprofessional collaboration | Improve clinical outcomes; address organizational issues (turnover, nurse satisfaction) |

TABLE 17.2  MODELS OF NURSING RESEARCH UTILIZATION: STRUCTURE, PROCESS, AND OUTCOMES *(continued)*

| Model | Target Population | Structure | Process | Outcomes |
|---|---|---|---|---|
| Goode Research Utilization Model | Group | Institution-based | 1. Inputs (information, knowledge, involvement, planning, value, consensus) | Outputs (change in policy, professional growth, procedure change, improved patient outcomes, feedback/ evaluation) |
| University of North Carolina | | Individual Caregiver Researcher Educator | 1. Topic selection 2. Call for abstracts 3. Research presentations 4. Publication of conference monographs | 1. Delivery of research-based care 2. Dissemination of research |

Completing an integrative review of the literature is another approach to research utilization. The Agency for Health Care Policy and Research has modeled an approach based on a critical, integrative review of literature conducted by a panel of experts. Several recently published articles on clinical practice guidelines (e.g., cancer pain management[10]) systematically evaluate the research and make specific recommendations for clinical practice.

Choosing a research utilization model or approach depends on the goals and resources of the individuals, professional groups, or institutions involved. No one model works for all clinicians or clinical situations. The different models provide various frameworks and implementation strategies. Regardless of the model, the person who uses the model must have a questioning mind, a willingness to use existing research, and a commitment to research-based practice. Research utilization is the responsibility of every nurse, whether working as an individual or within a group.

## RESEARCH UTILIZATION PROCESS

Research utilization involves a number of systematic, deliberate steps. Once a clinical problem is identified, research consumers must carefully evaluate the existing

**TABLE 17.3** STETLER MODEL OF RESEARCH UTILIZATION

| Phase | Activities |
|---|---|
| 1. Preparation | 1. Identify the purpose of the research review |
| 2. Validation | 1. Conduct utilization research critique |
| | 2. Identify the scientific merit and the applicability of the findings |
| 3. Comparative evaluation | 1. Assess the fit of the finding to the consumer's practice setting |
| |   a. Risk factors |
| |   b. Need for resources |
| |   c. Readiness |
| | 2. Assess current practice |
| | 3. Examine "substantiating evidence" |
| 4. Decision making | 1. Decide to: |
| |   a. Use |
| |   b. Consider use |
| |   c. Delay use |
| |   d. Reject findings or not to use |
| 5. Translation/Application | 1. Synthesize findings |
| | 2. Identify specific nature of practice implications |
| 6. Evaluation | 1. Specify expected outcomes |
| | 2. Implement evaluation plan (formally or informally) |
| | 3. Establish feasibility |

**EXCERPT 17.1**

## STETLER MODEL: PHASE I–PREPARATION

The task force decided that selecting a topic that was clinically relevant to all members and applicable in all practice settings throughout the oncology center was important. After much discussion, the group chose bereavement as a topic for its work because successful engagement in, and completion of, the grief process often is difficult.

The psychiatric liaison CNS and one other task force member conducted a literature search using the MEDLINE computerized data base. Five research-based articles were selected for evaluation. Originally, the task force decided that all members would read each of the five selected articles and, during the group's regularly scheduled bimonthly meeting, they would evaluate each article using the Stetler model criteria. The group also felt that its regularly scheduled meeting times should be preserved for information exchange, peer support, and discussion associated with the group's other identified goals. Consequently, the task force divided into four working groups, each of which conducted the Phase II (validation) portion of the model for one of the four remaining articles. The entire group then met to complete Phases III, IV, and V.

*Source: Hanson, JL, and Ashley, B: Advanced practice nurses' application of the Stetler model for research utilization: Improving bereavement care. Oncol Nurs Forum 21:720, 1994, with permission.*

Excerpt 17.2

## STETLER MODEL: PHASE II—VALIDATION

In this phase, each of the working groups sought to define the strengths, weaknesses, and overall scientific merit of its individual study. The first study was strongly grounded in the theoretical framework of Lazarus and Folkman. The investigators used two established instruments and two self-developed instruments to measure resources and nature of appraisal in a group of 159 widowed people from Catholic parishes in two midwestern cities. The study assessed the relationship between appraisal/coping/resources and psychosocial functioning using a complex causal model and path analysis techniques. Several significant findings emerged. Appraisal of the loss as highly threatening appeared to directly influence type of coping and to indirectly influence amount of psychosocial dysfunction. Problem-focused coping resulted in lower levels of psychosocial dysfunction, whereas emotions-focused coping resulted in more dysfunction. Nature of the subjects' resources directly influenced appraisal and indirectly influenced coping, and respondents with stronger resources reported less psychosocial dysfunction. Older, widowed people experienced more dysfunction than did younger ones, although they also had lower degrees of threat appraisal.

[The other four articles were critiqued as above.]

*Source: Hanson, JL, and Ashley, B: Advanced practice nurses' application of the Stetler model for research utilization: Improving bereavement care. Oncol Nurs Forum 21:720, 1994, with permission.*

research for its applicability. If changes are made in clinical practice, patient outcomes must be carefully evaluated. The first and perhaps most important step in the research utilization process is clarifying the clinical question or problem.

### Specifying the Clinical Problem

Most clinical problems are first identified by clinicians who ask, "Why do we do it this way?" or "Is there a better way to do this?" Questions or problems may also arise when new knowledge or technology emerges. Clinical issues may be generated from risk management data or from quality improvement studies, or they may emerge after the publication of national standards or clinical practice guidelines. Research utilization projects may also be initiated when policies and procedures are developed or revised.

Clinical questions, like researchable problems, need a specific focus. For example, quality improvement studies may indicate that patients' pain is poorly controlled in the medical-surgical units. Before starting a research utilization project, the specific nature of the question must be determined. Perhaps the problem is related to a specific age group (young, middle-aged, or elderly), the way pain is assessed, or the nurses' attitudes toward pain. As an example, narrowing the focus to address the assessment and management of pain in older adult patients makes the project more feasible.

**EXCERPT 17.3**

## STETLER MODEL: PHASE III—COMPARATIVE EVALUATION

The working groups reconvened to complete the remaining phases of the Stetler Model. In conducting Phase III, the group examined areas prescribed by the model. The bereaved population seen at the Johns Hopkins Oncology Center (JHOC) differed from the samples described in the studies, which were predominantly white females, the majority of whom had lost their husbands through a chronic illness and thus likely experienced some anticipatory grief. JHOC's bereaved population is more heterogeneous with regard to race, gender, and relationship to the deceased. The task force was of the opinion, however, that these differences in sample characteristics did not preclude use of study findings. In this comparative evaluation, the group eliminated Scruby and Sloan's (1989) study from potential use in decision making because its central hypothesis was that bereavement counseling provided to individuals in their homes would promote health. At JHOC, which has a broad catchment area, home counseling is not feasible. Additionally, Scruby and Sloan's small sample size was a serious concern. The four remaining studies were deemed applicable to an inpatient practice setting. Finally, the task force evaluated the feasibility, resources, readiness, and risks of implementing the studies' findings given JHOC practice setting constraints. Practitioners at the individual, departmental, and interdisciplinary levels were ready for a change in practice, and little resistance was anticipated.

*Source: Hanson, JL, and Ashley, B: Advanced practice nurses' application of the Stetler model for research utilization: Improving bereavement care. Oncol Nurs Forum 21:720, 1994, with permission.*

A research utilization project should potentially benefit as many patients as possible. Available resources must be considered before starting any project. With ever-decreasing clinical resources, it may not be cost-effective to conduct a research utilization project to benefit just one patient. Identifying clinical resources and the specific nature and magnitude of the problem will help direct the research utilization effort.

**EXCERPT 17.4**

## STETLER MODEL: PHASE IV—DECISION MAKING

In this phase, the task force determined that the findings of the three studies involving identification of risk factors associated with poor bereavement outcomes (Gass & Chang, 1989; Jacobs et al, 1990; Vachon et al, 1982) were applicable at both the cognitive and instrumental levels. The study that tested a self-help intervention for widows (Vachon et al, 1982) seemed to require further validation, so the task force postponed implementing this study's findings until more information could be gathered. Finally, as noted, Scruby and Sloan's (1989) study was eliminated from further consideration.

*Source: Hanson, JL, and Ashley, B: Advanced practice nurses' application of the Stetler model for research utilization: Improving bereavement care. Oncol Nurs Forum 21:720, 1994, with permission.*

**EXCERPT 17.5**

## STETLER MODEL: PHASE V—TRANSLATION/APPLICATION

In keeping with the Research Utilization Subcommittee's decision about how best to disseminate findings and recommendations based on the research utilization process, the task force presented a nursing grand rounds on bereavement for the entire Nursing Department. Because members of the social work department are integral members of the health-care team responsible for psychosocial assessment and intervention at JHOC, they also were invited to participate. During the grand rounds, the Stetler Model was reviewed and then applied using bereavement as the example.

The nursing grand rounds forum provided a means to educate nursing staff about the research utilization process as well as about current bereavement, assessment, and intervention practices. The nursing grand rounds also served as a vehicle for introducing the final recommendations of the task force to the entire Nursing and Social Work Departments. Recommended practice changes were considered applicable primarily at a departmental or programmatic level. Written recommendations also were submitted to the directors of Nursing and Social Work. The recommended changes, which are outlined below, were both organizational and clinical in nature.

*Source: Hanson, JL, and Ashley, B: Advanced practice nurses' application of the Stetler model for research utilization: Improving bereavement care. Oncol Nurs Forum 21:720, 1994, with permission.*

### Assembling the Research Literature

Once the clinical problem has been delineated, the next step is to visit the library and obtain articles related to the topic of concern. The librarian or *Medical Subject Headings (MeSH)* can help to identify search terms. Various indexes, computer-assisted searches, and on-line searches can be used to access the literature and identify articles related to the topic. Two indexes commonly used by nurses, *MEDLINE* and *Cumulative Index to Nursing and Allied Health Literature (CINAHL)*, are available in a variety of formats including print, CD-ROM, and on-line. Most medical and nursing librarians are expert at searching *CINAHL* and *MEDLINE* as well as other health-related indexes such as *Hospital Literature Index, PsychoINFO*, and

**EXCERPT 17.6**

## STETLER MODEL: PHASE VI—EVALUATION

Because the recommended practice changes were programmatic in nature and involved both the Nursing and Social Work Departments, the task force did not develop a formal evaluation plan. Once responsibility for implementation of the recommendations has been decided and changes are implemented, an evaluation strategy will be designed. The Nursing Research Committee, as part of its goals, will monitor progress in this area.

*Source: Hanson, JL, and Ashley, B: Advanced practice nurses' application of the Stetler model for research utilization: Improving bereavement care. Oncol Nurs Forum 21:720, 1994, with permission.*

*Nursing Studies Index.* Many nursing and health-related indexes are relatively easy to learn and, with practice, even a beginner can identify appropriate references.

Reference lists and bibliographies from books and journal articles can help identify other potential resources. Collaborating and networking with other nurses is another strategy to use for identifying appropriate references. One such strategy involves using the Internet to access a discussion group. Posting a query about a topic may produce information and answers from other nurse colleagues. Another approach is collaborating with nurses within one's specialty organization or at other clinical agencies.

Once references have been identified, the next step is to acquire the materials. Published summaries of the research, such as integrative reviews or meta-analyses, may also be helpful. Reading abstracts from on-line or computerized searches may help determine whether an article relates to the topic of interest. Electronic searches enable clinicians and researchers to obtain the most recent information from journal articles, research reports, and dissertations. Access to reference materials is ever-increasing with on-line search capabilities and interlibrary searching and loans. Many resources, including journal articles, can also be ordered on-line.

## Critiquing the Research

The next step is to read and analyze the research and synthesize the findings. General strategies when reading research articles include skimming the report and then reading it more thoroughly. It is often helpful to collaborate with someone with more research expertise. When nurses first start reading research, they may feel hesitant and unsure about their abilities. Inexperienced research readers often use their common sense and clinical expertise to critique the design and identify problems and issues.

Most experts advise readers to start by reading the title. The title provides information about the nature of the study and should interest the reader in reading the study. If the title is interesting and pertinent, the next step is to read the abstract. The abstract presents a brief summary of the research article. Reading the abstract will help determine whether the study is related to a specific clinical issue. If the abstract appears pertinent, the reader will find it useful to scan the entire article and review the major headings. Sometimes it is helpful to read the title, abstract, and discussion first. When those sections have been read, the reader should return to the introduction section. In this section, the research questions/hypotheses and the justification for the study are specified. The introduction may also include a review of the literature and a discussion of the theoretical framework. These sections provide a background of related research efforts and a framework for the research design.

The next section usually discusses the study's design. Research methods, including the design, sample size, data collection, and data analysis, are described. In this section, one can discover if the study is experimental or nonexperimental and whether it is qualitative (analyzing words) or quantitative (analyzing numbers). The researcher usually describes the sample and how and where research subjects were obtained. Usually the author discusses the characteristics of the sample (e.g., age, gender, health status), who was included/excluded in the study, and the practice setting.

In this section, the researcher also usually discusses issues of protection of human rights. The processes of informed consent, as well as the risks and benefits of the research, should be discussed. The researcher also describes the research protocol and the data collection instruments. The reader should ask whether the study environment approximates the real world and whether the study methods could have affected the outcomes.

The results section presents the research findings and analysis methods. Regardless of the type of research, descriptive information is provided about the sample and key variables. In quantitative studies, statistical analyses are presented. Reading and understanding statistics is difficult, but this section should be read carefully. The statistical results are explained in the discussion section, where the researcher interprets the results and discusses their significance. Limitations of the study are also explicated.

Critiquing research requires a systematic, consistent approach. Many groups develop their own critique instrument or use a published format. A number of specific guidelines exist to examine qualitative or quantitative research. Phillips[11] provides four basic criteria that should be met for any research study: clarity of presentation, logical progression of arguments, explicit rationale, and documentation of the research.

## Assessing the Applicability

When implementing research findings, three criteria to consider include scientific merit, need for replication, and potential risk factors.[12] In the process of critiquing, the researcher must evaluate the methods, including the sampling plan and research design; the reliability and validity of the measurement tools; the appropriateness of the statistical procedures; and the interpretation of the results.

Additionally, before any research can be adopted, the fit of the findings to the practice setting must be analyzed. What may be applicable in the hospital may not work in a community setting. Similarities of the study population to the practice setting must be evaluated. For example, results from an urban clinic may not have relevance to one in a rural setting. Understanding the characteristics of the sample and setting is critical to evaluating the applicability of the findings.

Other factors that must be considered include whether practitioners are willing to implement a change in a practice, policy, or procedure. Other considerations include client safety and the efficacy of the change in terms of equipment, time, and money. Sometimes a decision to replicate a research project may be the most appropriate step before incorporating the findings in practice. Regardless of the research findings, consideration must be given to each study. Each research report needs to be evaluated in relation to all other available data. Rarely is one isolated research report sufficient to change practice.

## Implementing the Innovation

Once the research has been critiqued and its applicability determined, a decision to implement an innovation may occur. Such a change in practice may be part of a policy, procedure, or clinical practice guideline. Prior to implementation, specific clinical outcomes are established. No change can occur without educating all involved personnel, a process that can be assisted by verbal and written communication. All staff members need to understand clearly the reasons for the change, the potential benefits, and the specific nature of the change.

Change occurs most effectively when staff members are committed and involved in the process. All involved need education, opportunities to have their questions answered, and a sense of support. They need to value the change and believe it is worthwhile. Realizing a change without considering the process can lead to problems during implementation. Any innovation can be undermined or resisted, especially when the stakeholders are not adequately prepared for the change.

## Evaluating the Innovation

When considering evaluation, it may be helpful to reexamine the original practice problem or issue. Improving care is usually the final goal. Specific objectives may include enhancing pain assessment or increasing patients' levels of comfort. Before implementing any change, it is essential to develop project-specific outcome measures that are realistic, measurable, and understandable.

Once the innovation is in effect, an ongoing evaluation process occurs. The implementation process and the outcome objectives should be evaluated. Knowledge gained from evaluating the implementation process may be helpful with future projects. Evaluation may be part of a quality improvement program. Another approach is to measure specific patient outcomes with a research instrument. Previously developed instruments can be used or an instrument can be developed specifically for the project. Interviews or chart reviews are another way to examine the results of the project.

## BARRIERS AND FACILITATORS TO RESEARCH UTILIZATION

Several factors are either barriers to or facilitators of research utilization. These factors have been described as social, political, organizational, economic, attitudinal, and environmental.[13,14] **Barriers** are influences that negatively affect clinicians' utilization of research. In contrast, **facilitators** are reasons clinicians adopt a research-based practice.

## Research and Researcher-Related Barriers

Barriers to research utilization are related to a number of issues. A major barrier is the absence of research on specific topics that helps explain clinical practice problems. In addition, published studies may have limitations in terms of sample size and design, thus limiting the generalizability of the results. Many clinicians lack experience reading research reports, have difficulty interpreting statistical findings and, as a result, think they lack the preparation and expertise to critique research reports.

Researchers do not always fully understand or approach practice issues from a clinical perspective. The research jargon that is often used may make it difficult for clinicians to understand or interpret research reports. Published research may have limited clinical application and rarely appears in clinical journals. The results of research studies are most often presented to audiences composed of other researchers. When this happens, pertinent findings never reach clinicians.

## Professional and Administrative Barriers

Many research utilization barriers result from the educational preparation of nurses and availability of administrative support. Traditionally, varying amounts of importance have been assigned to research and research utilization education during entry-level programs. Another problem is that many clinicians never receive research-related content during their basic program or continuing education programs. It is only since the late 1970s that most baccalaureate programs started including a specific research course in the curriculum. These professional and educational barriers are often compounded by several administrative barriers.

Administrative barriers include lack of time, money, or clinical resources for research utilization activities within the agency. Nurse administrators may not value or recognize the importance of research-based practice. The clinical environment may not support the research utilization process and the concept of change. Within the setting there may be limited access to individuals with expertise in research methods or minimal collaboration between academia and practice. Scarce availability of library resources, including journals and computerized searches, may affect the clinician's ability to access information.

## Clinician Barriers

A number of factors are identified as clinician barriers. Practicing nurses may not value using research or understand how it differs from conducting research. Nurses may not have the knowledge necessary to use research. Many traditions in clinical practice are accepted as fact and are rarely questioned, as questioning the traditions of practice may not be deemed appropriate. This can contribute to a limited identification of researchable problems. In addition, practice settings may offer few incentives for nurses to use research.

### Measuring Barriers

Since the late 1970s, many research studies have examined nurses', administrators', and researchers' perceptions of research utilization barriers. Early research findings found the most frequently reported barrier was an inability to access research findings of interest. Funk and colleagues[13] conducted a survey to determine barriers from the clinician's perspective. Results indicated insufficient authority and insufficient time as the two most frequently reported barriers. Other barriers included a lack of cooperation from physicians, administration, and other staff; inapplicability of the research to the setting; inadequate facilities for implementation; insufficient time to read research; lack of awareness of research findings by the clinician; difficulty understanding and interpreting statistics; and a sense of isolation from knowledgeable colleagues. Other concerns affecting nursing research utilization stemmed from the fact that nurses were not convinced of the need or benefit to practice and an unwillingness to try new ideas.

### Facilitators to Enhance Research Utilization

There are several factors that facilitate research utilization. Perhaps most critical is the identification of clinically relevant problems and issues. Another factor is an administration that is committed to the research utilization process and critical thinking. Provision of adequate resources, consisting of personnel, equipment, money, and time, is essential to the research utilization process. Staff nurses also benefit from having an increased knowledge of both research and research utilization.

Research utilization is facilitated when expectations are clearly communicated to staff and incentives for research utilization are provided. Establishing linkages between academia and practice, while supporting collaboration between novice and expert researchers, enhances research utilization activities. Easy access to the literature and literature reviews is critical to any research utilization project.

When barriers are identified, researchers, administrators, and clinicians can design and implement specific strategies that will facilitate research utilization. Such activities may be institution- or situation-specific. Strategies to address specific research utilization obstacles have been proposed by Lekander, Tracy, and Lindquist[14] (Table 17.4).

Some agencies may find it helpful to offer incentives such as pay increases within a clinical ladder program. Other agencies may form a committee. Additional strategies include providing staff with time to read research reports and having experts available to help interpret and critique the findings. Each clinical setting should identify barriers and solutions unique to that setting. For example, addressing a barrier such as inaccessibility to the literature by providing computerized searches via the Internet may assist a particular institution.

### STRATEGIES TO PROMOTE RESEARCH UTILIZATION

Simply sharing research-related information with nurse colleagues is one approach to research utilization. Involvement in research utilization can begin by forming a journal club and reading and critiquing research reports with others. Attending conferences where research is presented and discussed helps clinicians.

Additional strategies to promote research utilization include incorporating research findings into nursing textbooks, basic nursing education, continuing education programs, and policy and procedure manuals. Reading summaries or abstracts

TABLE 17.4 RESEARCH UTILIZATION: OBSTACLES AND RELATED STRATEGIES

| Obstacles | Strategies |
|---|---|
| Lack of perceived value of nursing research | • Support role modeling by nursing leadership<br>• Provide explicit sanction for research utilization activity<br>• Provide support through rewards/incentives<br>• Analyze how organizational environment can support research utilization<br>• Link research utilization to institutional goals and objectives |
| Lack of access to resources | • Circulate research journals, abstracts, and summaries<br>• Establish clinician access to health sciences libraries<br>• Provide education about performing literature searches<br>• Develop joint programs between schools of nursing and hospital departments of nursing<br>• Increase funding specifically for research utilization |
| Lack of preparation | • Establish journal clubs and unit-based research councils<br>• Develop a curriculum focus on implementing research findings into practice<br>• Implement mentoring by graduate nurses in research critique and innovation |
| Lack of availability of research findings | • Publish research results in clinical and research journals<br>• Promote teleconferences and satellite conferences to disseminate findings speedily<br>• Sponsor newsletters, presentations, and conferences devoted to research utilization |
| Lack of authority to change | • Target influential leaders to lead change process<br>• Determine stakeholders in change and involve them in change process |
| Patient care procedures | • Collaborate with other disciplines<br>• Develop education programs to promote individuals' roles and responsibilities |
| Lack of motivation to change practice | • Create rewards/recognition for implementing innovations |
| Insufficient methods for implementation/dissemination | • Promote careful preplanning for successful research utilization implementation<br>• Develop realistic implementation periods<br>• Develop appropriate evaluation programs to document results of research utilization<br>• Sponsor face-to-face/communication or telecommunication as possible alternatives to print media |
| Lack of clinician researcher | • Promote active, reciprocal exchange of ideas and information<br>• Develop formal, explicit relationships<br>• Encourage unit-based clinicians with research skills to communicate with peers |

*Source: From Lekander, BJ, Tracy, MF, and Lindquist, R: Overcoming the obstacles to research-based clinical practice, AACN Clinical Issues 5:115, 1994.*[14]

of research studies or working with colleagues within one's practice setting or professional organization often facilitates the research utilization process. Every patient deserves a nurse who uses research. Reading and using research must become integral parts of each nurse's practice.

## THE FUTURE OF RESEARCH UTILIZATION

The future of health care and research utilization will be collaborative and include researchers, educators, practitioners, and the organization. With the increasing interest in cost and quality in health care, research-based care will continue to be an important focus. Increasing opportunities to network, by using resources available on the Internet, will facilitate consultation and cooperation. References such as the *Online Journal of Knowledge Synthesis for Nursing* will enhance access to integrative reviews of research. Resources such as expert clinicians and specialty-based nurse researchers will facilitate research utilization efforts. In today's practice areas, research-based care is mandatory for all health-care workers.

## SUMMARY OF KEY IDEAS

1. Research utilization is an organized, deliberate process by which research findings are incorporated in practice.
2. The purpose of nursing research utilization is improved patient outcomes.
3. Research utilization models in nursing vary in terms of their purpose, organizing frameworks, target population, structure, and processes. Models such as the CURN Project[3] and the Iowa Model of Research in Practice[4] focus on research utilization, whereas the University of North Carolina Model[6] focuses on research dissemination.
4. Research utilization begins with identifying a clinical problem and initiating a process by which the literature is first assembled and critiqued. The next step requires that the applicability of the findings be evaluated. Once an innovation is designed, it must be implemented and then evaluated.
5. The gaps between research and practice can be explained by social, political, organizational, economic, attitudinal, and environmental barriers. Identifying barriers and developing strategies to minimize or eliminate them can facilitate research utilization.
6. Research-based care is mandatory in today's health-care market.

## LEARNING ACTIVITIES

1. Conduct a literature search on a research question or topic of interest. As you review the citations that you retrieve, identify which ones are research reports. Where are the research findings published? Within the citations, is there an example of findings published by the same researcher in both a research journal and a clinical journal? If so, obtain copies of both articles.

Read them to compare and contrast. How are they similar? How are they different? Is one more complete than the other? Does either article provide sufficient evidence for a research practice change?

2. What is the difference between a meta-analysis and an integrative research review? Conduct a literature search and find an example of each published in the nursing literature. Read each and compare and contrast. Why would an author choose to do one versus the other? Be specific.

3. Identify guidelines for a nursing procedure, either in a nursing text or a procedure manual on a clinical unit. Is there evidence of research being used to support the steps presented in the procedure? If so, where is the research documented? Do a literature search on the topic. Does research exist for this particular procedure? If so, is the procedure that you originally read congruent with the research presented? If research evidence is not presented, what rationale is provided for the steps of the procedure? Does this rationale seem scientifically sound?

## References

1. Rogers, EM: Diffusion of Innovations, ed 3. Free Press, New York, 1983.
2. Havelock, R: The knowledge perspective: Definition and scope of a new study domain. In Beal, GM, Dissanayake, W, and Knonshima, S (eds): Knowledge Generation, Exchange, and Utilization. Westview Press, Boulder, CO, 1986.
3. Horsley, JA, et al: Using Research to Improve Nursing Practice: A Guide. Grune & Stratton, New York, 1983.
4. Titler, MG, et al: Infusing research into practice to promote quality care. Nurs Res 43:307, 1994.
5. Dracup, KA, and Breu, CS: Using research findings to meet the needs of grieving spouses. Nurs Res 27:212, 1978.
6. Funk, SG, Tournquist, EM, and Champagne, MT: A model for improving the dissemination of nursing research. West J Nurs Res 11:361, 1989.
7. Stetler, CB, and Marram, G: Evaluation of research findings for applicability in practice. Nurs Outlook 24:559, 1976.

8. Stetler, CB: Refinement of the Stetler/Marram model for application of research findings to practice. Nurs Outlook 42:15, 1994.

9. Mitchell, PH, et al: American Association of Critical Care Nurses demonstration project: Profile of excellence in critical care nursing. Heart Lung 18:219, 1989.

10. Jacox, A, et al: Management of Cancer Pain. Clinical Practice Guideline No. 9, AHCPR Publication No. 94-0592. Rockville, MD: Agency for Health Care Policy and Research, US Department of Health and Human Services, Public Health Service, 1994.

11. Phillips, LR: A Clinician's Guide to the Critique and Utilization of Nursing Research. Prentice Hall, East Norwalk, CT, 1986.

12. Haller, KB, Reynolds, MA, and Horsley, JA: Developing research-based innovation protocols: Process, criteria, and issues. Res Nurs Health 2:45, 1979.

13. Funk, SG, et al: Barriers to using research findings in practice: The clinician's perspective. Appl Nurs Res 4:90, 1991.

14. Lekander, BJ, Tracy, MF, and Lindquist, R: Overcoming the obstacles to research-based clinical practice. AACN Clin Issues 5:115, 1994.

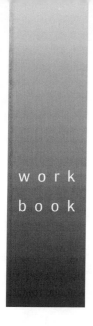

work
book

# Reading, Understanding, and Applying Nursing Research

# 1 Introduction to Nursing Research

**REVIEW QUESTIONS:**

1. In one or two sentences, state the importance of research in nursing.

---

2. Many students are uneasy about the idea of research. Why?

---

3. How is the research process different from the problem-solving process?

---

4. Can you think of some other ways of knowing besides those mentioned in this chapter? What are they? What, if any, are the limitations of these methods?

---

5. What makes scientific inquiry different from other types of inquiry?

_____

_____

_____

_____

_____

_____

_____

6. What types of research questions lend themselves to scientific inquiry?

_____

_____

_____

_____

_____

_____

7. What is expected of students in a baccalaureate versus those in a master's degree program in terms of research competencies as defined by the American Nurses Association?

_____

_____

_____

_____

_____

_____

_____

8. List two ways that you as a student can participate in research activities.

_____

_____

_____

_____

_____

_____

9. Based on your areas of interest, list a couple of specialty journals in which you might be interested.

_____

_____

_____

_____

## MULTIPLE CHOICE QUESTIONS:

1. Nursing research is the key to providing high-quality health care. Through the process of conducting research, nurses:

    a. ask questions that come up in daily nursing practice that need answers
    b. provide data that document the effectiveness of nursing care
    c. build a body of knowledge unique to the discipline of nursing
    d. all of the above

2. The scientific method incorporates those procedures used by researchers in the pursuit of new knowledge. The first step involved in the scientific method is:

    a. developing a framework
    b. reviewing the literature
    c. formulating a research problem and purpose
    d. formulating research objectives, questions, or hypotheses

3. Nursing has historically acquired knowledge from an assortment of methods. Which method has nursing used to generate new ideas and knowledge?

    a. tradition
    b. personal experience
    c. intuition
    d. all of the above

4. An approach used to acquire nursing knowledge that describes life experiences is classified as:

    a. qualitative research
    b. quantitative research
    c. experimental research
    d. quasiexperimental research

5. Triangulation refers to the process of:

    a. reaching agreement among three members of a research team on the identity of the concepts or themes
    b. collecting data through different research approaches
    c. abstracting themes into constructs
    d. examining problems to gain knowledge about improving patient care

# 2 Understanding the Research Process and Ethical Issues in Nursing Research

## REVIEW QUESTIONS:

1. Identify the five general phases of the research process.

_____

_____

_____

_____

2. What are the major categories of research discussed in this chapter? What are their special purposes? What are their major difficulties?

_____

_____

_____

_____

3. Distinguish between retrospective and prospective research.

_____

_____

_____

_____

4. Distinguish between cross-sectional and longitudinal research.

_____

_____

_____

_____

5. What purposes did the Nuremberg Code and Declaration of Helsinki serve in protecting individuals who participate in research studies?

_____

_____

_____

_____

_____

6. What three rights protect subjects participating in research?

_____

_____

_____

_____

_____

7. What is the difference between anonymity and confidentiality?

_____

_____

_____

_____

_____

8. The risk-benefit ratio is a standard by which researchers can judge the ethics of certain research procedures. What does *risk-benefit ratio* mean?

_____

_____

_____

_____

_____

9. What is informed consent?

_____

_____

_____

_____

_____

10. What different ethical committees or institutional review boards exist in your college, department, or institution? What functions and responsibilities do they serve?

_____

_____

_____

_____

_____

## MULTIPLE CHOICE QUESTIONS:

1. The research process may best be characterized as:

    a. a way of assigning people to groups
    b. a set of steps to be carried out one by one in the prescribed order
    c. a set of rules that must always be followed
    d. a decision-making process that attempts to guard against making false interpretations

2. In some situations, a researcher obtains informed consent without asking the subject to sign his or her name on a written consent form. This is done to protect the subject's:

    a. human dignity
    b. anonymity
    c. right to self-determination
    d. confidentiality

3. Which of the following potential research participants have diminished autonomy and are incompetent to give informed consent?

    a. cognitively impaired older adults
    b. mentally ill patients
    c. children
    d. all of the above

4. A researcher wants to determine if nurses' levels of empathy for patients change after graduation from nursing school. She measures new graduates, nurses who have worked for 2 years, and nurses who have worked for 4 years as regards to their empathy for patients and compares their scores. This study is:

    a. prospective
    b. retrospective
    c. cross-sectional
    d. longitudinal

5. A researcher is interested in why some elderly patients are discharged when considered not medically stable. The researcher reviews charts of patients who have been discharged in order to explore factors that occurred during the hospitalization and relate these to status at discharge. This study is:

    a. prospective
    b. retrospective
    c. cross-sectional
    d. longitudinal

# 3 Selecting and Defining the Problem

**REVIEW QUESTIONS:**

1. State the difference between a problem statement and a purpose statement.

2. List several characteristics of a good problem statement.

3. From where are a majority of research problems derived?

4. Why is replication of nursing research so important?

5. Why is it important for a researcher to do a literature review before planning a study?

6. Much information is found in nursing and social science journals. Identify three nursing research journals that contain empirical-based literature.

_____

_____

_____

_____

_____

7. Many published research reports include only a few references to related studies. Why?

_____

_____

_____

_____

_____

8. One rarely finds books cited in a literature review? Why? Is it a good idea to refer to books?

_____

_____

_____

_____

_____

9. What is meant by a *primary source of information?*

_____

_____

_____

_____

_____

10. List several print and computer-based indexes useful for searching the literature.

_____

_____

_____

_____

_____

## MULTIPLE CHOICE QUESTIONS:

1. The purpose of an operational definition is to:

    a. assign numerical values to variables
    b. specify how a variable will be defined and measured
    c. state the expected relations between the variables under study
    d. designate the overall plan by which the research will be conducted

2. A literature review serves several functions. They include:

    a. expanding or further defining the problem statement
    b. helping to establish a theoretical base
    c. identifying relationships between variables
    d. all of the above

3. A nurse decides to conduct a historical study about the care of chronically ill children in American frontier families between 1800 and 1820. Which of the following would be a primary source on this topic?

    a. Jones's *History of the American West,* published in 1930
    b. a previous historical study, *The Nature of Childhood Among Nebraska Settlers in the 1800s,* which was recently completed by a prominent nurse researcher
    c. a set of three letters written by a pioneer woman in Minnesota in 1811 and 1812 concerning the experiences of her family, which includes one child with asthma
    d. all of the above

4. As a nurse researcher, you are studying the evolution of nursing and read the English translation of a book written by a Russian nurse. This source is:

    a. primary
    b. original
    c. secondary
    d. tertiary

5. Reproducing or repeating a study to determine whether similar findings will be obtained is referred to as:

    a. secondary research
    b. replication
    c. secondary analysis
    d. meta-analysis

## CRITICAL THINKING QUESTIONS:

Read the following excerpt, and answer the questions below.

Excerpt 3.1

More than 700,000 pregnant women in the United States are placed on bed rest at home or in hospitals each year in an effort to reduce the prevalence of preterm birth. Despite the commonality of this practice, studying effects of activity restriction on the mothers has only recently begun.[1,2] There is even less information about how fathers respond to having a mate on bed rest during pregnancy. The only reported study to date[3] indicates that these men experience high levels of worry and an overload of responsibilities and that they receive little, if any, attention from health-care providers.

Paternal anxiety during a healthy pregnancy appears to be common.[4] A high-risk pregnancy, with the implied threat to well-being, appears to heighten paternal stress. Fathers experience anxiety about the outcome for the mother and fetus as well as guilt, fear, inadequacy, and powerlessness.[5-8] In a study[9] of men whose partners were at high risk, men exhibited depression and anxiety and reported little perceived support. Fathers whose partners delivered prematurely reported anger, distress, grief, and fear of the unknown.[10] Maternal ill health and hospitalization have also been associated with decreased marital well-being.[11,12]

Managing emotional responses to a high-risk pregnancy is a major problem. Gyves[13] reported that fathers often attribute the problem to something they did, such as jeopardizing his partner's health by impregnating her or jeopardizing fetal health by having intercourse. Likewise, a father may feel guilty about ambivalence toward the pregnancy or feel powerless to help his partner or fetus. Some researchers believe social support is a mediator of stress and anxiety and that it assists in coping.[14] Men frequently derive their primary source of support from their partners. However, during a high-risk pregnancy, the partner's support is often decreased at a time when the father's needs are increased. In contrast, health-care providers rarely focus attention on the father during a high-risk pregnancy.[15]

Although there are several studies of paternal responses to high-risk pregnancies, only one study of paternal responses to antepartum bed rest has been reported.[3] May's convenience sample consisted of two homogeneous groups: 15 fathers interviewed within 2 weeks of the start of their partner's activity restriction and once after birth, and 15 additional fathers participating in a focus-group interview, 1 to 2 years after the bed-rest experience. Fathers reported that an activity-restricted pregnancy was a major stress and left them overwhelmed because of "doing it all," meaning functioning in both paternal and maternal roles. Feelings of isolation predominated, yet fathers hid their distress from their partners to protect them.

In summary, studies of high-risk pregnancy suggest that fathers have increased stress, negative psychosocial responses, and decreased support. The only study of antepartum bed rest suggests that maternal activity restriction compounds paternal stress; however, this study used a small convenience sample. Further information is needed about the challenges posed by antepartum bed rest in order to guide interventions. Therefore, the purpose of this study was to describe the problems and stress of men whose pregnant partners are on bed rest and the assistance they received.

*Source: Maloni, JA, and Ponder, M: Fathers' experience of their partners' antepartum bed rest. Image J Nurs Schol 29:183, 1997.*

1. Identify pertinent background information leading to the proposed study.

2. Provide information on the significance or importance of the proposed problem in relation to nursing.

3. Based on the information provided within the problem statement and literature review, evaluate the existing knowledge on the proposed problem.

4. Identify the gaps that this study intends to fill.

5. What is the purpose of the study?

# 4 Applying Appropriate Theories and Conceptual Models

## REVIEW QUESTIONS:

1. What is a theory?

_____

_____

_____

_____

2. What is the relationship between research and theory?

_____

_____

_____

_____

3. Differentiate between an inductive and a deductive approach to discovering new knowledge.

_____

_____

_____

_____

_____

4. In your own words, define *metaparadigm*.

_____

_____

_____

_____

5. What are the characteristics of a useful theory?

_____

_____

_____

_____

_____

6. Distinguish between a grand theory and a middle-range theory.

_____

_____

_____

_____

7. What is the importance of using borrowed theories from other disciplines in nursing?

_____

_____

_____

_____

8. Explain the difference between a theoretical and an operational definition.

_____

_____

_____

_____

9. Distinguish between a theory and a conceptual model.

_____

_____

_____

_____

10. Are nursing's four metaparadigm concepts appropriate? Why or why not?

_____

_____

_____

_____

## MULTIPLE CHOICE QUESTIONS:

1. A theory generated and verified by research is useful because it:

    a. accounts for accumulated evidence
    b. provides an explanation of observed relationships
    c. is general enough to cover many individual cases and manifestations
    d. all of the above

2. The process of generating theory by beginning with known facts and moving to specifics is known as:

a. determinism
b. logical positivism
c. inductive reasoning
d. deductive reasoning

3. The building blocks of theory are:

a. concepts
b. hypotheses
c. models
d. observations

4. Which of the following is not one of the four metaparadigm concepts associated with nursing theory?

a. health
b. nursing
c. caring
d. person

5. The Uncertainty of Illness theory, which explains how clients cognitively process illness-related stimuli and construct meaning in these events, is best described as a:

a. grand theory
b. middle-range theory
c. practice theory
d. borrowed theory

## CRITICAL THINKING QUESTIONS:

1. Discuss with students their perception of grand nursing theories. Identify positive and negative aspects of studying grand theories. What is the value in extending nursing science?

2. Identify one or two research reports that present grand theories. Obtain the original work of the theorist and define the major concepts, assumptions, and relationships tested in the theory.

3. Select one of the middle-range theories covered in the chapter. Review several research reports cited for that theory. Was the theory clearly articulated in the research reports? Was there consistency in the various articles on the use of the theory? How did the studies contribute to the knowledge base of the theory?

# 5 Understanding Evidence-Based Practice

## REVIEW QUESTIONS:

1. Define evidence-based practice.

_____

_____

_____

_____

_____

_____

2. Idenitfy several critical features of evidence-based practice.

_____

_____

_____

_____

_____

3. List several reasons why there is a lack of implementation of research in nursing practice.

_____

_____

_____

_____

_____

4. What are some limitations of evidence-based practice?

_____

_____

_____

_____

_____

_____

5. What is the Cochrane Database of Systematic Reviews?

_____

_____

_____

_____

_____

_____

_____

6. What role does the Agency for Healthcare Research and Quality play within the evidence-based movement?

_____

_____

_____

_____

_____

_____

_____

7. Identify when a clinican would search the National Guideline Clearinghouse versus the ACP Journal Club.

_____

_____

_____

_____

_____

_____

_____

8. What is a meta-analysis?

_____

_____

_____

_____

_____

_____

_____

9. Discuss the level of evidence and grades of recommendation when reviewing research articles.

_____

_____

_____

_____

_____

_____

_____

_____

_____

10. Discuss some ethical concerns around the evidence-based movement.

_____

_____

_____

_____

_____

_____

_____

_____

_____

## MULTIPLE CHOICE QUESTIONS:

1. A distinguishing characteristic of evidence-based practice as compared with traditional nursing practice is the use of:

    a. innovative ideas
    b. scientific evidence
    c. problem-solving capabilities
    d. common sense

2. What type of studies are the basis for using the Cochrane Systematic Review?

    a. cohort
    b. case-control
    c. meta-analyses
    d. clinical trials

3. As a nurse practitioner, you see an adult who has a sore throat and needs an antibiotic. Where do you go for a treatment guideline on pharyngitis?

    a. MEDLINE
    b. MD Consult
    c. National Guideline Clearinghouse
    d. Best Evidence

4. As a nurse practitioner, you see a patient who has recently been treated for gastroparesis. You would like a current, broad overview on the topic. Which database would you consult?

    a. MEDLINE
    b. MD Consult
    c. National Guideline Clearinghouse
    d. Best Evidence

5. A hierarchy of research evidence is generally agreed on for the amount of confidence that may be placed in results of intervention testing. Which is the strongest evidence?

    a. small randomized experimental studies with control groups
    b. large randomized experimental studies with control groups
    c. meta-analysis of randomized clinical trials
    d. case studies

## CRITICAL THINKING QUESTIONS:

1. Can nurses actually practice evidence-based nursing? If so, how?

2. Outline how you would track down the best evidence to answer the following clinical questions:

    a. What are the effects of nutritional supplementation in elderly patients recovering from hip fractures?
    b. Does screening for colorectal cancer using the fecal occult blood test reduce colorectal cancer mortality?
    c. Can psychoeducational programs, such as stress management and health education, improve cardiac and physical health in patients with coronary artery disease?

# 6 Formulating Hypotheses and Research Questions

**REVIEW QUESTIONS:**

1. What is a hypothesis?

_____

_____

_____

_____

2. What are the major purposes of hypotheses?

_____

_____

_____

_____

_____

3. List the characteristics of a good hypothesis.

_____

_____

_____

_____

_____

4. What might cause a researcher to state a directional hypothesis rather than a nondirectional hypothesis?

_____

_____

_____

_____

5. Why do some studies contain research questions and not hypotheses?

_____

_____

_____

_____

6. "Hypotheses can never be proved, only supported." Is this true or false? Explain your answer.

_____

_____

_____

_____

_____

_____

7. How are hypotheses evaluated?

_____

_____

_____

_____

_____

8. Write the null (statistical) hypothesis for the following statement: A researcher believes that African-American and Caucasian clients with type 2 diabetes differ in self-reported dietary adherence.

_____

_____

_____

_____

_____

9. What type of hypothesis is the following statement: "Middle-aged adults who participated in an 8-week diet and exercise program had lower low-density lipoprotein and higher high-density lipoprotein levels and lower cardiovascular risk than middle-aged adults who did not participate in the program."

_____

_____

_____

_____

_____

10. What is an independent variable? a dependent variable? an extraneous variable?

_____

_____

_____

_____

_____

## MULTIPLE CHOICE QUESTIONS:

1. An example of a directional hypothesis is:

   a. persons with dementia who receive an orienting intervention will show less confusion and fewer problem behaviors than those who do not receive the orienting intervention
   b. there will be no difference in maternal and infant outcomes between women giving birth in a hospital and those giving birth at home while cared for by a midwife
   c. there will be a difference in weight among persons who have attended a nutrition program compared with those who have not attended such a program
   d. patients with a hydrocolloid dressing and those with a standard gauze dressing will show differences in the incidence of catheter-related infection and local inflammation at the insertion site of those receiving TPN

2. "Patients with type 2 diabetes who receive instruction on an individual basis will be more compliant than those who receive instruction in a group setting." Identify the dependent variable in this hypothesis.

   a. type 2 diabetes
   b. individual versus group setting
   c. compliance
   d. type of instruction

Questions 3 and 4 refer to the following:

You are concerned that subjects presenting to the emergency room with non-emergency problems are not following through on recommended referrals. You believe that you can influence this by incorporating systematic patient teaching into the visit, so you design a teaching intervention. Persons who present to the emergency room with urinary tract infection are randomly assigned to receive or not receive the teaching intervention; those not receiving the intervention are given a short written handout containing instructions to follow through on referral.

3. The independent variable is:

    a. urinary tract infections
    b. emergency room
    c. follow through on referral
    d. teaching intervention

4. From the list below, which would you suggest for use as a dependent variable in this study?

    a. education of the nurse
    b. education of the subject
    c. making an appointment with the referral agency
    d. presence or absence of urinary tract infection

5. Control techniques are introduced to reduce the contaminating effects of:

    a. independent variables
    b. extraneous variables
    c. dependent variables
    d. null hypotheses

## CRITICAL THINKING QUESTIONS:

Read the following excerpt, and answer the questions below.

Excerpt 6.1

In institutions, caregiving is generally focused on efficiency (getting the job done) rather than on identifying and supporting the cognitively impaired (CI) person's retained abilities with activities of daily living (ADLs). This practice accelerates the loss of abilities, induces excess disability, and poses a threat to autonomy and self-concept. To break this cycle, an urgent need exists to develop strategies that maintain or improve ADL independence in CI adults for as long as possible while meeting the institution's demands for efficiency.

   Previous studies have identified behavioral strategies used by caregivers during ADLs. Strategies to promote independence in dressing were used in the current study because dressing involves a predictable series of tasks and successful use of the strategies with dressing might encourage caregivers to generalize the strategies to other ADLs. A behavioral intervention, Strategies to Promote Independence in Dressing (SPID), was tested. In pilot studies, SPID was found to improve the dressing independence of CI nursing home residents. In SPID, the level of assistance provided by the caregiver is matched with the cognitive abilities and deficits of the resident. Two hypotheses were tested:

   I. There will be a significant improvement in the dressing independence of CI nursing home residents following implementation of SPID.

II. There will be no difference in the time required by nursing assistants to complete dressing activities with CI residents before and after implementing SPID.

*Source: Beck, C, et al: Improving dressing behavior in cognitively impaired nursing home residents. Nurs Res 46:126, 1997.*

1. Identify the independent variable and dependent variable in hypothesis I.

_____

_____

_____

_____

_____

_____

2. How would you classify hypotheses I and II?

_____

_____

_____

_____

_____

_____

3. Identify the population being studied in hypotheses I and II.

_____

_____

_____

_____

_____

_____

4. Rewrite hypothesis II to state a relationship between the variables.

_____

_____

_____

_____

_____

_____

# 7 Selecting the Sample and Setting

## REVIEW QUESTIONS:

1. What is the difference between a target population and an accessible population?

_____

_____

_____

_____

_____

_____

2. What does it mean when a researcher states that the sample is representative of a population?

_____

_____

_____

_____

_____

_____

3. How does a researcher ensure that the sample is representative of the population? Are there any guarantees?

_____

_____

_____

_____

_____

_____

4. What is a sampling frame?

_____

_____

_____

_____

_____

5. When does a researcher use a table of random numbers?

_____

_____

_____

_____

_____

_____

6. Does a researcher make inferences about a sample on the basis of knowledge of the population or about a population on the basis of the sample?

_____

_____

_____

_____

_____

_____

7. How is random selection different from random assignment?

_____

_____

_____

_____

_____

8. List several types of probability sampling.

_____

_____

_____

_____

_____

9. Do most published nursing research reports use probability or nonprobability sampling? Explain your answer.

_____

_____

_____

_____

_____

10. What is external validity?

_____

_____

_____

_____

_____

_____

_____

## MULTIPLE CHOICE QUESTIONS:

1. The population from which the researcher selects the research sample is commonly referred to as:

    a. target population
    b. universal population
    c. accessible population
    d. available population

2. Which of the following sampling methods provides a sample that is most representative of the target population?

    a. simple random sampling
    b. convenience sampling with random assignment to groups
    c. quota sampling
    d. purposive sampling

3. Another name for probability sampling is:

    a. accidental  - non probability
    b. random
    c. quota
    d. purposive

4. A nurse practitioner (NP) in a primary care clinic decides to study the health promotion practices of her patients. The NP makes a list of all adult patients seen in the clinic for the past 6 months. There are 475 patients on the list. By assigning a number to each name and using a table of random numbers, the NP selects 100 patients to be invited to participate in the study. What type of sample has been selected?

    a. simple random sample
    b. stratified random sample
    c. convenience sample
    d. purposive sample

5. You are shopping in the mall and are approached by an individual who identifies himself as a researcher for a local food chain. He asks you to participate in the study by answering a few questions. As a study participant, you were selected by which method of sampling?

   a. random
   b. convenience
   c. systematic
   d. network

## CRITICAL THINKING QUESTIONS

Read the following excerpt, and answer the questions below.

Excerpt 7.1

The sample included 79 women, recruited from a large urban tertiary care center in a mid-Atlantic state, who had been diagnosed and treated surgically for breast cancer within the previous 3 to 7 months. A total of 96 women were determined eligible for interview. Eligibility criteria included English-speaking women who received a first cancer diagnosis within the past 3 to 7 months and were older than 21 years of age. Eight women could not be reached, and another nine refused to participate. Demographic and clinical characteristics of the refusers were statistically similar to the study sample of the total 79 women who consented to participate in the study (82% of those eligible). The time from diagnosis to the time of interview ranged from 3 months to 7 months (M = 157 days, SD = 28.6). The sample ranged in age from 25 to 85 years (M = 54.9 years, SD = 12.7 years); 37% of the sample were older than 60 years. The majority of the sample was white (83.5%), married (70%), and well-educated (M = 14.7 years, SD = 2.4 years); all were ambulatory. Forty-four percent of the sample were employed outside the home, and 51% had annual incomes of about $50,000. Two subjects had no health insurance. Ninety-eight percent of the sample reported a religious affiliation.

    Ninety-six percent of subjects had surgery before the interview. Sixty-two percent had mastectomies; 34% had lumpectomies. Of the 39% of subjects who received radiation after surgery, 70% had completed it 1 month or more before the interview. Of the 41% of subjects who received chemotherapy after surgery, 33% of subjects were receiving tamoxifen at the time of interview. Seventy-five percent of subjects self-reported early-stage disease.

*Source: Pasacreta, JV: Depressive phenomena, physical symptom distress, and functional status among women with breast cancer. Nurs Res 46:215, 1997.*

1. What type of sampling technique was used in this study? Identify its strengths and weaknesses.

_____

_____

_____

_____

_____

_____

_____

2. Describe some of the sample characteristics.

_____

_____

_____

_____

_____

_____

_____

3. What was the general procedure for recruiting subjects into the study?

_____

_____

_____

_____

_____

_____

4. State the significance of the following statement: "Demographic and clinical characteristics of the refusers were statistically similar to those of the study sample."

_____

_____

_____

_____

_____

_____

# 8 Principles of Measurement

1. What is a nominal level of measurement? an ordinal level of measurement? an interval level of measurement? a ratio level of measurement?

_____

_____

_____

_____

_____

_____

2. As a researcher, you collect data on the blood type of your clients. What is the appropriate level of measurement for this variable?

_____ NOMINAL Level of Measurement ✓ _____

_____

_____

_____

_____

_____

3. Can observations on a nominal scale be converted to an interval/ratio scale? Can observations on an interval/ratio scale be converted to a nominal scale? Explain your answer.

_____

_____

_____

_____

_____

4. The basic idea of reliability is described by what word?

_____ Consistency _____

_____

_____

_____

_____

5. What type of reliability is referred to as a coefficient of stability?

_test - retest    behar_

_____

_____

_____

_____

_____

6. When would a researcher use Cronbach's alpha coefficient versus the Kuder-Richardson #20 (KR-20) to assess internal consistency reliability?

_____

_____

_____

_____

_____

7. What is Cohen's kappa?

_____

_____

_____

_____

8. How does a researcher define *validity?*

_____

_____

_____

_____

9. Use of factor analysis is associated with what type of validity check?

_____

_____

_____

_____

_____

10. Which do you think is harder to obtain, reliability or validity? Why?

_____

_____

_____

_____

_____

## MULTIPLE CHOICE QUESTIONS:

1. Which of the following measurements is at the ratio level?

   a. self-rating on the following scale: nonsmoker, light smoker, heavy smoker
   b. religious affiliation
   c. minutes of second-stage labor
   d. age defined as individuals < 25 years old and those > 26 years old

2. As a teacher, you rank a group of students from most competent to least competent. Which type of scale has been described?

   a. nominal
   b. ordinal
   c. interval
   d. ratio

3. Variables that consist of just two categories are referred to as:

   a. dichotomous
   b. continuous
   c. linear
   d. alpha

4. Cronbach's alpha is used to determine which of the following instrument attributes?

   a. test-retest reliability
   b. internal consistency reliability
   c. interrater reliability
   d. stability

5. Instrument reliability and validity are related to each other in which of the following ways:

   a. an instrument that is not valid cannot be reliable
   b. an instrument that is not reliable cannot be valid
   c. reliability and validity are completely independent characteristics
   d. reliability and validity are completely interdependent; that is, if an instrument is reliable, it is also valid

## CRITICAL THINKING QUESTIONS:

1. The following is a list of variables. The way each variable is defined is located within the brackets. Identify the appropriate level of measurement for each variable.

    a. Sleep problems: [absence/presence of sleep problems]
    b. Birthweight of a neonate: [in grams]
    c. Type of solution for intravenous replacement: [crystalloid versus colloid]
    d. Amount of vacation: [actual number of days]
    e. Height: [in terms of percentile]

Read the following excerpt, and answer the questions below.

Excerpt 8.1

An AIDS/HIV knowledge scale was constructed based on the number of correct responses to 21 knowledge questions. The AIDS/HIV knowledge scale had high internal reliability, as indicated by Cronbach's alpha scores of 0.85 at pretest, 0.93 at the immediate posttest, and 0.79 at the 2-month posttest. A scale evaluating the intent to decrease AIDS risk-taking behavior was based on the responses to four questions: subjects were asked if they had stopped having sexual intercourse, had sexual intercourse less often, had sexual intercourse with fewer people, and used condoms more during sexual intercourse because of the AIDS/HIV infection. This scale ranged from 0 to 4 and had Cronbach's alpha scores of 0.77 at pretest, 0.74 at the immediate posttest, and 0.73 at the 2-month posttest.

*Source: Ashworth CS, et al: An experimental evaluation of an AIDS educational intervention for WIC mothers. AIDS Educ and Prev 6:154, 1994.*

1. What type of reliability is discussed in the excerpt? Are the reliability coefficients at an acceptable level? Explain your answer.

_____

_____

_____

_____

_____

2. How would a researcher go about assessing content validity on the measures described in the excerpt?

_____

_____

_____

_____

_____

# 9 Data Collection Methods

## REVIEW QUESTIONS:

1. What type of data collection methods do researchers use to collect quantitative data? qualitative data?

_____

_____

_____

_____

_____

_____

2. When does a researcher use closed-ended questionnaires? open-ended questionnaires?

_____

_____

_____

_____

_____

3. What are some concerns that must be considered in designing a questionnaire?

_____

_____

_____

_____

_____

4. Why is response rate so important to a questionnaire? What response rates are generally acceptable?

_____

_____

_____

_____

_____

5. Define *response set bias.*

_____

_____

_____

_____

_____

_____

6. How are Likert scales and semantic differential scales similar?

_____

_____

_____

_____

_____

_____

7. Define *psychosocial instrument.*

_____

_____

_____

_____

_____

_____

8. What is meant by *reverse scoring of a psychosocial instrument?*

_____

_____

_____

_____

_____

9. What is a visual analogue scale?

_____

_____

_____

_____

_____

10. Identify several biophysical measures.

_____

_____

_____

_____

_____

## MULTIPLE CHOICE QUESTIONS:

1. Which of the following data collection procedures provides "richer" data?

    a. searches through medical records or files
    b. observational techniques
    c. self-administered questionnaires
    d. structured interviews

2. The use of questionnaires in research has many advantages. They include all of the following *except:*

    a. facilitates collecting data from large samples
    b. associated with good response rates
    c. easily coded and tabulated
    d. expense of printing is considerably less than interviewing

3. Several different response formats are available when using Likert's scales. The most popular response choices address issues of:

    a. agreement
    b. frequency
    c. importance
    d. all of the above

4. On a seven-point Likert scale, the response "undecided" would probably be scored as:

    a. 0
    b. 1
    c. 4
    d. 7

5. If subjects are not very verbal or articulate, which type of data collection method is most appropriate?

    a. open-ended questionnaire
    b. closed-ended questionnaire
    c. unstructured interview
    d. use of a diary to keep field notes

## CRITICAL THINKING QUESTIONS:

Read the following excerpt, and answer the questions below.

Excerpt 9.1

### Purpose of the Study

The purpose of this study was to examine the relationship between self-blame and illness adjustment in women with breast cancer.

### Setting and Sample

The convenience sample comprised women receiving treatment for breast cancer in the medical oncology or radiation therapy departments in two metropolitan medical centers. The women had to be able to read and write English to be included in the study. Women with previous malignancies, late-stage breast cancer, diagnosed psychological disorders, or other major illnesses, such as heart disease, were excluded.

Research nurses in the oncology and radiation therapy departments screened the records of potential subjects for appropriateness for entry into the study. At their regularly scheduled clinic appointments, a nurse interviewer approached women who fit the criteria or contacted them by telephone to explain the study and ask for signed consent to participate. She told consenting patients that they would receive a phone call to schedule an interview at their next clinic visit. Researchers interviewed subjects using the Psychosocial Adjustment to Illness Scale (PAIS) and an attributions-and-blame interview. They also asked several questions about control over the cause and course of the cancer. They conducted the interviews, which took about 45 minutes to complete, in a private area adjacent to the clinic.

### Instruments

Subjects first responded to the PAIS, a 46-item semistructured interview. The interviewer codes the PAIS items on a 4-point scale. The potential range for the scale is 0 to 184, with higher ratings indicating poor adjustment. In addition to a total adjustment score, the PAIS provides subscores in seven different areas: health-care orientation, vocational environment, domestic environment, sexual relationships, extended family relationships, social environment, and psychological distress. Derogatis reported relatively high internal consistencies of 0.63 to 0.67 and provided evidence of construct validity with a factor analysis and convergent validity with measures such as the Affect Balance Scale ($r = 0.69$).

*Source: Houldin, AD, Jacobsen, B, and Lowery, BJ: Self-blame and adjustment to breast cancer. Onc Nurs Forum 23:75, 1996.*

1. Were the steps in collecting data described clearly and concisely? Explain your answer.

_____

_____

_____

_____

_____

_____

_____

_____

2. Was the instrument (PAIS) used to collect data appropriate based on the purpose of the study? Explain your answer. Were issues of reliability and validity discussed?

_____

_____

_____

_____

_____

_____

_____

_____

3. Was the PAIS scoring system described? its range of possible scores? What does a high score mean? a low score?

_____

_____

_____

_____

_____

_____

_____

_____

# 10 Analyzing the Data

1. Name the three most commonly used measures of central tendency. Which one is most sensitive to outliers?

_____

_____

_____

_____

2. Name the three most commonly used measures of dispersion. Which one is the simplest to calculate?

_____

_____

_____

_____

3. Would it be possible for two distributions to have the same means but different standard deviations? Explain.

_____

_____

_____

_____

4. Define *probability* as it refers to inferential statistics.

_____

_____

_____

_____

5. Explain what is meant by *0.05 level of confidence.*

_____

_____

_____

_____

6. What is a Pearson Product-Moment Correlation (r)? What is an acceptable range for correlational coefficients?

_____

_____

_____

_____

_____

7. Which correlation is more indicative of a strong relationship, $r = -0.78$ or $r = +0.53$? Why?

_____

_____

_____

_____

_____

8. Distinguish between an independent and a dependent t-test.

_____

_____

_____

_____

9. How are t-tests and analyses of variance similar?

_____

_____

_____

_____

10. Name the two types of chi-square.

_____

_____

_____

## MULTIPLE CHOICE QUESTIONS:

1. As a researcher, you collect data on the marital status of your clients. The appropriate measure of central tendency to use for this variable is the:

   a. mean
   b. median
   c. mode
   d. standard deviation

2. The appropriate measure of dispersion for the above example is:

   a. range
   b. variance
   c. standard deviation
   d. none of the above

3. On what basis does the t-test compare groups?

   a. frequency distributions
   b. mean score
   c. alpha level
   d. confidence intervals

4. Which of the following correlation coefficients give you the most precise prediction?

   a. $r = 0.80$
   b. $r = -0.60$
   c. $r = 0.45$
   d. $r = -0.85$

5. For the F ratio to be significant in an analysis of variance, the between-group variances should be:

   a. about the same as the within-group variance
   b. about the same as the probability level
   c. larger than the within-group variance
   d. smaller than the within-group variance

## CRITICAL THINKING QUESTIONS:

1. As a researcher, you are interested in using the Jalowiec Coping Scale (JCS). The JCS consists of a list of 20 coping behaviors derived from a comprehensive literature review. Ten items are classified as "problem-oriented," and 10 items are classified as "affective-oriented" behaviors. Extent of use of behaviors is rated on a 1-to-5 Likert scale with descriptive endpoints of "never" and "almost always." Subjects are asked to estimate how often they use various behaviors to cope with stress. You

pilot the JCS on a group of graduate students. The following data represent the students' scores on the JCS:

$$61, 58, 22, 96, 95, 21, 20, 35, 22, 92, 26, 42, 52, 26$$

a. Calculate the following descriptive statistics with respect to the above distribution of JCS scores: mean, median, mode, range, variance, standard deviation.

---

b. Using the data calculated above, write three or four sentences describing the JCS scores using measures of central tendency and dispersion.

---

Read the following excerpt, and answer the questions below.

Excerpt 10.1

Subjects were recruited from a list of patients who had undergone a cardiac catheterization after being admitted to the hospital with a diagnosis related to cardiac disease. Two groups of patients were identified: those who attended a postdischarge coronary artery disease (CAD) education class held at the institution during an 8-month period of time immediately before data collection (intervention group) and those who had not attended the class (comparison group). Health-promoting behavior was measured with the Health-Promoting Lifestyle Profile (HPLP). The HPLP is a 48-item questionnaire composed of six subscales that measure the frequency of self-reported health-promoting behaviors in several domains. Total scores and subscale scores are derived by summing the respective responses. Higher scores indicate more frequent performance of health-promoting behavior. Means and standard deviations (SDs) for the HPLP total score and subscales by each group are presented in the table that follows.

*Source: Plach, S, Wierenga, ME, and Heidrich, SM: Effect of postdischarge education class on coronary artery disease knowledge and self-reported health-promoting behaviors. Heart Lung 25:367, 1996.*

1. What type of t-test was computed in the previous example, independent or dependent? Explain your answer.

_____

_____

_____

_____

_____

TABLE 10.1  MEAN AND SD OF HEALTH-PROMOTING BEHAVIOR SCALES BY GROUP

|  | Intervention | | Comparison | | |
|  | Mean | SD | Means | SD | t |
|---|---|---|---|---|---|
| Total HPLP | 140.7 | 20.57 | 129.64 | 22.24 | 2.55* |
| Subscales |  |  |  |  |  |
| Self-actualization | 41.76 | 6.83 | 39.31 | 7.93 | 1.69 |
| Health responsibility | 27.75 | 5.22 | 24.25 | 6.06 | 3.11* |
| Exercise | 12.02 | 4.41 | 11.30 | 4.41 | 0.87 |
| Nutrition | 19.42 | 3.47 | 17.29 | 3.68 | 3.10* |
| Interpersonal support | 21.57 | 3.94 | 20.16 | 4.18 | 1.78 |
| Stress management | 19.69 | 3.91 | 18.38 | 3.85 | 1.60 |

* $p < 0.01$

2. Based on t-test analyses shown in the above table, describe the findings in two or three sentences.

_____

_____

_____

_____

_____

3. Is the following hypothesis supported or not supported based on the findings presented in the table: "Patients who attend the CAD education class will report more interpersonal support compared with patients who do not attend the CAD education class?" Explain your answer.

_____

_____

_____

_____

_____

# 11 Selecting a Research Design: Quantitative Versus Qualitative

## REVIEW QUESTIONS:

1. What is the difference between quantitative research and qualitative research?

_____

_____

_____

_____

_____

_____

2. List several characteristics of a good research design.

_____

_____

_____

_____

_____

_____

3. Is the concept of control important in quantitative research? in qualitative research? Explain your answer.

_____

_____

_____

_____

_____

_____

4. What are the differences between true experiments and quasiexperiments? Are true experiments better than quasiexperiments? Explain your answer.

_____

_____

_____

_____

_____

5. Describe the most basic type of quasiexperimental design.

_____

_____

_____

_____

_____

_____

6. What is the difference between a control group and an experimental group?

_____

_____

_____

_____

_____

7. In an experiment, is the independent or dependent variable manipulated by the researcher?

_____

_____

_____

_____

8. The concept of *internal validity* is sometimes confused with the idea of *instrument validity*. Explain the difference between the two.

_____

_____

_____

_____

9. State the strengths and weaknesses of descriptive designs.

_____

_____

_____

_____

_____

10. Distinguish between secondary analysis and meta-analysis.

_____

_____

_____

_____

_____

## MULTIPLE CHOICE QUESTIONS:

1. A concern researchers have about a qualitative approach to research is:

    a. the need for larger sample sizes
    b. the lack of fit with questions relevant to nursing
    c. the lack of rigor in its methodology
    d. the time-consuming nature associated with its methodologies

2. In choosing a quasiexperimental design over a true experimental design, the researcher realizes that the study involves less:

    a. bias
    b. control
    c. rigor
    d. significance

3. What threat to internal validity is controlled when a researcher completes an experiment in a relatively short period to minimize developmental changes?

    a. history
    b. maturation
    c. testing
    d. instrumentation

4. What threat to internal validity is controlled when a researcher uses reliable and valid assessment tools or scales for rating or scoring to avoid biases?

    a. history
    b. maturation
    c. testing
    d. instrumentation

5. In meta-analysis, the sample consists of:

    a. incidents occurring to a single subject
    b. research instruments
    c. previous studies
    d. human subjects

## CRITICAL THINKING QUESTIONS:

Read the following excerpt, and answer the questions below.

Excerpt 11.1

### Purpose of the Study

After reviewing the results of previous studies, we believed that additional research was indicated to evaluate and describe the recovery course of short-stay patients undergoing laparoscopic cholecystectomy procedures, comparing their experiences to those reported in the literature. We addressed these specific research questions in our study.

1. What is the pattern of occurrence of symptoms (i.e., pain, vomiting, nausea, fatigue, loss of appetite), and how do these symptoms change during the perioperative and recovery periods?

2. How many patients require analgesic medications, and for how long after surgery?

3. How quickly after surgery do patients resume normal eating and living patterns?

*Source: Cason, CL, et al: Recovery from laparoscopic cholecystectomy procedures. AORN 63:1099, 1996.*

1. Describe the type of research design that is appropriate for this study based on the research questions posed. Explain your answer.

_____

_____

_____

_____

_____

_____

_____

2. What are the advantages and disadvantages of the design you described in question 1?

_____

_____

_____

_____

_____

_____

# 12 Phenomenological Research

1. What is phenomenology?

_____

_____

_____

_____

_____

_____

2. Describe what is meant by *bracketing* and *intuiting.*

_____

_____

_____

_____

_____

_____

3. What is the role of the researcher in phenomenological research?

_____

_____

_____

_____

_____

4. Describe the type of sampling most commonly used in phenomenological inquiry. What is meant by *saturation?*

_____

_____

_____

_____

_____

_____

5. Identify the primary data collection techniques used in phenomenological research.

_____

_____

_____

_____

_____

6. Do qualitative researchers need to be concerned about ethical considerations and informed consent? Explain your answer.

_____

_____

_____

_____

7. How is scientific rigor in qualitative research documented?

_____

_____

_____

_____

8. How are data analyzed in phenomenological research?

_____

_____

_____

_____

9. Assumptions on which phenomenological studies are based come from the philosophy of Heidegger. His philosophy focused on language through hermeneutic analysis. Define *hermeneutics*.

_____

_____

_____

_____

_____

10. What do you see as the greatest strength of phenomenological research?

_____

_____

_____

_____

_____

## MULTIPLE CHOICE QUESTIONS:

1. The basic aim of a phenomenological study is to:

   a. study individuals, artifacts, or documents in their natural setting
   b. study social data for the purpose of explaining some phenomenon
   c. study the nature or meaning of everyday experiences
   d. study the cause-and-effect relationships among variables

2. In phenomenological research, researchers must acknowledge any previous information, ideas, or beliefs about a particular phenomenon before proceeding with the study. This is referred to as:

   a. bracketing
   b. intuiting
   c. confirmability
   d. intentionality

3. Sampling in phenomenological research is:

   a. random
   b. purposive
   c. stratified
   d. quota

4. Data are collected in a phenomenological study by a variety of techniques that include:

   a. observation
   b. descriptions written by subjects
   c. unstructured interviews
   d. all of the above

5. The process of analyzing data associated with phenomenological research involves:

   a. computation
   b. thinking
   c. enumeration
   d. analytic memos

## CRITICAL THINKING QUESTIONS:

Read the following excerpt, and answer the questions that follow.

Excerpt 12.1

### Data Generation

In-depth, face-to-face audiotaped interviews were conducted by the researcher with each of the participants in an interview room on the psychiatric unit. The interviews lasted 1 to 2 hours, although the interview was broken into shorter segments and completed over 2 or 3 days for some participants. This was necessary because of the frail condition and fatigability of some of the participants. Follow-up interviews were performed with five individuals to provide support and to clarify meanings of significant statements.

The very nature of phenomenological questioning makes it difficult to design a structured questionnaire because questions emerge and are derived as the understanding of the phenomenon emerges. However, Van Manen's method points out that the interview process needs to be disciplined by the fundamental questions that prompted the need for the interview in the first place. Van Manen suggests that researchers often give in to temptation to let the method rule the question rather than let the research questions determine what kind of (interview) method is most appropriate for its imminent direction. To avoid this pitfall, four research questions are posed to serve as a general interview guide:

I. I'm interested in what people see as important or meaningful experiences in their lives. As you reflect back over your life, what are some of these for you?

II. What would you say have been some of the successes in your life? disappointments? What were you doing at those times?

III. If you were to tell your life story, how would you describe the things, events, and so on that have given you a sense of meaning and purpose in your life? How did these influence or relate to your feeling that life is not worth living?

IV. Has your sense of meaning or purpose changed over the years? In what way? How do you experience meaning in your life now?

In addition to the taped interviews, detailed field notes and a methodological journal are used to keep track of the researcher's observations, decisions, feelings, and thoughts either during or immediately after the interviews.

### Data Analysis

The data were analyzed using components of Van Manen's methodological approach, which included description and interpretations. The audiotapes were transcribed verbatim, and a thematic analysis was conducted by reflecting and intuiting on each of the transcripts. Several levels of coding of significant statements and key words were performed as the individual transcripts and codings were examined in light of all the transcripts. From this process, general themes emerged across the data.

At this point, a collaborative analysis team of four nursing doctoral students with backgrounds in gerontology and mental health was formed to assist with interpretation of the texts. The team members were asked to read and reflect on the text individually and then meet together with the researcher, at which time "collaborative discussions or hermeneutic conversations" helped to generate deeper insights and understandings about the text and the emergent themes. As these deeper insights and meanings emerged, the investigator returned to the writing of the interpretive, thematic descriptions that were then brought back to the analysis team for further interpretive discussions and validation.

Watson stresses that in striving for understanding in the hermeneutical sense, we must try to see the object of interpretation in its larger context since a phenomenon takes its inner or true meaning only in relation to the whole of which it forms a part. In this research study, the reflective process was used to assist the researcher and the analysis team to understand and reveal the essential meaning of how meaning in life was experienced by older persons who felt suicidal. The collaborative discussions relied on interpreting current meaning in relation to the context of the older person's life.

*Source: Moore, SL: A phenomenological study of meaning in life in suicidal older adults. Arch Psych Nurs 11:29, 1997.*

1. Describe how the researcher became immersed in the data. What techniques did the researcher use to help participants describe meaning in their lives?

_____

_____

_____

_____

2. The issue of trustworthiness in qualitative research is a concern for researchers engaging in these methods. How did the researcher address trustworthiness and authenticity of data?

_____

_____

_____

_____

3. What is meant by the phrase "collaborative discussions or hermeneutic conversations"?

_____

_____

_____

_____

# 13 Ethnographic Research: Focusing on Culture

## REVIEW QUESTIONS:

1. What is an ethnography?

2. As a qualitative research method, ethnographic research developed its roots in what particular social science?

3. Where does all ethnographic research take place? Explain your answer.

4. Who was one of the first nurse researchers to become interested in ethnography as a research method?

5. Why is the role of participant observer so critical in ethnographic research?

_____

_____

_____

_____

_____

_____

6. What is considered an average amount of time to reside "in the field" while conducting ethnographic research?

_____

_____

_____

_____

_____

_____

7. Identify the stages in an ethnographic research study.

_____

_____

_____

_____

_____

_____

8. Identify the primary data collection techniques used in ethnographic research.

_____

_____

_____

_____

_____

_____

9. List several other techniques used for data collection in ethnographic research.

_____

_____

_____

_____

_____

_____

_____

10. What do you see as the greatest strength of ethnographic research?

_____

_____

_____

_____

_____

_____

## MULTIPLE CHOICE QUESTIONS:

1. Ethnographic research can be characterized as a means of:

   a. studying the sociopsychological problems present within human interactions
   b. studying the life, ways, or patterns of groups of individuals
   c. studying events, ideas, institutions, or people to assess historical meaning
   d. all of the above

2. The planning and implementing of an ethnographic study takes place in three stages. During phase 1 of fieldwork, the researcher focuses on:

   a. developing trust and acceptance
   b. forming long-term relationships
   c. gathering information as it relates to the problem
   d. obtaining large amounts of information

3. What group of social scientists has the greatest interest and commitment to discovery of cultural knowledge?

   a. anthropologists
   b. psychologists
   c. sociologists
   d. philosophers

4. Observations recorded about the people, places, and things that are part of the ethnographer's study of a culture are referred to as:

a. ethnographic styles
b. genealogies
c. field notes
d. participant observers

5. The phrase "researcher as instrument" is a fundamental characteristic of ethnography. This refers to:

a. the researcher's focusing on a combination of quantitative and qualitative methods of data collection
b. the researcher's becoming immersed in direct observation and learning from members of cultural groups
c. the process of data analysis whereby statements are grouped and given codes for ease of identification
d. the amount of dedication a researcher commits to analyzing data collected during a qualitative study

## CRITICAL THINKING QUESTIONS:

Read the following excerpt, and answer the questions that follow.

Excerpt 13.1

Three families, all residing in a large metropolitan area, participated in the study. Each father was 30 years old, the mothers were between 26 and 30 years old, and the boys with Duchenne's muscular dystrophy were between 7 years, 10 months and 9 years, 11 months of age. All were natural parents to the child with Duchenne's muscular dystrophy. Two of the boys were only children; only three had sisters. Two mothers had no family history of Duchenne's muscular dystrophy; one mother had a 21-year-old brother suffering from the disease who lived with the family and participated in the study.

The naturalistic case-study method involves both participating and observing, providing an opportunity for an in-depth understanding of events and interactions. This investigator engaged in play activities; trips to summer camps, restaurants, and parks; watching television; family conversations; and picking up children at school bus stops. The researcher's feelings while observing the activities, participants, and physical aspects of the family were used as a source for reflection and, in turn, helped formulate questions used to verify aspects of the subjects' experience. Bias, the "hidden ghost" of the researcher, is difficult and painful to confront. Keeping a log of such feelings, including biases, was one way to confront the "ghost."

The researcher visited each family weekly for 10 weeks. A log focusing on family events of each participant observation was kept. Key words were recorded during family visits. After each visit, the researcher wrote observations in an ethnographic log. These logs used a wide margin to record speculations regarding what was happening, codes for emerging patterns, and connections between pieces of data. Periodically, the researcher wrote analytic memos (comments on insights and suggestions for future action in the research) that also became part of the log and were used to examine the researcher's emotions, biases, and conflicts.

In-depth taped (and later transcribed) interviews, conducted twice over the 10-week period and a third time 1 year later, provided detailed information and verified data shaped by the interviewer's perception. The precise number of participant observations and interviews was not preset; rather, the study continued until saturation. Saturation was achieved when, after studying logs and memos and listening to taped interviews of all three families, it was clear that data had become repetitive and no new themes emerged.

Multiple analysis techniques were used to identify and describe the important themes in the data. These techniques were used in the context of the constant comparative method, a continuous process of refining from the first data collection until the final data analysis. The refining process consisted of several steps. First, in addition to transcribing field observations and interviews, transcripts and memos were examined for a preliminary set of content codes to identify common patterns of interaction within and among families. Then, after completion of the data collection phase for the first family, a primary list of 30 codes was made. This list was used and revised during data collection for the next two families, allowing for additional codes, collapsing of overlapping codes, and clarifying of ambiguous codes. A final list of 17 codes was made.

*Source: Gagliardi, BA: The family's experience of living with a child with Duchenne muscular dystrophy. Appl Nurs Res 4:159, 1991.*

1. How did the researcher gain access to the "culture" being studied?

_____

_____

_____

_____

_____

_____

_____

2. Describe the various types of techniques used to collect data.

_____

_____

_____

_____

_____

_____

# 14 Grounded Theory Research

## REVIEW QUESTIONS:

1. What is grounded theory?

_____

_____

_____

_____

_____

2. As a qualitative research method, grounded theory developed its roots in what particular social science?

_____

_____

_____

_____

_____

3. Identify the three major sources of data generation in grounded theory research.

_____

_____

_____

_____

4. Describe the process of theoretical sampling.

_____

_____

_____

_____

5. Discuss the constant comparative method of data analysis. What is substantive coding? open coding? selective coding?

_____

_____

_____

_____

6. What is a core category?

_____

_____

_____

_____

7. When is the literature review conducted in a grounded theory study? Why?

_____

_____

_____

_____

8. When does a researcher use memos in a grounded theory study?

_____

_____

_____

_____

9. What criteria are used to judge scientific rigor in grounded theory research?

_____

_____

_____

_____

10. What do you see as the greatest strength of grounded theory research?

_____

_____

_____

_____

## MULTIPLE CHOICE QUESTIONS:

1. Grounded theory is an important research method in that:
   a. a theory is discovered to explain a particular phenomenon
   b. an accurate interpretation describes a particular phenomenon under study
   c. the meanings of actions and events are described by researchers seeking to understand a particular phenomenon
   d. all of the above

2. In grounded theory research, the research question is:

a. refined by the researcher as data emerge
b. identified by the researcher after the problem statement
c. identified by an existing theory
d. formulated based on the focus of the study

3. Data gathered in grounded theory research using field techniques, observational methods, and documents are examined and analyzed through a system referred to as:

a. selective coding
b. constant comparative method
c. memoing
d. trustworthiness

4. The process of data analysis in grounded theory whereby statements are grouped for ease of identification is referred to as:

a. categorizing
b. memoing
c. coding
d. theoretical analysis

5. The process of selecting concepts that have proven relevance to the evolving theory is known as:

a. categorizing
b. memoing
c. coding
d. theoretical analysis

## CRITICAL THINKING QUESTIONS:

Read the following excerpt, and answer the following questions.

Excerpt 14.1

The ways parents cope with their child's diagnosis and treatment for cancer may influence the child's treatment-related morbidity, quality of life, and even treatment outcome. Parental coping and other psychosocial aspects of childhood cancer have been extensively studied for the past two decades. Most studies have focused on three phases of care: diagnosis, active treatment, and terminal care. Information from these studies has contributed to the development of interventions designed to foster and maintain successful coping efforts in pediatric oncology patients and their parents. A phase of treatment that has received minimal systematic study is relapse or recurrence. Greater knowledge of the psychosocial aspects of this phase of treatment could also contribute to the design of interventions to foster coping skills.

The first recurrence of cancer can occur after apparently successful treatment or even during initial therapy. The definition of recurrence used in this study was "a reappearance of cancer at the same site (local), near the initial site (regional), or in other areas of the body (metastatic)." Recurrence has been carefully studied from the biologic perspective, but little has been written regarding its impact on parents and patients. Anecdotal reports suggest that recurrence is a particularly difficult time for parents, in part because of their realization that the probability of cure is dramatically decreased. Staff describe parents as fluctuating between accepting and avoiding the reality of recurrence. These descriptions are based on limited clinical observations and impressions, most documented retrospectively. In addition, they were gathered at a time when cure rates and remission duration had not reached their current levels. Therefore, a systematic prospective study is needed to identify how parents cope with cancer recurrence in their child.

The purpose of this study was to identify and describe coping processes (meaning the behaviors and thoughts) used by parents of pediatric oncology patients to deal with the stress of a first cancer recurrence in their child. The authors' intent was to develop a substantive level theory of parental coping processes.

*Source: Hinds, PS, et al: Coming to terms: Parents' response to a first cancer recurrence in their child. Nurs Res 45:148, 1996.*

1. What is the substantive area of study in this grounded theory research study?

_____

_____

_____

_____

_____

2. Why does the phenomenon of interest require a qualitative approach?

_____

_____

_____

_____

Excerpt 14.2

A multisite approach was chosen to facilitate theory-generation processes and enrollment of study participants. Theory generation was aided by the backgrounds of the three primary investigators, who were experienced in different areas of pediatric oncology nursing research (the family's coping with initial diagnosis, adolescent's coping with cancer diagnosis and treatment, and family's coping with the death of a child).

The primary research techniques were semistructured interviews (conducted by the principal investigators), observations of parents interacting with staff or other parents, and medical record review to determine eligibility. With the parents' permission, interviews were tape-recorded and subsequently transcribed. When parents preferred not to be recorded, interview responses were handwritten and then typed. The typed version was given to the parent to check accuracy before the analysis was done. Six parents were interviewed a second time to validate study findings as they evolved.

The three principal investigators routinely shared the transcribed interviews completed at their respective study sites. Monthly conference calls and two face-to-face meetings occurred during the 17 months of data collection and validation. This approach permitted the interviewers to jointly develop and refine the data-gathering techniques. A process of reviewing major themes; using open, axial, and selective coding; and creating theoretical memos was established from each interview. This process helped identify and define core concepts of the developing theory and hypotheses for future testing. After each interview, a table that included open and axial codes, the interviews in which the codes occurred, and their conceptual definitions was completed and updated.

*Source: Hinds, PS, et al: Coming to terms: Parents' response to a first cancer recurrence in their child. Nurs Res 45:148, 1996.*

1. What strategies did the researchers use to analyze the data?

_____

_____

_____

_____

_____

_____

_____

_____

2. How did the researchers address the fit, credibility, and relevance of the research?

_____

_____

_____

_____

_____

_____

_____

# 15 Interpreting and Reporting Research Findings

## REVIEW QUESTIONS:

1. Is it possible for the results of a study to be of practical importance even though they are not statistically significant? Why or why not?

_____

_____

_____

_____

_____

_____

2. Why is it especially important to provide a detailed description of the characteristics of the sample in a research report?

_____

_____

_____

_____

_____

_____

3. What is the major goal when preparing a research report?

_____

_____

_____

_____

_____

_____

4. Name the major headings associated with a typical research report.

_____

_____

_____

_____

_____

5. What type of information is usually found in an abstract?

_____

_____

_____

_____

_____

6. If an author has done a good job of writing the "Methods" section of a research report, what should the reader of the report be able to do?

_____

_____

_____

_____

_____

7. List some common mistakes that should be avoided in preparing a research report.

_____

_____

_____

_____

_____

8. Identify several ways to disseminate research findings.

_____

_____

_____

_____

_____

9. What purpose does a query letter serve?

_____

_____

_____

_____

_____

10. What is meant by *refereed journal?*

_____

_____

_____

_____

_____

## MULTIPLE CHOICE QUESTIONS:

1. Generalizability refers to:

    a. the extent to which findings from an analysis are unlikely to be the result of chance

    b. the extent to which research findings are reported objectively

    c. the extent to which statistical significance is related to clinical significance

    d. the extent to which results of a study can be applied to other people, instruments, and settings

2. Name the place in the research report where you could find the following statement: "The purpose of this study was to examine the relationship between caregiver burden and social support among spouses of individuals with multiple sclerosis."

    a. introduction

    b. methods

    c. results

    d. discussion

3. Name the place in the research report where you could find the following statement: "Caregiving burden was measured using the Caregiving Burden Scale (CBS). The CBS is a list of 14 tasks that may be required of caregivers. These tasks are divided into three areas: direct care tasks, instrumental care tasks, and interpersonal care tasks."

    a. introduction

    b. methods

    c. results

    d. discussion

4. Name the place in the research report where you could find the following statement: "Subjects were 49 caregivers (25 women and 24 men) who were caring for adult family members receiving outpatient chemotherapy at a Midwestern cancer center."

    a. introduction

    b. methods

    c. results

    d. discussion

5. Disseminating nursing research findings can be accomplished through:

   a. publications
   b. oral presentations
   c. poster presentations
   d. all of the above

## CRITICAL THINKING QUESTIONS:

Read the following excerpt, and answer the questions below.

Excerpt 15.1

The purpose of this study was to describe the association between the marital relationship and the health of the wife with chronic fatigue and immune dysfunction syndrome (CFIDS). The convenience sample of 131 wives with CFIDS and their spouses reported their marital relationships similarly, but the wives reported higher CFIDS symptom scores. Marital adjustment scores, wives' conflict scores, and husbands' self-empathy scores were associated with wives' CFIDS symptom scores. Hierarchical multiple regression models showed that couples with higher marital adjustment and wives with higher education, lengthier marriages, less conflict, and less support were predictive of lower problematic CFIDS symptoms.

*Source: Goodwin, SS: The marital relationship and health in women with chronic fatigue and immune dysfunction syndrome: Views of wives and husbands. Nurs Res 46:138, 1997.*

1. How concise and succinct is the abstract?

_____

_____

_____

_____

_____

2. Does the title of the article capture the essence of the study? Explain your answer.

_____

_____

_____

_____

_____

_____

# 16 Critiquing Research Reports

## REVIEW QUESTION:

1. What is the difference between a research review and research critique?

_____

_____

_____

_____

_____

_____

_____

_____

_____

_____

_____

## MULTIPLE CHOICE QUESTIONS:

1. Critiquing published research reports is important because it helps to:

   a. provide an increased understanding of the research process
   b. determine whether findings associated with a study are suitable for use in practice
   c. learn from other researchers and build on previous research
   d. all of the above

2. Individuals who critique published research reports should attempt to:

   a. focus on the inadequacies inherent in the study
   b. be as objective as possible
   c. evaluate the scientific merit of a study based on the researcher's credentials
   d. restrict the amount of critical comments that would discourage the researcher

3.  A reviewer asks the question, "Is the problem being studied conceived as a nursing problem?" Where in the research report should this question be addressed?

   a. problem statement
   b. methodology
   c. results
   d. discussion

4.  A reviewer asks the question, "Are the analysis and interpretation of data adequate for the problem being studied?" Where in the research report should this question be addressed?

   a. problem statement
   b. methodology
   c. results
   d. discussion

5.  A reviewer asks the question, "How will the results of this study be incorporated into practice?" Where in the research report should this question be addressed?

   a. problem statement
   b. methodology
   c. results
   d. discussion

# 17 Research Utilization

1. What is research utilization?

_____

_____

_____

_____

_____

_____

2. Why is disseminating research findings so important?

_____

_____

_____

_____

_____

3. Why were nursing research utilization models developed?

_____

_____

_____

_____

_____

4. Describe "knowledge diffusion."

_____

_____

_____

_____

_____

_____

5. Identify two models of nursing research utilization and the purpose(s) for which they were developed.

_____

_____

_____

_____

_____

6. Identify the phases associated with the research utilization process.

_____

_____

_____

_____

7. What is meant by "the gap between research and practice"?

_____

_____

_____

_____

8. List several barriers to research utilization.

_____

_____

_____

_____

9. List several facilitators of research utilization.

_____

_____

_____

_____

10. What is the future of research utilization?

_____

_____

_____

_____

## MULTIPLE CHOICE QUESTIONS:

1. Research utilization is a process by which:

    a. information generated from research becomes incorporated into practice
    b. researchers critically evaluate the importance of the phenomenon being studied
    c. researchers recognize the effectiveness of collaborating on research-related issues
    d. researchers develop project-specific outcome measures that are measurable

2. The Stetler Model of research utilization primarily focuses to facilitate application of research findings at what level?

    a. systems-based
    b. practitioner
    c. institution-based
    d. professional organization

3. Regardless of which nursing research utilization is chosen, the first step in the research utilization process is:

    a. critiquing the literature
    b. identifying the problem
    c. implementing a change
    d. evaluating the change

4. Which of the following strategies for utilization is *most* amendable for students and staff nurses?

    a. replicating previous research studies
    b. reading and understanding published research reports
    c. prepare an integrative literature review or meta-analysis
    d. devoting a specific amount of time working with an established researcher

5. Which of the following are barriers to research utilization?

    a. absence of research that explains practice
    b. time, money, and clinical resources
    c. attending conferences where research is presented that are outside your institution
    d. establishing linkages between academics and practice

# index

*Page numbers followed by "e" denote excerpts, "f" denote figures, and "t" denote tables.*

Abstract, 56, 293, 294e
Abstract journals, 56
Accessible population, 105
Accidental sampling, 112
ACP Journal Club, 80–81
Across-group comparison, 205
ADAS, 133e
Adult consent form, 33–34f
Advance directive attitude survey (ADAS), 133e
*Advances in Nursing Science,* 10
Agency for Healthcare Research and Quality (AHRQ), 81
AIDSLINE, 55, 80
Alpha coefficient, 130
Alternative hypothesis, 94
American Association of Critical Care Nurses model, 329t, 332t
*American Journal of Maternal Child Nursing,* 10
Analysis of variance (ANOVA), 181–184
Analytic epidemiological studies, 213
Analyzing the data, 165–189
    ANOVA, 181–184
    chi-square, 184–186
    correlations, 177–179
    critiquing, 186–187
    descriptive statistics, 167–174
    inferential statistics, 174–176
    mean, 167
    measures of central tendency, 167–172
    measures of dispersion, 172–174
    median, 167–170
    mode, 170–171
    parametric *vs.* nonparametric tests, 176–177
    Pearson *r,* 178
    probability, 175–176
    purpose, 166
    range, 172
    standard deviation, 172, 173
    t-test, 179–181
    variance, 172
Anonymity, 31
ANOVA, 181–184
ANOVA summary table, 183t
*Applied Nursing Research,* 10
Applied research, 19, 20e
*Association of Operating Room Nurses Journal,* 10
Assumptions, 192
Attrition, 208
Audio-taped interviews, 161e

Auditability, 233
Authorship of published papers, 10t

Barriers, 340–342, 343t
Basic research, 19
Basic social processes (BSPs), 275–276
Beck, Cheryl Tatano, 265
Before-and-after experimental design, 201
Behavior Test of Interpersonal Skills (BTIS), 131
Between-group variance, 183
Beyea, Suzanne C., 327
Biophysical measures, 158–159
Blinding, 205
Blumer, Herbert, 266
Borrowed theories, 69, 70t
Bracketing, 222
Bretano, Franz, 221
BSPs, 275–276
BTIS, 131

Call for Papers, 302
CANCERLIT, 80
Categorical response, 148–149
Category, 272
Census taking, 258t
CHID, 55
Child's assent form, 35f
Chi-square analysis, 184–186
CINAHL, 55, 337
Circular nature of research, 17
Clinical questions, 78
Clinical trial, 205
Clinically significant, 291
Closed-ended question, 146t
Cluster sampling, 110–111
Cochrane Database of Systematic Reviews, 80
Cochrane Library, 80
Cochrane Review of Methodology Database, 80
Coding, 272–275
Coding families, 275t
Coefficient alpha, 130
Cohen's kappa, 130, 131, 132e
Colaizzi's method, 231t
Communicating research findings. *See* Disseminating research findings; Interpretation of research findings
Comparison group, 204
Complex hypothesis, 91, 92t
Concepts, 69–71

Conceptual framework, 65
Conceptual model, 65, 70–71
Conceptual models of nursing, 71
Concurrent validity, 133–134
Conduct and Utilization of Research in Nursing (CURN), 329t, 331t
Conference on Nursing Research Priorities, 11
Confidence interval, 175
Confidence levels, 175, 176f
Confidentiality, 31, 227
Confirmability, 233
Confounding variable, 201
Consensus family, 275t
Constant comparative method of data analysis, 272
Construct validity, 134–135
Constructs, 70
Content validity, 132–133, 134e
Contingency table, 185
Continuous responses, 149
Continuous variable, 127
Control, 197–198
Convenience sampling, 112, 113e, 114e, 115e
Core category, 274, 276
CORP # 2, 11
Correlated t-test, 180
Correlation, 177
Correlation coefficient, 177
Correlation matrix, 178
Correlational design, 209–210
Correlational research, 21
Credibility, 233 ✓
Crisis at John Hopkins University, 27
Criterion variable, 98
Criterion-related validity, 133–134
Critiquing
    data collection methods, 161–163
    descriptive/inferential statistics, 186–187
    ethnographic research, 259–260
    grounded theory research, 283–284
    hypothesis/research questions, 98–99
    instruments, 137–139
    interpretation of research findings, 302–303
    levels of measurement, 137
    literature review, 57–58
    phenomenological research, 236–237
    reliability/validity, 137
    research designs, 214–215
    research reports, 307–325. See also Critiquing research reports
    research utilization, 338–339
    sampling, 119
    theories/conceptual models, 71–72
Critiquing research reports, 307–325
    critical components to be evaluated, 309t
    critique vs. review, 307–308
    do's/dont's, 309t
    example (qualitative study), 320–323

example (quantitative study), 312–320
    research appraisal checklist, 311–312, 313–315
    suggested questions, 308–311
Cronbach's alpha, 130
Cross-sectional research, 22, 23e
Cultural family, 275t
Cumulative Index to Nursing and Allied Health Literature (CINAHL), 55, 337
CURN, 329t, 331t
Cushing, Frank, 248
Cutting point family, 275t

Data analysis. See Analyzing the data
Data collection methods, 143–164
    biophysical measures, 158–159
    critiquing, 161–163
    focus groups, 160–161, 162e
    instruments, 157–158
    interviews, 159, 161e
    Likert scales, 150–154
    participant observation, 159–160
    PRQ, 150–151, 152t
    Q Methodology, 156–157
    qualitative measures, 159–161
    qualitative methods, 144–159
    qualitative vs. quantitative data, 144
    RQ, 153–154
    scales, 149–158
    semantic differential scale, 154–155
    surveys/questionnaires, 144–149
    VAS, 156
Databases, 54–55, 79–80. See also Searching databases
Declaration of Helsinki, 25–26
Declarative hypothesis, 94
Deductive approach, 65
Deductive hypothesis, 94, 95e
Degree family, 275t
Dependent t-test, 180
Dependent variable, 98
Descriptive correlational design, 210
Descriptive designs, 208–209, 209e
Descriptive epidemiological studies, 213
Descriptive research, 21
Diabetes Educator, The, 10
Dichotomous variables, 125
Dimension family, 275t
Directional hypothesis, 92–93, 93e
Disproportional stratified sampling, 109
Disseminating research findings, 299–303
    oral presentation, 301–302
    poster presentation, 302, 303f
    publication, 299–301
    research report. See Research report
Distribution-free tests, 176
Document analysis, 258t
Double-blinded study, 205

Dracup-Breu Model, 329t, 331t

EBH, 76
EBM, 76
EBMR, 79
EBN, 76
EBP. *See* Evidence-based practice (EBP)
Electronic databases, 54–55, 55t
Empirical data, 5
Empirical literature, 53
Entering the field, 248
Environment, 67t
Epistemology, 222
ERIC, 55
Essences, 221
Ethics, 23–28
    developing guidelines, 24–26, 28
    EBP, 81–82
    human rights, 28–36. *See also* Human
        rights
    phenomenological research, 226–227
    research scandals, 26–28
Ethnograph, 247
Ethnographic interview, 247
Ethnographic research, 243–263
    characteristics, 247–248
    critiquing, 259–260
    data collection techniques, 258, 258t
    ethnographic styles, 249
    field notes, 256–258
    fieldwork, 252–259
    historical overview, 245–247
    overview, 225t
    post-fieldwork, 259
    pre-fieldwork, 250–252
    stages, 249t
Ethnographic styles, 249
Ethnography, 245
Event analysis, 258t
Evidence-based health care (EBH), 76
Evidence-based medicine (EBM), 76
Evidence-Based Medicine Reviews
    (EBMR), 79
Evidence-based nursing (EBN), 76
Evidence-based practice (EBP), 75–86
    appraising the evidence, 81
    asking clinical questions, 78
    characteristics, 77
    ethical concerns, 81–82
    evidence databases, 79–80
    information sources, 79–81
    limitations, 77–78
    steps in process, 78
    tracking down best evidence, 79
    what is it, 76–77
Evidence databases, 79–80
Expedited review, 35–36
Experimental designs, 200–203

Experimental group, 201
Experimental research, 19–20
External validity, 118
Extraneous variable, 201
Extraneous variables, 98
Eyeballing, 256

Facilitators, 340, 342
Fain, James A., 3, 15, 43, 63, 75, 87, 103, 123,
    143, 165, 307
Family Stressors Index (FSI), 131e
Farmer, Bonnie, 244, 245e
Field notes, 256–258, 270e
Fieldwork, 245, 252–259
Findings. *See* Disseminating research findings;
    Interpretation of research findings
Fittingness, 234
Focus groups, 160–161, 162e
Formal theory, 266
Framework, 65
FSI, 131e
Fundamental research, 19

GAIS, 132e
Genealogies, 258t
Generalizability, 291
Giorgi's method, 230t
Glaser, Barney, 266
Global Adjustment to Illness Scale (GAIS),
    132e
Goode Research Utilization Model, 329t, 333t
Goodness-of-fit test, 184
Grand theories, 67, 68t
Grounded theory, 266
Grounded theory research, 265–286
    application of, in nursing, 278–283
    BSPs, 275–276
    clinical research examples, 279–283
    coding, 272–276
    critiquing, 283–284
    data collection, 268–270
    judging grounded theory, 277–278
    literature review, 277
    memos, 277, 281e
    overview, 225t
    research problem/questions, 268
    sorting memos to produce outline, 277,
        281t
    symbolic interaction, 266–268
    theoretical sampling, 271–272
*Guidelines for the Investigative Function of
    Nurses,* 7

$H_a$, 94
$H_o$, 93
$H_1$, 94

Health, 67t
Health-related Internet directories, 55t
HealthSTAR, 55, 79
*Heart & Lung,* 10
Hegel, Georg Wilhelm Friedrich, 221
Heidegger, Martin, 222
Hermeneutics, 222
Hierarchy of research evidence, 82f
Historic overview
    ethnographic research, 245–247
    phenomenology, 221–223
    unethical research studies, 24–28
Historical research, 211–213
History, 207
Holistic ethnography, 249
Homogeneity of variance, 180
*Hospital Literature Index,* 56
Human rights, 28–36
    evaluating evidence for protection
        of, 36, 37t
    guidelines, 30t
    informed consent, 31–34
    IRB, 34–36
    right to anonymity and confidentiality, 31
    right to freedom from injury, 28–30
    right to privacy and dignity, 30–31
Human science, 223
Husserl, Edmund, 221–222
Hypothesis
    characteristics, 88–91
    critiquing, 98–99
    defined, 88
    directional, 92–93, 93e
    examples, 90e, 91e
    nondirectional, 92
    null, 93
    purposes, 88
    research (alternative), 94, 94e
    simple, 91, 92t
    testing, 95
Hypothesis testing, 95, 175

*Image: Journal of Nursing Scholarship,* 10
In-class questionnaire, 146–147f
Independence samples of chi-square
    test, 185
Independent t-test, 180
Indexes, 56
Inductive approach, 65
Inductive reasoning, 94
Inferential statistics, 166, 174–176
InfoPOEMS, 81
Information sources. *See* Sources of
    information
Informed consent, 31–34, 226
Institutional review board (IRB), 34–36, 227
Instrument, 127–128
Instrument development, 128–138

Instrumentation, 207–208
Intentionality, 221
Interactive family, 275t
Internal consistency reliability, 129–130
Internal level of measurement, 125–127
Internal validity, 198, 207
*International Nursing Index,* 56
Internet resources, 55t
Interpretation of research findings, 290–292
    critiquing, 302–303
    drawing conclusions, 292
    examining the meaning of results,
        290–291
    generalizing the findings, 291–292
    implications, 292
    limitations, 292
    significance of findings, 291
Interrater reliability, 130–131
Intersubjectivity, 221
Interval estimate, 175
Intervening variable, 201
Interviews, 159, 161e
Intuiting, 222
Investigative functions, 8t
Iowa Model of Research in Practice,
    329t, 332t
IRB, 34–36, 227

John Hopkins, crisis at 27
Journals, 10
    abstract, 56
    nursing, 53, 53t
    refereed, 53, 301
    research, 10
    specialty, 10

Kant, Immanuel, 221
Kappa statistic, 130, 131, 132e
Knowledge diffusion, 328
Kuder-Richardson 20 reliability, 131e

Leache, Edmund, 248
Leininger, Madeline, 246, 246e
Level I coding, 273
Level II coding, 273
Level III coding, 273
Level of confidence, 175, 176f
Life histories, 258t
Life world, 221
Likert scales, 150–154
Literature review
    critiquing, 57–58
    defined, 50
    grounded theory research, 277
    outline, 57t
    purpose, 50, 51t

research report, 295, 295e
scope, 50–51
searching the literature, 51–52, 52t
source of research problems as, 48, 49e
sources of information, 53–56
writing the review, 56–57
Lived experience, 220
Longitudinal research, 23, 24e
Lusardi, Paula T., 191
Lyder, Courtney, 289

Mailed questionnaires, 144, 145e
Mainline family, 275t
Mapping, 258t
Matched t-test, 180
Maturation, 207
Maximal inspiratory pressure, 159, 159e
MD Consult, 81
Mead, George Herbert, 266
Mead, Margaret, 245
Mean, 167
Measurement, 124. *See also* Principles of measurement
Measurement error, 127
Measurement scales, 127–128
Measures of central tendency, 167–172
Measures of dispersion, 172–174
Median, 167–170
Medical Literature On-Line (MEDLINE), 55
Medical Subject Headings (MeSH), 337
MEDLINE, 55, 79, 337
Memos, 277, 281e, 281t
Merleau-Ponty, Maurice, 222, 223
MeSH, 337
Meta-analysis, 80, 212
Metaparadigm, 66
Metaparadigm concepts, 67t
MFSC, 158e
Middle-range theories, 67–69
Midwest Nursing Research Society guidelines, 7
Mode, 170–171
Modified Fatigue Symptom Checklist (MFSC), 158e
Morgan, S., 234
Mortality, 208
Multistage sampling, 110–111

National Center for Nursing Research (NCNR), 10–11
National Guideline Clearinghouse, 81
National Institute of Nursing Research (NINR), 11
National Nursing Research Agenda, 11
Natural sciences, 224
NCNR, 10–11
Negative correlation, 177

Negatively skewed distribution, 168, 169f
Network sampling, 114, 115e
Neuman Systems Model, 67
Nicoll, Leslie H., 327
NINR, 11
NINR research priorities, 12t
NINR-supported research, 11–12
Nominal level of measurement, 124–125
Nondirectional hypothesis, 92
Nonequivalent control group design, 204f
Nonexperimental designs, 208–210
Nonexperimental research, 21
Nonparametric test, 176–177, 184–186
Nonprobability sampling, 105, 112–116
Nonrandom sampling, 112
Null hypothesis ($H_o$), 93
Numerical data, 144
Nuremburg Code, 25
Nursing, 67t
Nursing Child Assessment Satellite Training Project, The, 329t, 331t
Nursing journals, 53, 53t
Nursing research. *See also* Research
defined, 4, 6
promoting, 10–12
scientific research, contrasted, 6
*Nursing Research,* 10
Nursing research utilization models, 329–333
*Nursing Scan in Critical Care,* 308
Nursing science, 7
*Nursing Science Quarterly,* 10
Nursing theory, 65–69
borrowed theories, 69, 70t
defined, 65–66
grand theories, 67, 68t
middle-range theories, 67–69
practice theories, 69

Objectivity, 5
Observational studies, 213
Ocular scan, 256
*Oncology Nursing Forum,* 10
One sample chi-square test, 184
One-way ANOVA, 181
*Online Journal of Knowledge Synthesis for Nursing,* 344
Ontology, 222
Open coding, 272
Open-ended question, 146t
Open-ended questionnaires, 145
Open-ended responses, 148
Operational definitions, 45, 70, 125
Oral presentations, 301–302
Ordering or elaboration family, 275t
Ordinal level of measurement, 125
Outcome variable, 98
Outlier, 167
OVID, 54

Pallikkathayil, L., 234
PaperChase, 54
Paradigm, 193
Parameter, 174
Parameter estimation, 174
Parametric procedures, 176
Parse's method, 233t
Participant observation, 31, 159–160, 258, 270
Participant observer, 247
Patterson and Zderad's method, 231t
Pearson product-moment correlation,
    178, 179e
Pearson r, 178
Perception, 223
Person, 67t
Personal Resource Questionnaire (PRQ),
    150–151, 152t
Phenomenological reduction, 222
Phenomenological research, 219–241
    clinical research example, 234–235
    content outline (report), 236t
    critiquing, 236–237
    data analysis, 229–233
    data collection, 227–229
    definition/purpose, 220–221
    ethical considerations, 226–227
    historical overview, 221–223
    overview, 225t
    sample, 226
    scientific rigor, 232–234
    when appropriate, 225–226
    writing the findings, 234
Phenomenology, 211t, 220
PKPCT, 155e
Point estimate, 174
Pooled t-test, 180
Population, 104
Positive correlation, 177
Positively skewed distribution, 168, 169f
Poster presentation, 302, 303f
Post-fieldwork, 259
Posttest-only control group, 202, 202f, 203e
Power as Knowing Participation in Change Test
    (PKPCT), 155e
Practice theories, 69
Predictive validity, 134
Pre-fieldwork, 250–252
Prescriptive theories, 69
Presentations, 301–302
Pretest-posttest comparisons, 180
Pretest-posttest control group design, 201, 202f
Primary source, 53
Principles of measurement, 123–141
    critiquing, 137–139
    errors, 127
    instrument development, 128–138
    interval measurement, 125–127
    measurement scales, 127–128
    nominal measurement, 124–125
    ordinal measurement, 125

psychometric properties, 136–137
    ratio measurement, 127
    reliability, 128–131
    validity, 131–135
Print databases, 55t
Probability, 175–176
Probability sampling, 105, 106–112
Problem statement, 44–46
Proportional stratified sampling, 109, 110e
Prospective research, 21–22, 209–210
PRQ, 150–151, 152t
Psychometric evaluation, 136
Psychosocial instruments, 157
Psychosocial measures, 128
PsycINFO, 55
Publication, 299–301
Pure research, 19
Purpose statement, 46–47
Purposive nonprobability sampling, 109, 110e
Purposive sampling, 116, 117e

Q Methodology, 156–157
Q sort, 156–157
QOL Index, 129e, 130
Qualitative data, 144
Qualitative data collection methods, 159–161
Qualitative designs, 210–211
Qualitative research, 6, 193
Quality Assurance Model Using Research,
    329t, 332t
Quality of Life (QOL) Index, 129e, 130
Quantitative data, 144
Quantitative data collection methods, 144–159
Quantitative designs, 200–205
Quantitative nursing research, 6
Quantitative research, 6, 193
Quasiexperimental before-and-after design, 205
Quasiexperimental designs, 203–205
Query letter, 301
Questionnaires, 144–149
Questions to ask. See Critiquing
Quota sampling, 114–115, 116e

Ragucci, Antoinette, 243–244, 244e, 251, 251e,
    253, 254, 254e, 255, 255e, 256, 256e, 258
Random assignment, 107, 109f
Random numbers, 108t
Random sampling, 106–110
Random selection, 107, 109f
Randomized clinical trials (RCTs), 205–206
Range, 172
Ratio level of measurement, 127
RCTs, 205–206
Reading family, 275t
Red books, 55t
Refereed journals, 53, 301
Reliability, 128–131
Reliability coefficient, 128

Reliability testing, 128
Replication, 6, 49
Research. *See also* Nursing research
    circular nature, 17
    defined, 4–5
    hierarchy of research evidence, 82f
    importance of, 4
    types, 19–21
Research appraisal checklist, 311–312,
    313–315
Research-based nursing journals, 296
Research consumer, 7
Research critique, 307
Research design, 191–218
    assumptions, 192
    characteristics, 195–199
    choice of design, 214
    control, 197–198
    correlational designs, 209–210
    critiquing, 214–215
    defined, 194–195
    descriptive correlational design, 210
    descriptive designs, 208–209, 209e
    epidemiological research, 213
    experimental design, 200–203
    historical research, 211–213
    nonexperimental designs, 208–210
    qualitative designs, 210–211
    quantitative designs, 200–205
    quantitative *vs.* qualitative approaches,
        193–194
    quasiexperimental design, 203–205
    RCTs, 205–206
    researcher/participant relationship, 199
    trustworthiness of findings, 198
    validity, 206–208
Research findings. *See* Disseminating research
    findings; Interpretation of research findings
Research hypothesis, 94
*Research in Nursing and Health,* 10
Research journals, 10
Research-practice gap, 77
Research priorities, 12t
Research process, 16–19
Research questions, 95–96, 96e, 97e
Research-related activities, 9t
Research report, 293–300
    abstract, 293, 294e
    critiquing, 307–325. *See also* Critiquing
        research reports
    discussion, 299, 300e
    introduction, 293–294, 294e
    literature review, 295, 295e
    methods, 296, 297–298e
    references, 299
    results, 296, 298e
    statement of purpose, 294e
    theoretical framework, 295, 295e
    title, 293
Research review, 308

Research scandals, 26–28
Research team, 7
Research utilization, 327–346
    assembling research literature, 337–338
    assessing the applicability, 339
    barriers/facilitators, 340–342, 343t
    critiquing the research, 338–339
    defined, 327–328
    evaluating the innovation, 340
    future of, 344
    implementing the innovation, 340
    process of, 333–340. *See also* Stetler
        model of research utilization
    promoting, 342, 344
    purpose/scope, 328
    research process, contrasted, 328
    specifying the clinical problem, 335–336
    utilization models, 329–333
Research utilization process, 333–340
Resilience, 71e
Resilience Scale (RS), 71e
Response set bias, 150
Retrospective research, 21, 22e, 209
Review of literature. *See* Literature review
Right to privacy and dignity, 30–31
Rigor, 6
Risk-benefit ratio, 29, 30
Robust, 182
Role ambiguity, 153
Role conflict, 154
Role Questionnaire (RQ), 153–154, 154e
Rorschach ink-blot test, 258
RQ, 153–154, 154e
RS, 71e
Russell, Gail E., 219

Sample, 104
Sample size, 116–118
Sampling, 103–121
    adequacy of sample, 116–118
    cluster, 110–111
    convenience, 112, 113e
    critiquing, 119
    defined, 105
    external validity, 118
    network, 114, 115e
    nonprobability, 112–116
    population, 104–105
    probability, 106–112
    purposive, 116, 117e
    quota, 114–115, 116e
    random, 106–110
    sample size, 116–118
    simple random, 106–108
    snowball, 113, 114e
    stratified random, 108–109
    systematic, 111, 112e
    types, 105t
Sampling frame, 106–107

Sartre, Jean-Paul, 222, 223
Saturation, 226
Scales, 149–158
*Scholarly Inquiry for Nursing Practice,* 10
Scholarly publications, 8, 10
Schwartz-Barcott, Donna, 243
Scientific hypothesis, 94
Scientific inquiry, 5
Scientific integrity guidelines, 7, 9t
Scientific literature, 53
Scientific method, 5–6
Scientific research, 6
Scientific rigor, 232–234
Searching databases, 82t
Secondary analysis, 212
Secondary source, 53, 54e
Selecting research problem
    guidelines, 46t
    identify a general problem, 50
    review of related literature, 50–58. *See
        also* Literature review
    where to look, 47–49
Selective coding, 272
Semantic differential scale, 154–155
Semiotic ethnography, 249
Separate t-test, 180
SilverPlatter, 54
Simple hypothesis, 91, 92t
Simple random sampling, 106–108
Single-blinded study, 205
Skewed distribution, 169, 169f
Snowball sampling, 113, 114e
Solomon Four-Group design, 203, 204f
Sorting memos, 277, 281t
Sources of information
    abstracts, 56
    databases, 54–55
    EBP, 79–81
    indexes, 56
    Internet resources, 55t
    journals. *See* Journals
    literature review. *See* Literature review
Specialty journals, 10
Stability, 128
Standard deviation, 172, 173
Standardized instruments, 158
Statistical regression, 208
Statistical significance, 291
Stetler model of research utilization,
    329t, 330, 331t
    overview, 334t
    phase I (preparation), 334e
    phase II (validation), 335e
    phase III (comparative evaluation), 336e
    phase IV (decision making), 336e
    phase V (translation/application), 337e
    phase VI (evaluation), 337e
Stetler/Marram Model, 329t
Strategy family, 275t
Stratification, 109, 110e

Stratified random sampling, 108–109
Strauss, Anselm, 266
Stumpf, Carl, 221
Substantive coding, 272, 273e
Substantive theory, 266
Summative scales, 150
Survey, 144
Sutherland, Dorothy, 246
Symbolic interaction, 211t, 266–268
Symmetrical distribution, 168, 169f
Systematic sampling, 111, 112e

Target population, 104
Testing, 207
Test-retest reliability, 128–129
Theoretical coding, 274
Theoretical definition, 70
Theoretical family, 275t
Theoretical framework, 65, 72
Theoretical literature, 53
Theoretical sampling, 116, 271–272
Theoretical sampling memo, 272e
Theory, 48–49, 64–65. *See also* Nursing theory
Triangulation, 6
True experimental design, 200–203
Trustworthiness of findings, 198
t-test, 179–181
t-test for paired comparisons, 180
Turnbull, Colin, 243, 244e
Tuskegee Syphilis Study, 26
2 X 2 contingency table, 185
Two-way ANOVA, 181
Type family, 275t

Unethical research studies, 26–28
Unit family, 275t
University of North Carolina Model, 329t,
    330, 333t
Utilization models, 329–333
Utilization of research. *See* Research utilization

Validity
    concurrent, 133–134
    construct, 134–135
    content, 132–133, 134e
    criterion-related, 133–134
    critiquing, 137
    defined, 131
    external, 118
    internal, 198
    predictive, 134
    research design, 206–208
Van Kaam's method, 230t
Van Manen's method, 232t
Variable
    continuous, 127
    defined, 96

dependent, 98
dichotomous, 125
extraneous, 98, 201
independent, 97
Variance, 172
Visual analogue scale (VAS), 156

Ways of knowing, 5
Websites
associations, etc., 12–13
directories, 55t

Western Interstate Commission for Higher
Education model, 329t, 331t
*Western Journal of Nursing Research,* 10
Willowbrook Study, 26–27
Within-group comparison, 205
Within-group variance, 183
Women's Roles Interview Protocol
(WRIP), 160e

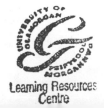

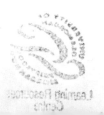